The Tracks We Leave

ETHICS & MANAGEMENT DILEMMAS IN HEALTHCARE

Second Edition

The Tracks We Leave

ETHICS & MANAGEMENT DILEMMAS IN HEALTHCARE

Second Edition

Frankie Perry

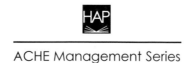

ACHE Management Series

Your board, staff, or clients may also benefit from this book's insight. For more information on quantity discounts, contact the Health Administration Press Marketing Manager at (312) 424-9470.

This publication is intended to provide accurate and authoritative information in regard to the subject matter covered. It is sold, or otherwise provided, with the understanding that the publisher is not engaged in rendering professional services. If professional advice or other expert assistance is required, the services of a competent professional should be sought.

The statements and opinions contained in this book are strictly those of the author(s) and do not represent the official positions of the American College of Healthcare Executives or the Foundation of the American College of Healthcare Executives.

Reprinted March 2019

Library of Congress Cataloging-in-Publication Data
The tracks we leave : ethics and management dilemmas in healthcare / [edited by] Frankie
Perry.—Second edition.
    pages cm
    Includes index.
    ISBN 978-1-56793-578-3 (alk. paper)
1. Managed care plans (Medical care)—Moral and ethical aspects. 2. Medical ethics. I. Perry,
Frankie, editor of compilation.
    RA413.T73 2014
    174.2—dc23

                                    2013027747

The paper used in this publication meets the minimum requirements of American National Standard for Information Sciences—Permanence of Paper for Printed Library Materials, ANSI Z39.48-1984. ⊚™

Acquisitions editor: Carrie McDonald; Project manager: Andrew Baumann; Cover designer: Marisa Jackson; Layout: Fine Print, Ltd.

Found an error or a typo? We want to know! Please e-mail it to hapbooks@ache.org, and put "Book Error" in the subject line.

For photocopying and copyright information, please contact Copyright Clearance Center at www.copyright.com or at (978) 750-8400.

Health Administration Press
A division of the Foundation of the American
    College of Healthcare Executives
One North Franklin Street, Suite 1700
Chicago, IL 60606-3529
(312) 424-2800

We will be known forever by the tracks we leave.

—*Native American proverb*

Contents

Foreword

FRANKIE PERRY HAS succeeded in creating an ethics book that is practical, pragmatic, and thought provoking. The judicious use of actual cases, issue discussions, and thoughtful brief essays on related topics makes for interesting and meaningful reading. This book not only serves the individual reader, but also provides the basis for roundtable and classroom discussions. An epilogue, rare in books of this type, provides some closure on each of the cases. This is real life tied together with solid contributions to our literature to help all of us improve our perspective on ethical situations.

This book is quite timely. Complications in healthcare delivery, complex business transactions, conflicts of interest, and the vastly expanding list of issues relating to bias confound our daily life as healthcare executives. Every organization faces these and other ethical problems constantly. Understanding these problems and acting proactively to prevent them is a critical skill of any executive. The breadth of this book goes far beyond the cases and provides a foundation for enhancing existing ethics education programs or creating new ones. Once read, this book will be a very useful reference tool for any institution's effort to deal with and prevent ethical dilemmas. Furthermore, this book should find a home in many graduate and undergraduate classes as both a text and a foundation for case discussions.

Creating a book of this type requires a special person. Frankie Perry approached this effort with outstanding preparation. Ms. Perry has held hospital positions from staff nurse through nursing supervision to top hospital management. From her hospital executive role, she joined the staff of the American College of Healthcare Executives (ACHE). Once again, she rose through the ranks to serve the professional society as executive vice president and as staff representative to the ACHE ethics committee. Implementing and preserving the ACHE *Code of Ethics* is the focus of the work of the ethics committee, which in turn becomes a major part of the role of the staff representative. This includes extensive analysis and action over violations of the *Code*. This is the exceptional perspective of Frankie Perry, which serves as a key to the value of this excellent book.

I have high hopes for this book and its effect on our profession, both in the practice and academic communities. I know it will assist all readers to more effectively fulfill their responsibilities as healthcare executives, as professionals in other healthcare roles, or as students aspiring to leadership and service roles in healthcare.

Stuart A. Wesbury, Jr., PhD, LFACHE

Preface

EVOLUTION IS A progression of interrelated phenomena. Society is continuously evolving, and as an institution of society, healthcare is evolving as well. Thoughtful men and women have studied this evolution and helped develop rules of conduct for each new paradigm. Our sense of morality also changes, and the old rules of moral behavior do not always apply. On a fundamental level, people need and want guidance and standards to help them "do the right thing."

Nowhere is this evolution more evident than in the complex field of healthcare management. Healthcare as a microcosm of society reacts and responds to societal events. Continual advances in technology, changes in healthcare financing, increasing consumer needs and expectations, the proliferation of socioeconomically induced health problems, ever-expanding public scrutiny and litigation, and the healthcare reform mandate all contribute to the significant complexity of healthcare. The decision-making process in healthcare management has become more complicated, and healthcare executives may sometimes waver in their confidence that they are making ethically responsible decisions.

Amid this turmoil of constant change, healthcare executives frequently find themselves in uncharted waters where the ethical "rules" may be unclear. Real-life ethical dilemmas are complex. Rarely do such dilemmas involve a single ethical issue. More often, numerous intertwined issues involving many stakeholders with diverse values clamor for attention. Ambiguities abound; resolutions to ethical dilemmas do not come easily. The implementation of the Patient Protection and Affordable Care Act will present new ethics issues and will pose new ethical challenges. Friedman (2012) suggests that these future ethics issues will surround access to care; informed consent for participation in "health policy trials," such as accountable care organizations; insurance discrimination; power shifts; scope-of-practice issues; the drive to maximize profits; end-of-life issues; privacy and security of health information; and a focus on thinking communally. Friedman tells us that we need ethical leadership to address these issues head-on and that "being able to justify one's decisions on ethical grounds as well as fiscal ones will be essential to success."

PART I

Part I of this book deals with ethics as a leadership imperative. Zenger and Folkman (2002, 12) report that "character is at the center of leadership" and is "the core of all leadership effectiveness." Indeed, when we hear of the leadership failures of industry titans, corporate executives, politicians, religious leaders, and others, we find these failures are often ones of character and ethics. Healthcare executives are not exempt from such failures. Part I discusses the ethical responsibilities of healthcare executives and makes the case for committing resources to establish an ethical culture and infrastructure in one's organization.

PART II

Part II presents cases that reflect the realities of healthcare management, the diversity of special interests, and the competing values and moral conflicts that challenge the healthcare executive. Many of the cases examine the ethical responsibility of managers as stewards of valuable organizational and community resources. Each case is followed by a description of the ethics issues inherent in the situation presented and a discussion of these interrelated issues. These cases and discussions are intended to stimulate thoughtful analysis and reflection that will help readers successfully navigate the quagmire of ambiguity that ethical dilemmas can present.

The Paradise Hills Medical Center case in Chapter 3 focuses on medical errors, truth telling, and autonomy. In Chapter 4, the Qual Plus HMO case appears to focus on conflict-of-interest issues but actually explores the issue of conflicting moral demands when an individual is asked to do something he believes to be unethical or observes someone in authority behaving in an unethical way. In Chapter 5, the Rolling Meadows Community Hospital case discusses the issues surrounding mentorship, sexual harassment, and gender discrimination and highlights some of the ambiguities of wrongdoing. In Chapter 6, the University Hospital case examines some of the pitfalls of professional impairment and shows how impairment can compromise patient safety, employee morale, and graduate medical education.

The Hillside County Medical Center case by Glenn A. Fosdick, FACHE, in Chapter 7 focuses on the ethical implications of workforce reductions. Hospitals under financial stress sometimes use the euphemism "rightsizing" to describe such reductions, but to the employee being laid off and the ones left behind to pick up the slack, a workforce reduction can be a disaster. This case looks at the issues involved and the leadership required to make ethically sound decisions when a hospital is in financial crisis.

The Metropolitan Community Hospital case (Chapter 8) is an example of the failure of leadership to effectively address a nursing shortage and the disruptive behavior of physicians. The Heartland Healthcare System case (Chapter 9) examines the ethical issues surrounding a major information technology setback. The Richland River Valley Healthcare System case (Chapter 10) explores the ethics issues surrounding a failed hospital merger and takes a closer look at administration–board relationships. The Hurley Medical Center case (Chapter 11) is ripped right from today's headlines; both timely and challenging, it involves a situation where workforce diversity, patient demands, and hospital policies collide. The issues this dilemma presents are far-reaching and have unanticipated consequences.

Chapter 12 provides a legal perspective on each of the preceding cases by attorney Walter P. Griffin, JD, who also discusses the differences between "illegal and unethical" and "legal but unethical" behaviors.

PART III

Part III looks at the importance of establishing policies and infrastructure components that support an ethical culture and integrate ethical decision making into the way of doing business. For most of the cases in Part II, a relevant chapter can be found in Part III that expands on the issues in the case and enriches the discussion. In Chapter 13, Joan McIver Gibson, PhD, describes a values-based ethical decision-making model and a process that leads to decisions made with integrity that are comprehensive, coherent, and transparent. In Chapter 14, I discuss the ethics of managing people and examine the different values, special interests, and goals that each person brings to the workplace and the conflicts and ethical dilemmas that may ensue. Management style, role modeling, mentoring, and ethical human resources policies and practices are also addressed. In Chapter 15, Richard H. Rubin, MD, examines from a physician's perspective both the ethical issues and the legal ramifications faced by physicians and managers of managed care organizations. In Chapter 16, Rebecca A. Dobbs, RN, PhD, outlines strategies for evaluating healthcare ethics committees to determine if they are meeting the needs of the organization and the patients and clients served. In Chapter 17, J. Mitchell Simson, MD, explores the prevalence, prevention, and treatment of substance abuse and addiction among healthcare professionals. In Chapter 18, Clinton H. Dowd, MD, looks at unique considerations that must be given attention in teaching hospitals.

Make no mistake about it—our society has undergone major change since September 11, 2001, and the burden on healthcare to be able to plan for and respond appropriately to disasters, whether the result of nature or terrorism, has never been greater. The 2013 Boston Marathon bombing brought high praise to Boston hospitals and healthcare workers for their successful medical response to the mass casualties of that day, a response attributed to their ability to build and practice state-of-the-art emergency preparedness programs (Biddinger et al. 2013). With this enormous responsibility come ethical issues that must be anticipated and addressed. Rebecca A. Dobbs, RN, PhD, who is a national expert on planning and evaluating healthcare's response to disasters, shares her expertise in Chapter 19.

EPILOGUE

Finally, for those who wish to know if and how the ethical issues in the case studies were resolved and what happened subsequently, the epilogue provides follow-up on each case presented in Part II.

I have drawn all of the cases from real-life experiences. They represent the kinds of management dilemmas and moral challenges that confront a healthcare manager on a day-to-day basis. Thoughtful analysis of these cases, and exploration of strategies that deal effectively with the issues they present, will better prepare healthcare managers to successfully address similar issues in the future. If anticipating and forestalling situations comparable to the ones presented in this book is the result of your thoughtful reflection here, then this work will have served its purpose. If, having read this book, you are more apt to add a discussion of ethical implications to your decision-making process, then even better. And finally, I hope that you will become ever more aware that good management requires morally sound management decisions. Ignoring the ethical implications of management decisions can be disastrous—to the organization, to the community, to patients and clients, and to the careers of healthcare managers.

INSTRUCTOR RESOURCES

Instructor resources—including PowerPoints, a quiz, additional cases, case-analysis instructions, and websites of interest—are available to instructors who adopt this book. Please e-mail hapbooks@ache.org for more information.

REFERENCES

Biddinger, P. D., A. Baggish, L. Harrington, P. d'Hemecourt, J. Hooley, J. Jones, R. Kue, C. Troyanos, and K. S. Dyer. 2013. "Be Prepared—the Boston Marathon and Mass-Casualty Events." *New England Journal of Medicine* 368 (21): 1958–60.

Friedman, E. 2012. "The Ethics of Change: Making the Right Decisions in a Shifting System." *Hospitals & Health Networks Daily* October 2. www.hhnmag.com/hhnmag/HHNDaily/HHNDailyDisplay.dhtml?id=8200007092.

Zenger, J., and J. Folkman. 2002. *The Extraordinary Leader: Turning Good Managers into Great Leaders.* New York: McGraw-Hill.

Acknowledgments

MUCH HAS BEEN written in the past decade about ethics and how it applies to healthcare management and delivery, for which I am grateful.

My 28 years of hospital experience, first as a nurse and then as an administrator, and several years as staff to the American College of Healthcare Executives Ethics Committee made it clear to me that much still needed to be written to help healthcare managers successfully navigate the sometimes murky paths to ethical decisions.

Significant contributions to the literature have been made by John Griffith, Austin Ross, John Worthley, Laura Nash, Paul Hofmann, Emily Friedman, and others whose valuable work has found its way into this book. To them I owe a debt of gratitude.

I humbly submit this work to the collection of ethics literature in the field for healthcare managers, knowing that much has been written, but also knowing there can never be too much written on this important subject.

PART I

The Leadership Imperative

CHAPTER 1

Understanding Your Ethical Responsibilities

HEALTHCARE LEADERS AND those aspiring to be leaders must recognize first and foremost that character and integrity constitute the very cornerstone of leadership. Organizations have failed and promising careers have been derailed when ethics have been relegated to secondary importance or, worse yet, ignored in the pursuit of more bottom-line considerations. Healthcare managers must understand their role and responsibility in creating an ethical healthcare environment that is honest, just, and always in the best interests of those being served. Whether you are the CEO, an assistant administrator, a department head, a program manager, or a clinician, if you are "in charge," you have the ultimate responsibility for establishing the culture and setting the standards of conduct in your sphere of influence.

This task is not always an easy one. Nor is it easy for well-intentioned managers to always make ethical decisions themselves.

BARRIERS TO ETHICAL DECISION MAKING

In our book *Healthcare Leadership Excellence: Creating a Career of Impact*, James Rice and I identify some of the common barriers to ethical decision making and seven pitfalls for managers to avoid (Rice and Perry 2013, 29–37). We then make recommendations for building a solid culture and infrastructure to support ethical decision making throughout the organization. The following summarizes those pitfalls and our recommendations for overcoming them:

1. **Failing to recognize that ethics and management decisions are interrelated.** Management decisions are too often based solely on financial data, market share, and other bottom-line considerations without regard to ethical implications. Ethics and management are, in fact, closely related (Exhibit 1.1).

Exhibit 1.1: Relationship Between Ethics and Management

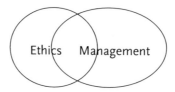

2. **Failing to recognize that management decisions directly affect clinical care.** Operational decisions must take into account how actions affect patient safety and healthcare needs.

3. **Failing to integrate ethics into the way of doing business.** Ethical standards must be more than a well-crafted values statement published in the annual report. They must be incorporated into the work life of every staff member throughout the organization, from the boardroom to housekeeping.

4. **Failing to understand that just because something is legal does not mean it is ethical.** Pushing legal boundaries does not build leadership character. Wise leaders recognize that the role of the attorney is to advise regarding the law; the healthcare leader must decide what is morally right.

5. **Believing you are above the rules and laws of "ordinary men."** Hubris is often at the root of unethical behavior. Leaders cannot operate by one set of standards and expect their employees to function under different, higher ones.

6. **Rushing to judgment.** Ethical mistakes are often the result of hasty decisions made without reflection and consultation with others. Aspiring leaders may mistakenly believe that rapid, independent decisions are expected of them and are the mark of a leader. Technology has further compounded our time crunch. Healthcare managers who are hard pressed for time suffer from information overload. Always-on, multitasking work environments leave little time for thoughtful analysis of ethical dilemmas and the implications of decisions (Dean and Webb 2011).

7. **Believing that when everyone else does it, you can do it, too.** The creep of moral relativism, in which the standards of right and wrong are mere products of time and culture, may have become more pronounced through the economic downturn and new challenges in healthcare. If everyone is bending the rules, don't we need to do the same to remain competitive? Experienced healthcare leaders know that bending the rules for short-term gains may have long-term negative consequences. Inevitably, questionable

legal or ethical behavior has a price. Actions will come to light and competitive gains will be lost.

So, how do you avoid these pitfalls and build an ethical infrastructure and an organizational culture that make ethics the only acceptable way of doing business?

OVERCOMING BARRIERS TO ETHICAL DECISION MAKING

To quote ethics leader Paul Hofmann, "organizational culture always has been and always will be largely determined for better or worse by the CEO" (quoted in Rice and Perry 2013, 26). While this is certainly true, middle managers, supervisors, and other staff have a responsibility to promote and role-model ethical decisions in their sphere of influence and to advocate for an infrastructure that supports ethics in their corporate organization. Managers must encourage leadership to promote ethical conduct in the organization by taking the following steps (Rice and Perry 2013, 38–44):

1. Establish ethical standards, expectations, and a written code of conduct. Rethink the code of conduct regularly, to ensure that it is current with ethical demands.
2. Hire ethical people. Consider presenting ethical dilemmas as part of your organization's interview process.
3. Cultivate a relationship with a trusted colleague within or outside your organization who can provide candid, honest feedback regarding the appearance of your personal and professional conduct. Invite colleagues to continually review and enhance your ethical culture.
4. Serve as a role model of ethical standards.
5. Complete an ethics self-assessment from time to time and address areas that need improvement (see Appendix A for the "Ethics Self-Assessment" of the American College of Healthcare Executives).
6. Establish an ethics committee to address both clinical and business ethics issues.
7. Require ethics training and education of all employees and staff. Ensure that training and education are up to date and widely disseminated. Use of real-life cases has proven to be an especially effective teaching methodology.
8. Ensure compliance with ethical standards that includes enforcement, reprimands for improper actions, and rewards for ethical conduct.

9. Create an ethical environment with fair and equitable personnel practices and workforce reduction policies—one that is free from harassment, discrimination, or pressure to perform or ignore illegal or unethical actions.
10. Address impairment in the workplace with education, reporting mechanisms, counseling, and treatment options.
11. Integrate patients' rights into operations. Implement patient advocacy and customer service programs as needed.
12. Adopt a framework for ethical decision making consistent with the mission, vision, and values of the organization.

Freund (2010, 32) tells us that "an organization's policies and practices, allocation of resources and expectations for its leaders are indicators of its culture. Equally telling is what the organizational leaders encourage and reward, discourage and punish and what they tolerate."

THE IMPORTANCE OF CULTIVATING A "LEARNING ORGANIZATION"

As the case studies in Part II of this book demonstrate, many moral dilemmas are the result of management mistakes and the reluctance of executives, managers, or employees to own up to these mistakes and be accountable for their actions. Many organizations retain a "blame and shame" culture, where the punishment may far outweigh the mistake and where organizations fail to learn from their missteps. In such a culture, employees learn very quickly to hide their mistakes and thus compound potential ethical dilemmas.

In contrast, a "learning organization" takes a systems approach rather than a personal one and, through such mechanisms as root-cause analysis, attempts to locate the cause of errors and make changes in the system to prevent errors from occurring again. A learning organization provides venues for employees to candidly explore ethical concerns and conflicts and ask questions without fear of retribution or scorn. In such an organization, under-recognized ethical issues may come to light. Hofmann identifies three such issues that warrant attention and discussion (summarized in Buell 2009, 56):

1. **Promoting unrealistic expectations on the part of the public that an organization can do more than it can deliver.** Promoting unrealistic expectations is an issue that calls for organizations to closely examine their marketing and advertising claims to make certain they are valid. Gershon and Buerstatte (2003) recommend that healthcare organizations develop internal marketing and advertising guidelines and share them with everyone

who develops these materials. They suggest that the guidelines address such practices as "use of actors or models instead of actual patients and staff; inclusion of awards information and patient satisfaction surveys; avoidance of unsupported claims that create unrealistic expectations; and addition of messages that create a demand for unnecessary services." Van Hook (2013) tells us that "ethical public relations is not an oxymoron"—public relations professionals can be "a company's conscience" stressing honesty above all else.

2. **Rationalizing inappropriate or incompetent behavior.** Rationalizing inappropriate or incompetent behavior can have a negative effect on patient safety and quality of care. It certainly has a demoralizing effect on staff morale and productivity.

3. **Failing to acknowledge mistakes.** Failing to acknowledge mistakes is not only unethical in and of itself; it also means that the mistake cannot be corrected or, in the case of medical errors, that the information is withheld from the patients affected.

ADOPTING AN ETHICAL DECISION-MAKING FRAMEWORK

Employees must be able to recognize an ethical problem and be encouraged to question the ethics of actions and decisions—both their own and those of others. If an ethical issue is not recognized, it cannot be addressed. Decision-making frameworks are especially helpful in this regard.

A healthcare manager is confronted with ethical dilemmas on a daily basis. Most of the time, the manager makes the right decisions unconsciously and does the right thing. For the most part, those involved in healthcare are decent, moral individuals who are attracted to the healthcare field because they wish to contribute something of value to society. Nevertheless, they occasionally make errors in judgment, detrimental decisions, and unintentional mistakes. More often than not, mistakes are the result of the barrage of decisions that must be made by managers who are pressed for time and strained by the demands of the job. Decisions are frequently made without the benefit of thoughtful reflection or consultation with others.

Theoretical constructs and ethical decision-making frameworks abound, but as the busy practitioner knows only too well, the exigencies of time and place sometimes preclude their proper usage. The healthcare manager is expected to know the answers, to make decisions quickly and authoritatively, and to lead the staff down a path of moral integrity.

This book is intended to provide some practical guidance to healthcare managers who are confronted with these challenges. What useful thought process can healthcare managers employ to make this task easier? What steps can they take to move staff in the direction of ethically sound decisions?

The process suggested here to arrive at such decisions is a relatively simple one—a series of questions that the healthcare manager can ask to determine if additional time or resources need to be brought to bear on the decision-making process and the situation at hand. These questions focus on identifying the issues in any particular situation as well as the stakeholders, the organizational impact, the colleagues, and the resources surrounding those issues (Exhibit 1.2).

- **Issues.** What are the ethical issues in this situation? Relatively few situations involve a single issue. More often, the ethical dilemma comprises a number of interrelated issues. Each issue must be isolated and thoughtfully explored.
- **Stakeholders.** What persons or groups will be affected by this situation and the actions taken? What will each feel is in his or her best interest?
- **Organizational impact.** What will be the effect on the organization that pays the executive's salary and has expectations that the executive will act in its best interests?
- **Colleagues.** Which trusted colleagues may have insights, experiences, and knowledge to offer and can be consulted about this matter? Can they be consulted in confidence?
- **Resources.** What resources are available? Does the organization have a mission statement? Values statement? Ethics committee? Ethics officer? Code of conduct? Compliance officer? Guiding principles? Policies? Laws? Regulations? Decision-making models? Legal counsel?

Exhibit 1.2: Issues Wheel

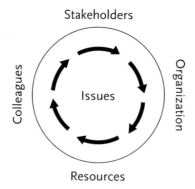

Leaders must exercise caution, however, to avoid assuming that if no law, rule, regulation, or policy addresses an action, then the action must be ethical. This is not true. Moral men and women do not need situations to come with written instructions to do the responsible thing.

Nash (2009) offers the following 12 questions for examining the ethics of a business decision:

1. Have you defined the problem accurately?
2. How would you define the problem if you stood on the other side of the fence?
3. How did this situation occur in the first place?
4. To whom and to what do you give your loyalty as a person and as a member of the corporation?
5. What is your intention in making this decision?
6. How does this intention compare with the probable results?
7. Whom could your decision or action injure?
8. Can you discuss the problem with the affected parties before you make your decision?
9. Are you confident that your position will be as valid over a long period of time as it seems now?
10. Could you disclose without qualm your decision or action to your boss, your CEO, the board of directors, your family, or society as a whole?
11. What is the symbolic potential of your action if understood? If misunderstood?
12. Under what conditions would you allow exceptions to your stand?

Hosmer (1995) discusses ten ethical principles that healthcare executives can use to determine an ethical course of action:

1. **Self-interests.** Never take any action that is not in the long-term self-interests of yourself and the healthcare organization to which you belong.
2. **Personal virtues.** Never take any action that is not honest, open, and truthful and that you would not be proud to see reported widely in national newspapers and on television.
3. **Religious injunctions.** Never take any action that is not kind and that does not build a sense of community.
4. **Government requirements.** Never take any action that violates the law.
5. **Utilitarian benefits.** Never take any action that does not result in greater good than harm.

6. **Universal rules.** Never take any action that you would be unwilling to see others take in similar situations.
7. **Individual rights.** Never take any action that abridges the agreed-on rights of others.
8. **Economic efficiency.** Always act to maximize profits, subject to legal and market constraints and with full recognition of external costs.
9. **Distributive justice.** Never take any action in which the least among us is harmed in some way.
10. **Contributing liberty.** Never take any action that will interfere with the rights of others for self-fulfillment.

Nelson (2005, 10–13) provides an eight-step process reflecting procedural justice:

1. Clarify the ethical conflict. What is the specific ethical question or conflict? If the question or conflict is not an ethical one, it should be referred to another person or process.
2. Identify all of the affected stakeholders and their values. Who are the individuals or programs affected by the ethical question?
3. Understand the circumstances surrounding the ethical conflict. Identify the economic, patient care, legal, and community concerns.
4. Identify the ethical perspectives relevant to the conflict. Refer to professional codes, ethics literature, and the organization's policies and procedures.
5. Identify different options for action. What is the ethical reasoning for each?
6. Select among the options. Is the selected option practical? Does it have a clear ethical foundation? Does one ethical concept or stakeholder value appear to be stronger than the others?
7. Share and implement the decision.
8. Review the decision to ensure it achieved the desired goal.

In Chapter 13, Joan McIver Gibson provides detailed guidance and a helpful elliptical diagram for identifying values and applying values-based decision making to the analysis of ethics situations. She also provides a tool for a "values analysis on the fly" when time is short but values still must be considered.

Before codes of conduct and ethical frameworks for decision making were available, the young hospital administrators who reported to me looked to me for sage advice on how to do the right thing when they were on call. They knew that they could call me if they really got into trouble, but they also knew I expected them to have a plan of action when they did call. To help them formulate this plan of action, I gave them four simple questions to apply to any situation:

1. What action is in the best interests of the patient(s) involved?
2. What action is in the best interests of the organization?

3. If this action is taken, what is the worst possible thing that can happen?
4. What is my contingency plan to deal with all possible ramifications of the action?

Although this thought process did not easily solve every problem, my objective was to focus the administrator's thinking on what was best for the patient and the organization (instead of on subjective concerns, such as personal power, authority, or control) in solving the problem at hand. For the most part, it worked—the process did lend itself to the quick resolution of the kinds of problems an administrator tends to see at three o'clock in the morning.

Whichever strategy the healthcare manager uses to arrive at a sound ethical decision, the manager must examine all of the consequences of each action considered. The key to ethical decisions is an awareness of the need to ask thoughtful questions and to take the time to formulate ethically sound answers. Doing so will help healthcare managers avoid hasty decisions that are not always attentive to the ethical implications of actions taken. Aristotle considered contemplation the best activity, remarking that "it is also the most continuous since we can contemplate truth more continuously than we can do anything" (Crisp 2000, 195).

Hofmann reminds us that managers of character and integrity demonstrate certain behavioral traits (Buell 2009, 54). They are ethically conscious of ethical dimensions and implications. They are ethically committed to doing the right thing. They are ethically competent, possessing the knowledge and understanding required to make ethically sound decisions. They are ethically courageous even when actions may not be accepted with enthusiasm or endorsement. They are ethically consistent without making inconvenient exceptions. They are ethically candid, open, and forthright and are active advocates of ethical analysis and conduct. A wise and experienced healthcare executive whom I know once observed that "working in healthcare gives you the opportunity to do something ethical every day."

TOOLS

To further assist healthcare managers in future decision making, the appendixes at the end of the book include the following:

- American College of Healthcare Executives "Ethics Self-Assessment" (Appendix A)
- American College of Healthcare Executives *Code of Ethics* (Appendix B)
- American College of Healthcare Executives Ethical Policy Statements (Appendix C)
- American College of Healthcare Executives Policy Statements (Appendix D)

REFERENCES

Buell, J. M. 2009. "Ethics and Leadership." *Healthcare Executive* 24 (3): 54–56.

Crisp, R. (ed.). 2000. *Aristotle: Nicomachean Ethics*. Cambridge, UK: Cambridge University Press.

Dean, D., and C. Webb. 2011. "Recovering from Information Overload." *McKinsey Quarterly* January. Accessed July 3, 2012. www.mckinseyquarterly.com/article _print.aspx?L2=18&L3=31&ar=2735.

Freund, L. 2010. "Creating a Culture of Accountability." *Healthcare Executive* 32 (1): 30–36.

Gershon, H., and G. Buerstatte. 2003. "The E in Marketing: Ethics in the Age of Misbehavior." *Journal of Healthcare Management* 48 (5): 292–94.

Hosmer, L. T. 1995. "Brief Summaries of Ten Ethical Principles." *Academy of Management Review* 20 (2): 396–97.

Nash, L. 2009. *Ethics Without the Sermon*. Boston: Harvard Business School Publishing.

Nelson, W. A. 2005. "An Organizational Ethics Decision-Making Process." *Healthcare Executive* 20 (4): 9–14.

Rice, J., and F. Perry. 2013. *Healthcare Leadership Excellence: Creating a Career of Impact*. Chicago: Health Administration Press.

Van Hook, S. 2013. "Ethical Public Relations: Not an Oxymoron." All About Public Relations. Accessed April 30. www.aboutpublicrelations.net/aa052701a.htm.

CHAPTER 2

The Business Case for Ethics Management

HEALTHCARE LEADERS KNOW that ethics management is not merely a nice thing to do. Ethics management has a business case. McNamara (2013) says that managing ethics in the workplace

- improves society;
- helps maintain a moral course in turbulent times;
- cultivates teamwork and productivity;
- supports employee growth and meaning;
- helps ensure policies are legal;
- helps prevent criminal acts and lowers fines if such acts occur;
- helps with quality management, strategic planning, and diversity management;
- promotes a strong public image;
- strengthens organizational culture, trust, quality of service, and sensitivity to values; and
- is the right thing to do.

McNamara does not mention in this list that morally sound management decisions are also financially prudent. Doing the right thing to begin with is much less costly than cleaning up the mess—and sometimes the litigation—that unethical behavior leaves in its wake. Morally sound management decisions save time, effort, and resources in the long run.

In 1991, the US Congress passed the Federal Sentencing Guidelines for Organizations, which apply to all profit or not-for-profit organizations with ten or more employees, including healthcare organizations. The guidelines hold an organization responsible for the wrongful acts of its employees if they are acting in their official capacities, whether the manager or the organization knew about the illegal action or not. Fines and jail sentences can be handed down to the organization, the employees involved, and the managers and executives as well. If the organization has an effective ethics and compliance program, fines and penalties may be significantly reduced. Criteria for an effective program include

- compliance standards and procedures,
- oversight by high-level personnel,
- due care in delegating authority,
- ethics training programs,
- internal auditing and reporting systems,
- consistent enforcement of standards through disciplinary actions, and
- measures to prevent reoccurrences of offenses.

Revisions made in 2004 to the Federal Sentencing Guidelines required organizations to "heighten their efforts to detect and prevent violations of law and to implement efforts to establish an ethical culture" (USSC 2012). The guidelines now require measurement of program effectiveness—specifically, that organizations have an effective compliance and ethics program, periodically evaluate the program's effectiveness, and periodically assess the risk of criminal conduct and take appropriate steps to modify each requirement as necessary to reduce any risk of criminal conduct identified through this process. To measure and evaluate program effectiveness, organizations need to determine employees' knowledge of the organization's standards of conduct through the collection of data.

An additional benefit of ethics management is that it saves the organization time, effort, and resources in the recruitment and retention of talent. Competent physicians and employees want to work with ethical managers who inspire them and challenge them to achieve high levels of ethical performance. They do not want to follow leaders who do not demonstrate strong character and integrity and who are less than worthy of their loyalty and commitment (Zenger and Folkman 2002, 79). The ability to attract and retain a quality workforce will become increasingly important to the viability of organizations because of the labor shortages predicted in the future. Patients, too, value honest and trustworthy care and will seek organizations and clinicians they feel they can trust. Likewise, vendors and insurers want to do business with reputable organizations and credible administrators they can trust. Wise healthcare executives know that they must be personally and professionally ethical to enjoy and prosper in their many business and professional relationships (Perry 2012, 16).

Simply put, managing ethics in the workplace is good management. It saves time, effort, and resources in the long run. The wise stewardship of resources is a paramount responsibility of leadership in any organization, but especially in a healthcare organization whose mission is to serve humanity.

In a recent address to an assembly of healthcare executives, noted journalist and political analyst Juan Williams (2010) challenged healthcare leaders to extend their leadership role and work at changing society to make it a more ethical, more civil environment in which people are more concerned for one another. Such an effort will advance productivity and the responsible stewardship of valuable resources throughout organizations and make society a better place for all.

REFERENCES

McNamara, C. 2013. "Complete Guide to Ethics Management: An Ethics Toolkit for Managers." Free Management Library. Accessed April 26. http://managementhelp.org/businessethics/ethics-guide.htm.

Perry, F. 2012. *Healthcare Leadership That Makes a Difference: Creating Your Legacy.* Self-study course. Chicago: Health Administration Press.

US Sentencing Commission (USSC). 2012. "Sentencing of Organizations." Chapter 8 of the USSC *Guidelines Manual.* www.ussc.gov/Guidelines.

Williams, J. 2010. "American Leadership: The Inspiration and Power Behind Proven Leaders." Malcolm T. MacEachern Memorial Lecture presented at the American College of Healthcare Executives Congress on Healthcare Leadership, Chicago, March 23.

Zenger, J., and J. Folkman. 2002. *The Extraordinary Leader: Turning Good Managers into Great Leaders.* New York: McGraw-Hill.

PART II

Case Studies and Moral Challenges

CHAPTER 3

Medical Errors:
Paradise Hills Medical Center

PARADISE HILLS MEDICAL CENTER is a 500-bed teaching hospital in a major *Case* metropolitan area of the South. It is known throughout a tri-state area for its com- *Study* prehensive oncology program and serves as a regional referral center for thousands of patients suffering from various forms of malignant disease.

Paradise Hills is affiliated with a major university and has residency programs in internal medicine, surgery, pediatrics, obstetrics and gynecology, psychiatry, radiology, and pathology, all fully accredited by the Accreditation Council for Graduate Medical Education. In addition, Paradise Hills has an oncology fellowship program, a university-affiliated nursing program, and training programs for radiology technicians and medical technologists. All of these teaching programs are highly regarded and attract students from across the nation.

Paradise Hills enjoys an enviable reputation throughout the area. It is known for its high-quality care, its state-of-the-art technology, and its competent, caring staff. Although Paradise Hills is located in a highly competitive healthcare community, it boasts a strong market share for its service area. Its patients provide significant referrals to the surgery, pediatrics, and radiology programs as well.

Paradise Hills is a financially sound institution with equally strong leadership. Its past successes can be attributed in large part to its aggressive, visionary CEO and his exceptionally competent management staff.

But all is not as well as it seems at Paradise Hills. Although the oncology program still enjoys a healthy market share of 75 percent, it has been slowly and steadily declining from a peak of 82 percent two years ago. In addition, the program's medical staff is aging, and some of its highest admitting physicians are contemplating retirement. The oncology fellowship program was established a few years ago to address this situation, but unfortunately the graduates of this program have so far elected not to stay in the community. Of most concern to the CEO and his staff is the fact that the hospital's primary competitor has recently recruited a highly credentialed oncology medical group practice from the Northeast and has committed enormous resources to strengthening its own struggling oncology program.

Last week Paradise Hills's board of trustees had its monthly meeting, with a fairly routine agenda. However, during review of a standard quality assurance report, one of the trustees inquired about a section of the report indicating that 22 oncology patients had received radiation therapy dosages in excess of what had been prescribed for them. It was explained that the errors had occurred as a result of a flaw in the calibration of the linear accelerator and that the medical physicist responsible for the errors had been asked to resign his position. Another trustee then asked if the patients who had received the excessive radiation had been told about the errors. The CEO responded that it was the responsibility of the medical staff to address this issue, and they had decided not to inform the patients about the errors. The board did not agree that the medical staff were solely responsible for informing the patients about the errors and requested that the administrative staff review both the hospital's ethical responsibility to these patients and its liability related to this incident, and report back to the board within two weeks.

The CEO and his management staff responsible for the radiology department and the oncology program met with the medical staff department chairmen for internal medicine and radiology, the program medical directors for oncology and radiation therapy, and the attending oncologists. The CEO related the board's discussion about the errors and the board's request that the actions taken be reviewed, specifically the decision not to inform the affected patients.

All of the physicians agreed that the adverse effects of the accidental radiation overdose on the patients were unknown. The oncologists argued that the patients should not be told of the incident, asserting that the cancer patients did not want or need any more bad news. "Let's face it, these patients are terminal," they said. "Informing them about this error will only confuse them and destroy their faith and trust in their physicians and in the hospital." Furthermore, they claimed, informing the patients of the errors could unnecessarily frighten them to the extent that they might refuse further treatment, which would be even more detrimental to them. Besides, the physicians argued, advising the patients of potential ill effects just might induce those symptoms through suggestion or excessive worry. Every procedure has its risks, the radiology department chairman insisted, and these patients signed an informed consent.

Physicians know what is best for their patients, the attending oncologists maintained, and they would monitor the patients in question for any ill effects. The department chairman for internal medicine was of the opinion that the incident was clearly a patient–physician relationship responsibility and not the business of the hospital. Besides, the radiology chairman added, informing the patients would "just be asking for malpractice litigation."

The medical director for the oncology program then suggested that the board of trustees and the management staff "think long and hard" about the public relations effect this incident would have on the oncology program. "Do you really think patients will want to come to Paradise Hills if they think we're incompetent?" he asked.

The CEO conceded that he supported the position of the medical staff in this matter and that he, too, was concerned about preserving the image of the oncology program. But "his hands were tied" because the board clearly considered this an ethical issue that would have to be referred to the hospital's ethics committee for its opinion.

The physicians noted that if indeed the ethics committee subsequently recommended that the patients be informed, then realistically that responsibility would rest with the patients' primary care physicians and not with any of them.

ETHICS ISSUES

Truth telling: Is there a difference between lying to a patient and withholding the truth? Does it matter to the patient whether the act is one of omission or commission?

Justice and fairness: Is it fair to these patients to withhold information about their clinical treatment and any potential risks inherent in the accidental overdose?

A patient's right to know: Do these patients have a right to know about this incident? Do these patients have a right to know so that they may make informed therapeutic choices? Can not informing the patients affected by this radiation overdose be reconciled with the patients' bill of rights?

Adherence to the organization's mission statement, ethical standards, and values statement: Are the actions being considered in this incident consistent with the hospital's mission statement, ethical standards, and values statement?

Adherence to professional codes of ethical conduct: Are the actions being considered in this incident consistent with the codes of ethical conduct promulgated by the professional organizations and associations representing physicians, healthcare executives, and hospitals?

Discrimination against a class of patients: Does labeling these patients as "terminal" invalidate their self-determination? Does it limit their ability to participate in their choice of treatment options? Does discrimination against terminal patients give tacit permission to discriminate against other diverse groups, such as the aged, immigrants, or gays and lesbians?

Hospital management's role and responsibility: What are the hospital management's role and responsibility in this matter? What are the role and responsibility of the hospital CEO specifically?

Legal implications: What are the legal implications of the actions being considered for the hospital? For the physicians involved? Does withholding information about this medical treatment and its potential risks from the patients involved constitute medical malpractice? In the view of the legal system, is this action indeed fraud? Has the hospital's management considered the liability exposure for fraud that is not covered under medical malpractice insurance?

Other legal aspects to be considered relate to specific liability and employment issues. Who employs and supervises the medical physicist? Who pays the medical physicist, and who asked him to resign? Is the medical director for radiation oncology, who typically prescribes radiation therapy dosages, an employee of the hospital or an independent contractor? If the medical director is a contract physician, does the contract stipulate that he hires and pays the medical physicist? Should it? Is the medical director responsible for the actions of the medical physicist whether the medical physicist is employed by the medical director or not? Finally, who owns the linear accelerator used in this case?

Organizational implications: How will the actions being considered in this incident affect the oncology program? The hospital as a whole? The hospital staff?

Ethical decision-making framework: Can the actions being considered in this incident be justified within an acceptable ethical decision-making framework?

DISCUSSION

Truth Telling and Justice and Fairness

The fundamental issue in this case seems to be one of truth telling. Is it not a basic tenet of all ethical relationships that individuals and organizations tell the truth? Is it not the "right" thing to do?

The physicians in this case have argued that telling the truth would cause more harm than good—not sharing this incident with their patients is, in fact, in their patients' best interest. This position, of course, assumes that the patients will never find out about the incident or that they will die without the incident ever coming to light. From a practical standpoint, this eventuality may indeed be the case. But on closer examination, is this scenario likely? Consider the number of health-care workers who interact with a patient on any given day and have access to the patient's medical record. In a teaching hospital, that number is likely to be higher. The prescribed radiation therapy and the received radiation therapy are a matter of medical record. Incident reports and quality assurance reports are also a matter of record. Is it realistic to believe that staff will not have questions about the incident and, worst-case scenario, inadvertently discuss it with the affected patient? Given the great number of staff, physicians, and trustees who are privy to this information, is maintaining a "conspiracy of silence" even possible? Is it right for the hospital to attempt to cover up the error?

In the event that the patients or their families find out about the incident after the fact, what then? What effect will this knowledge have on their opinions of the physicians and the hospital?

Clearly, human relationships are built on the communication of information. If the information shared is not truthful, there can be no trust. Unfortunately, not telling the entire truth in a situation usually means additional shading of the truth or outright lying when questions arise. An individual or institution that betrays the trust on which relationships are built is no longer credible. This betrayal of trust can be especially problematic in healthcare, where patient compliance and positive health outcomes depend on the patient's trust in his healthcare provider.

In the Paradise Hills case, lying or withholding the truth carries enormous risk for undermining the image of the physicians and the hospital. If the incident is discovered by the patients or their families, the physicians and the hospital could be accused of attempting to cover up the incident, which could prove disastrous both in the judgment of the community and in a court of law. Recent political scandals are a tragic reminder that the public will not quietly stand for deceitfulness.

However, the intent in withholding information could arguably be to protect the patients from unnecessary stress and anxiety, not unlike the "white lies" used to spare someone's feelings in everyday life. Is this a fair comparison? Using the Golden Rule as a guide, if you or a loved one were the patient, would you want to know the truth about the incident? Or would you wish to be spared the anxiety?

In the assessment of Elisabeth Kübler-Ross (1969, 32), the psychiatrist renowned for her theory of the five stages of grief, "the question should not be stated, 'Do I tell my patient?' but should be rephrased as, 'How do I share this knowledge with my patient?'" Kübler-Ross believed that "the way in which the bad news is communicated is . . . an important factor which is often underestimated and which should be given more emphasis in the teaching of medical students and supervision of young physicians." Does her assessment apply in this case?

Much in the literature supports the notion that what matters is not so much what is said as how it is said and in what context. Medical information should be presented by a physician with whom the patient has a trust relationship, and nursing staff should be in attendance so that they can prompt the patient to ask questions of the doctor before he leaves or answer such questions after he has gone. While this solicitude may seem like a small thing to do, in today's rushed environment nurses may not be expected or have time to make rounds with physicians. To further compound the situation, in teaching hospitals the patient may feel overwhelmed by a large entourage of house staff, and in non-teaching hospitals a hospitalist whom the patient does not know well may be designated to inform the patient about the medical error. Some might suggest that the risk manager or hospital attorney should be in attendance when a patient is informed about an error. This consideration must be weighed against any alarm or apprehension their presence may generate. When multiple patients need to be informed individually about an error, using scripted information—or at least talking points—may be wise to ensure all patients receive the same information.

A recent study by Iezzoni and colleagues (2012) presented some startling revelations about physician attitudes:

> Approximately one-third of physicians did not completely agree with the need to disclose serious medical errors to patients, almost one-fifth did not completely agree that physicians should never tell a patient something untrue, and nearly two-fifths of physicians did not completely agree that they should disclose their financial relationships with drug and device companies to patients. . . . Just over one-tenth said they had told patients something untrue in the previous year.

The researchers concluded:

> Our findings raise concerns that some patients might not receive complete and accurate information from their physicians, and doubts about whether patient-centered care is broadly possible without more widespread physician endorsement of the core communication principles of openness and honesty with patients.

The study suggests that healthcare professionals could use more education and training about truth telling in patient-centered care. Patients need information and to have all of their questions answered in a straightforward, concerned manner to be able to participate appropriately in their treatment options and to comply with medical instructions. The increasing diversity of both patient populations and healthcare professionals further complicates communications. For more on managing diversity and the ethical implications it presents, see Chapter 14.

A Patient's Right to Know

Do the patients in the Paradise Hills case have a right to know about the error and how it may potentially affect them? The "Patient Care Partnership" of the American Hospital Association (AHA 2003) states:

> Our hospital works hard to keep you safe. We use special policies and procedures to avoid mistakes in your care and keep you free from abuse or neglect. If anything unexpected and significant happens during your hospital stay, you will be told what happened, and any resulting changes in your care will be discussed with you.

How does this standard of conduct apply to the radiation therapy incident at Paradise Hills? The management team and the physicians involved should review its applicability. Their review should consider the patients' and their family members' interpretation of the standard as well.

As healthcare becomes more outcomes driven, "transparency is not only the right thing to do, but also the pragmatic thing to do" (Cosgrove 2013). At Cleveland Clinic, patients have "a clear window into their medical information" through universal access to medical records during their entire care process. After they go home, patients can sign in to MyChart to review all of their care, renew prescriptions, make appointments, and consult with their doctor's office. When patients have such immediate and ongoing access to their medical records, physicians and other clinicians have no choice but to keep patients informed of all aspects of their care, including medical errors. This access makes patients active partners in the care process and provides them with the information they need to make informed decisions about their care and treatment, including what actions to take when medical errors occur. The staff at Cleveland Clinic believe that patients have a right to know and that this kind of transparency holds the staff accountable and makes them better (Cosgrove 2013).

Do patients and their families have a right to know when a medical error has occurred during the course of their treatment? As the following section discusses, the federal government seems to think so as well.

Adherence to the Organization's Mission Statement, Ethical Standards, and Values Statement

The Institute of Medicine report *To Err Is Human: Building a Safer Health System* (Kohn, Corrigan, and Donaldson 1999) claimed that medical errors in the nation's hospitals, clinics, and physician offices account for the deaths of nearly 100,000 Americans each year. Not surprisingly, this landmark report was covered extensively by the media, which in turn prompted a rapid political response.

Congressional hearings, a report from the Quality Interagency Coordination Task Force (2000) titled *Doing What Counts for Patient Safety: Federal Actions to Reduce Medical Errors and Their Impact,* and a major policy speech by President Bill Clinton on reducing medical errors soon followed.

In his speech, President Clinton introduced a national action plan to reduce preventable medical errors by 50 percent within five years (Pilla 2000). This action plan called for

- $20 million for the creation of a Center for Quality Improvement and Patient Safety to sponsor research and education in reducing errors;
- new regulations requiring all 6,000 hospital participants in the Medicare program to implement patient safety programs to reduce medical errors;
- development of a national, state-based system for reporting medical errors, which includes mandatory reporting of preventable errors causing death or serious injury and voluntary reporting of other medical errors such as "near misses";
- support of legislation that protects provider and patient confidentiality without undermining existing tort remedies; and
- new steps to specifically reduce medication errors.

This national action plan signaled government intervention in a domain that previously had been notorious for "policing its own," where medical errors had been held in secret for fear of malpractice litigation, where those committing medical errors were blamed and punished, and where the prevailing standard for prevention of medical errors was to educate those involved in the hope that such errors would not happen again.

To change what some have called a "conspiracy of silence," the Institute of Medicine and the Quality Interagency Coordination Task Force (2000) recommended further actions, including the following:

- Health plans involved in the Federal Employees Health Benefits Program were required to implement patient safety programs.
- Employers were to incorporate patient safety performance into their health-care purchasing decisions.
- Periodic relicensing and reexamination of physicians and nurses by state boards would include knowledge of and competence in patient safety practices.
- Healthcare organizations would establish a goal of continually improved patient safety.
- Healthcare organizations would implement proven medication safety practices.

- Accrediting bodies such as The Joint Commission would review organizational efforts to minimize errors and promote patient safety.
- Computerized medical records that are integrated with drug ordering and administrative systems would be implemented.

For healthcare providers, perhaps the most disconcerting of these recommendations was the mandatory reporting of medical errors to patients and their families. No responsible healthcare professional will argue about the need for strategies to reduce medical errors and ensure patient safety, but the notion of placing the organization and its staff at risk for malpractice litigation gives one pause.

Yet, in his policy address, President Clinton stated, "People should have access to information about a preventable medical error that causes serious injury or death of a family member, and providers should have protections to encourage reporting and prevent mistakes from happening again" (Pilla 2000). Is the expectation that healthcare institutions and medical professionals will report their errors unreasonable? More to the point, is the fear of litigation sufficient justification for withholding the truth from those affected by medical errors? Any reasonable healthcare manager will respond, "Of course not." The patient must always be the first priority. And yet, knowing the right thing to do may be easier than actually doing the right thing.

The Institute of Medicine report *To Err Is Human* had recommended that Congress create a Center for Patient Safety within the Agency for Healthcare Research and Quality (AHRQ 2003) to

- set the national goals for patient safety, track progress in meeting these goals, and issue an annual report to the president and Congress on patient safety; and
- develop knowledge and understanding of errors in healthcare by developing a research agenda, funding centers of excellence, evaluating methods for identifying and preventing errors, and funding dissemination and communication activities to improve patient safety.

In addition, AHRQ was authorized to establish a comprehensive patient safety initiative to

- identify the causes of preventable healthcare errors and patient injury in healthcare delivery;
- develop, demonstrate, and evaluate strategies for reducing errors and improving patient safety; and
- disseminate such effective strategies throughout the healthcare industry.

AHRQ's Center for Quality Measurement and Improvement was renamed in 2001 as the Center for Quality Improvement and Patient Safety (AHRQ 2012), which now

- conducts and supports user-driven research on patient safety and healthcare quality measurement, reporting, and improvement;
- develops and disseminates reports and information on healthcare quality measurement, reporting, and improvement; and
- collaborates with stakeholders across the healthcare system to implement evidence-based practices, accelerating and amplifying improvements in quality and safety for patients.

Despite these agencies' best efforts, little has changed to stem the tide of medical errors. Murphy (2013) tells us that "when patient-first priorities break down, quality, safety, coordination, satisfaction, and profit all decline." As Murphy points out, the Institute of Medicine now reports that more than 80 percent of unnecessary patient deaths are the result of not putting the patient first. Recent studies suggest that the problem has only gotten worse. A US Department of Health & Human Services (HHS) report found that one in seven Medicare patients died or was harmed by hospital care (Greider 2012). Even more disconcerting, another HHS report said that 86 percent of harm to Medicare patients from errors goes unreported. This failure to report errors is not surprising, given that many hospitals have been unwilling or unable to transform their facilities into learning organizations rather than punitive ones. No wonder *American Medical News* has claimed that a "fear of punitive response to hospital errors lingers" (O'Reilly 2012a), citing an AHRQ survey that found 67 percent of healthcare professionals said they are concerned that mistakes are held in their personnel files, and fewer than 50 percent feel free to question decisions or actions of superiors.

The cost of medical errors has received an increasing amount of media attention in recent years, and the numbers are staggering: One study puts the annual cost of medical errors in the United States near $1 trillion (Goedert 2012). In 2008, in an effort to reduce the cost of medical errors to the government, Medicare adopted a policy of "no pay for never events" (medical errors that should never happen). This "ethical and patient safety imperative" seems to have induced hospital leaders to focus more on patient safety and fostered more collaboration among healthcare professionals (O'Reilly 2008, 2012b).

Despite all of the pressures to disclose medical errors so that they can be analyzed and prevented in the future, an overriding fear of litigation still exists. Citing a study that found that 43 percent of 127 families who sued their healthcare providers after perinatal injuries were motivated by suspicion of a cover-up or revenge, Kraman and Hamm (1999) argued in an oft-cited scholarly article that honesty is the best policy in risk management. The authors reported on the experiences of one Veterans Affairs Medical Center that implemented a policy of full disclosure of medical errors to patients and families (in the presence of a family attorney, if the family so desired). The medical center initiated this practice because staff believed it was "the right thing to do." They also found that this honest approach resulted in unanticipated financial benefits to the medical center when lower-cost settlements began replacing higher-cost litigation. This study remains the definitive scholarly work that provides evidence supporting full disclosure of medical errors.

A word about transparency may be in order here. *Transparency* has become the buzzword during the past decade for all that is right. Transparency is advocated in business, government, and healthcare, especially recently. Much media attention has been given to the book *Unaccountable: What Hospitals Won't Tell You and How Transparency Can Revolutionize Health Care* by Marty Makary, a surgeon and professor of public health at Johns Hopkins. Makary (2012) advocates making more hospital performance metrics public and cautions that lack of transparency leaves flaws unchecked and systems uncorrected.

What kind of information, and how much, is appropriate to disclose? And to whom should it be disclosed? A political commentator recently questioned the wisdom of too much transparency—so much transparency that the public is getting bogged down in the minutiae, backdoor bickering, and grandstanding that are obscuring the real issues the public needs to grapple with. Transparency needs to be tempered with judgment. The CEO of one not-for-profit organization spoke with pride of his philosophy that "dirty laundry needs to be aired," but some influential members resigned from the organization because they believed he was publicly sharing too much detail about internal staff conflicts that leadership should have quietly handled.

A case can be made that the greatest positive effect of transparency is that the mere idea of it directs an organization's culture and activities in ways that can withstand public scrutiny whether the public needs to know about them or not. Transparency should lead to resources being committed to activities that are in the best interests of patients and the community being served. As a physician once put it during a discussion about transparency, "If you're going to be naked, you'd better be buff." Although the language may be brash, the advice is good.

Today's management must consider more than just how their actions would play on CNN. Advances in technology and social networking mean that an organization's actions may immediately become a viral Internet sensation with a series of unintended consequences.

Adherence to Professional Codes of Ethical Conduct

Do the existing codes of ethical conduct promulgated by the professional organizations and associations representing physicians, healthcare executives, and hospitals require that the incident at Paradise Hills be fully disclosed to the patients?

The *Code of Medical Ethics* of the American Medical Association (AMA) states:

> A physician shall uphold the standards of professionalism, be honest in all professional interactions, and strive to report physicians deficient in character or competence, or engaging in fraud or deception, to appropriate entities. (AMA 2001, II)

> The patient has the right to receive information from physicians and to discuss the benefits, risks, and costs of appropriate treatment alternatives. Patients should receive guidance from their physicians as to the optimal course of action. Patients are also entitled to obtain copies or summaries of their medical records, to have their questions answered, to be advised of potential conflicts of interests that their physicians might have, and to receive independent professional opinions. (AMA 1993)

The *Code of Ethics* of the American College of Healthcare Executives (ACHE 2011) states:

> The healthcare executive shall conduct professional activities with honesty, integrity, respect, fairness and good faith in a manner that will reflect well upon the profession. (Section I, B)

> The healthcare executive shall, within the scope of his or her authority, work to ensure the existence of a process that will advise patients or others served of the rights, opportunities, responsibilities and risks regarding available healthcare services. (Section II, C)

The AHA's (1999) "Principles of Accountability for Hospitals and Health Care Organizations" states:

> The organization's primary focus is the care of individuals and their families with the goal of maintaining and improving health, alleviating disability, and preventing illness. The organization's policies and procedures should emphasize and the organization's employees and clinical staff must continually demonstrate respect for the individual patient, their values, and their privacy. These policies and procedures should also reinforce the right of patients to be provided information, in understandable language and terms, that relate to their health care and to participate in decisions affecting their health care.

Although the language in these ethical standards is general, the standards nevertheless provide guidance to those wrestling with the ethical dilemma at Paradise Hills. As professionals, the physicians and executives must determine if their actions are consistent with the ethical standards that apply to them.

The AHA's (1999) "Principles of Accountability for Hospitals and Health Care Organizations" make it clear that the governing board and leadership of the organization are responsible for the quality and safety of patient care:

> The organization's governing body and leadership, in conjunction with the clinical staff, are responsible for developing and implementing, in a comprehensive manner, systems and procedures for safeguarding and enhancing the quality of patient care and services. The governing body and leadership, in conjunction with the clinical staff, are also responsible for actively monitoring and immediately acting upon, where appropriate, the results derived from those systems and procedures such that patient/staff safety is ensured and/or improvements in patient care occur.

This guidance supports the argument that ethical matters involving patient–physician relationships are, in fact, the business of the hospital and cannot be relegated to the medical staff alone.

Understanding the Medical Staff Perspective

That the physicians at Paradise Hills take a different view is not surprising. A basic understanding of the medical staff orientation helps explain why physicians adamantly protect what they consider to be their professional province.

The physician typically enjoys a supreme position in the hospital's organizational hierarchy. She generally establishes and maintains the rules that regulate most patient care in the hospital, and she serves as a gatekeeper in admitting patients to the healthcare system. Once patients are admitted for care, they and their caregivers are required to follow "doctor's orders." The physician thus sets the standards for patient care and defines illness.

The physician is granted the authority to define illness because he possesses "a body of knowledge that defines and constructs the roles to be played in the context of the institution" (Berger and Luckmann 1967, 67). Roles make it possible for institutions to exist. The role the physician plays inducts him into specific areas of knowledge, not only in the narrower cognitive sense but also in the sense of norms, values, and even emotions. This knowledge may become so internalized that the physician considers the role "an inevitable fate for which [he] may disclaim responsibility." Thus, he might say, "I have no choice in the matter, I have to act this way because of my position" (Berger and Luckmann 1967, 76).

The physician learns his role through a complex socialization process that begins when he enters medical school. The rigors and expense of medical school, the admission requirements, the protégé system, and the collegial bonds of the medical profession all reflect occupational socialization. On completion of medical school, the symbolic universe of the physician includes elaborate rights, obligations, standard practices, and a role-specific vocabulary. The physician is now socialized to play the role as definer of reality for the patient (Berger and Luckmann 1967, 91).

The effects of this socialization on the moral reasoning of medical students was the subject of an important study conducted by Hébert, Meslin, and Dunn (1992) at the University of Toronto. Their research instrument presented four clinical vignettes, and respondents were asked to list the ethical issues in each. The study assumed that physicians must recognize issues before they can behave appropriately. Students in all four years of medical school participated in the study. The first-year students completed the survey during their medical school orientation. The fourth-year students identified far fewer ethical issues than did the first-year students. The researchers concluded that "these studies show a disturbing pattern; the ethical sensitivity of medical students seems to decrease with more time in medical school. Is this the consequences of medical socialization and is it harmful?"

Thus, physicians approach the world very differently than hospital administrators do. "Physicians tend to be doers, reactive, independent, solo decision makers, business owners," whereas hospital administrators "tend to be planners, proactive, participative, collaborative problem solvers, business stewards" (Peck 2012). Physicians tend to focus on individual patients, whereas administrators focus on the overall organization. To work together successfully, they must reach agreement that what is good for individual patients and what is good for the organization are one and the same.

In any discussion of the role of the physician, some attention must be given to professionalism. Professionals, such as physicians, lawyers, accountants, and healthcare executives, have a number of characteristics in common. They typically form associations, establish licensing or certifications, require specialized education, establish standards of conduct, have their own language, and promote professional autonomy and self-regulation. These characteristics tend to foster exclusivity and place professionals in a position of dominance in society. Some will argue that the physician's position of dominance is justified because she must make life-and-death decisions. Advocates of patient self-determination, however, claim that physician dominance is detrimental—the health status of individuals or populations can only improve when they have a better understanding of health promotion, disease prevention, and disease management.

The occupational socialization and professional dominance that the Paradise Hills physicians enjoy is the reason they believe that matters of patient care fall strictly in their domain.

Discrimination Against a Class of Patients

Labeling the patients in the Paradise Hills case as "terminal" and treating them differently from the way other groups in similar situations are treated is arguably a form of discrimination. Situations where withholding information because of class distinctions appears to be the norm can place decision makers on a slippery slope, because allowing this action with one group may be taken as permission to replicate it among other groups. Treating certain patients differently can be especially dangerous in healthcare organizations, whose patient, employee, and professional populations are becoming increasingly diverse.

Who decides if withholding information from a particular patient or group is appropriate? As resources become increasingly scarce and the population ages, the debate about limiting treatment options for the aged will rage on. This issue is not new—when dialysis and kidney and heart transplants were introduced in the 1960s, the same discussions took place. Around the same time, ethics committees were finding their way into the hospital setting. However, costs are now central to the discussions, so more conflicts are likely to occur. When the issues at stake involve "priceless" lives and the cost-benefit analysis of treatments, the following questions are likely to come into consideration:

- Does the extended quality of life for the individual matter?
- Does the individual's contribution or future contribution to society matter? For example, is treating a rocket scientist different from treating a homeless person?
- Where does self-determination fit into the equation?
- Do "believers" get priority over "nonbelievers"?
- Do patients born in the United States get priority over immigrants?
- What about those who have abused their bodies—substance abusers, alcoholics, smokers, or the obese?
- Does it matter who is paying the bill—government, insurance, or private pay?
- When dealing with the aged, are all 75-year-olds equal physically, mentally, emotionally, and intellectually?
- Who should participate in these decisions?

These same questions may be asked in the future to determine whether costly medications or procedures should be part of the treatment plan for any patient, not just those of a particular group. Clearly, the ethical implications of these decisions will weigh heavily on the minds of healthcare managers faced with the responsibility of developing organizational structures to deal with such issues. A national conversation about this topic is necessary, one that does not allow political interests and hysteria to influence the discussion. Healthcare executives must take the lead in framing the discussion and in developing language and terminology that allow the discussion to take place without talk of "death panels."

Management's Role and Responsibility

What are the hospital management's role and responsibility in the Paradise Hills case? What are the role and responsibility of the hospital CEO specifically? A literal interpretation of the standards of ethical conduct promulgated by ACHE and the AHA (see above) would indicate that the role of the CEO in this case is indeed burdensome because the CEO must balance complex needs and conflicting interests. In fulfilling all his duties, the CEO has responsibilities to the governing board, the institution, the medical staff, the employees, the community, the patients, the profession, and himself.

The CEO's mandate is to carry out the policies of the governing board, which include ensuring compliance with the board-approved ethical standards for the practices of the institution. The CEO is likewise charged with the responsibility of ensuring that the institution operates in ways that are consistent with its mission and values statements.

Partnering with the Medical Staff

The management staff at Paradise Hills have a strong working relationship with the medical staff. The oncology physicians have been especially loyal and committed to Paradise Hills, and in return hospital management has provided them with the resources and technology they need to practice state-of-the-art medicine. It has been a win–win situation for Paradise Hills. The CEO is determined to arrive at a solution to this problem that will preserve the existing medical staff–management relationship. Not incidentally, he knows he must avoid alienating these community-based physicians whose patients are vital to the financial viability of the hospital.

Leadership hospitals generally embrace the core belief that medical staff participation is essential to the successful operations and strategic planning of the institution. Management in such an institution enthusiastically integrates medical staff participation into its way of doing business, fosters ongoing dialogue with physicians, and recognizes the medical staff as a needed resource. The CEO at

Paradise Hills has worked to develop such an environment and is staunch in his resolve that the medical staff must be full and active participants in this ethical decision making. The CEO believes that a satisfactory solution to this incident must not violate confidentiality of patient information, must not infringe on or threaten patient–physician relationships, and must not precipitate a lawsuit. He knows that to secure these objectives he must work closely with the medical staff and avoid an adversarial confrontation. The physicians must be full partners in the analysis and resolution of the problem. Their voice in the proceedings must be heard and attended to. The outcome must be one in which they have been allowed to exercise some element of control.

Fortunately, the CEO at Paradise Hills is armed with the primary prerequisite to successful partnering with the medical staff: They trust him. To solve this ethical problem successfully, he must be well prepared with solid facts, a well-thought-out rationale for actions, and a commitment and plan to deal with all consequences of the actions taken.

The CEO and management staff must also recognize that medical errors take their toll on the physicians and other staff who are involved in an incident. In an organizational culture that emphasizes perfection, self-reproach, and accountability, guilt can affect a clinician's effectiveness in future patient care. Management must therefore take measures to assist staff in appropriately coping with medical errors (Morreim 2000, 56).

Leadership

In this case, as in all ethical matters, the CEO has enormous leadership responsibility. The CEO is responsible for the ethical culture in the organization, implementing the standards of ethical conduct, and serving as an ethical role model for staff. While clinical professionals may bring their own codes of conduct to the workplace, management must set the tone for how business is conducted, how professionals interact, and how patients are served.

Bennis and Namus (1985, 186) are clear on this point: "The leader is responsible for the set of ethics or norms that govern the behavior of people in the organization. Leaders set the moral tone." Nancy Schlichting, CEO of Henry Ford Health System, says, "The greatest deterrent to unethical behavior is values-driven leadership. When people stand for something and there are visible symbols of those values for all to see, they hold it up and measure against it. Employees look at what the leaders are doing and they feel free to come forward and challenge behaviors that do not meet that standard" (quoted in Rice and Perry 2013, 33).

According to Hofmann, "the consistent and absolute intolerance of unethical behavior" is a leadership responsibility. "A policy of zero tolerance means swift action is taken when it occurs, regardless of organizational status. Prerequisites include a comprehensive and unambiguous code of conduct that is well disseminated and understood; no disconnect between the rhetoric and reality of organizational values; [and] behavior of all organizational leaders and staff members that is always above reproach" (quoted in Rice and Perry 2013, 38). The significance of the leader as a role model should not be underestimated. Through their behavior, leaders define what is acceptable and what is not. Others in the organization will seek to emulate those behaviors to gain favor or status.

Ethical problems are a true managerial dilemma because they often represent conflict between an organization's financial performance and its responsibilities to the community and the patients it serves. In the Paradise Hills case, will telling the patients about the errors reduce the public's trust in the organization and dissuade patients from being treated there? Will telling the patients about the errors alienate the physicians and induce them to admit their patients to another facility? This case, like all ethical problems, requires that the CEO, his management team, and the medical staff think through the consequences of their actions on multiple dimensions using ethical analysis as well as bottom-line considerations. While the task is complex and the conflicts may appear insurmountable, Bennis and Namus (1985, 186) remind us that "leaders are persons who are able to influence others; this influence helps to establish the organizational climate for ethical conduct; ethical conduct generates trust; and trust contributes substantially to the long-term success of the organization."

The Betsy Lehman Case

A real-life case that is strikingly similar to the Paradise Hills incident is the one involving Betsy Lehman and the Dana-Farber Cancer Institute. This case underscores the interrelatedness of management, clinical care, and ethics and drives home the point that leadership cannot delegate risk management but must make risk management its own responsibility.

For those who may be unfamiliar with this case, Betsy Lehman was a health news reporter for the *Boston Globe*, and her husband was a scientist at the Dana-Farber Cancer Institute. She died in December 1994 while undergoing chemotherapy at Dana-Farber. Her overdose error was discovered in February 1995 during a medical records review. The *Boston Globe* broke the story in March 1995 with the headline "Doctor's Orders Kill Cancer Patient." An ABC News special with Barbara Walters and Dr. Timothy Johnson, "Betsy Lehman and Medical Errors in U.S. Hospitals," aired in July 1995 and is still timely today.

A root-cause analysis of this case revealed the breakdown of a complex medication process compounded by a lack of communication, illegible physician handwriting, and professional arrogance. Although the human loss in this case was immeasurable, the organization also suffered a public relations crisis that had an extensive negative impact on merger negotiations, staff morale, clinical trials, donations, and the recruitment of physicians, nurses, and researchers. Both The Joint Commission and the state of Massachusetts placed Dana-Farber on probation, affecting both its Medicare reimbursement and its ability to treat patients. This case has been published by Harvard Business School and is used as a teaching tool in university programs throughout the United States (Bohmer and Winslow 1999).

REFERENCES

Agency for Healthcare Research and Quality (AHRQ). 2012. "Center for Quality Improvement and Patient Safety." Posted in October. www.ahrq.gov/cpi/centers/cquips/index.html.

————. 2003. "AHRQ's Patient Safety Initiative: Breadth and Depth for Sustainable Improvements." Chapter 3 in *AHRQ's Patient Safety Initiative: Building Foundations, Reducing Risk.* Interim report to the Senate Committee on Appropriations. Updated December. www.ahrq.gov/research/findings/final-reports/pscongrpt/index.html.

American College of Healthcare Executives (ACHE). 2011. *Code of Ethics.* Updated November 14. www.ache.org/abt_ache/code.cfm.

American Hospital Association (AHA). 2003. "The Patient Care Partnership: Understanding Expectations, Rights and Responsibilities." Accessed July 1, 2013. www.aha.org/advocacy-issues/communicatingpts/pt-care-partnership.shtml.

————. 1999. "Principles of Accountability for Hospitals and Health Care Organizations." Approved November 11–12. www.aha.org/content/00-10/AHAPrinciples Accountability.pdf.

American Medical Association (AMA). 2001. "Principles of Medical Ethics." Preamble to the AMA *Code of Medical Ethics.* Revised June. www.ama-assn.org/ama/pub/physician-resources/medical-ethics/code-medical-ethics/principles-medical-ethics.page.

————. 1993. "Fundamental Elements of the Patient-Physician Relationship." Opinion 10.01 of the AMA *Code of Medical Ethics.* Accessed July 1, 2013. www.ama-assn.org/ama/pub/physician-resources/medical-ethics/code-medical-ethics/opinion 1001.page.

Bennis, W., and B. Namus. 1985. *Leaders: The Strategies for Taking Charge.* New York: Harper and Row.

Berger, P. L., and T. Luckmann. 1967. *The Social Construction of Reality.* Garden City, NY: Anchor Books, Doubleday and Co.

Bohmer, R. M. J., and A. Winslow. 1999. "The Dana-Farber Cancer Institute." Harvard Business School Case 699-025. Revised July. www.hbs.edu/faculty/Pages/item.aspx?num=304.

Cosgrove, T. 2013. "Transparency: A Patient's Right to Know." Institute of Medicine commentary. Published May 17. www.iom.edu/Global/Perspectives/2013/RightToKnow.aspx.

Goedert, J. 2012. "Study Pegs Cost of Medical Errors Near $1 Trillion Annually." HealthData Management. Published October 19. www.healthdatamanagement.com/news/medical-errors-economic-cost-study-hospitals-45134-1.html.

Greider, K. 2012. "The Worst Place to Be If You're Sick." *AARP Bulletin* March, 10–14. http://pubs.aarp.org/aarpbulletin/201203_DC?pg=10.

Hébert, P. C., E. M. Meslin, and E. V. Dunn. 1992. "Measuring the Ethical Sensitivity of Medical Students: A Study at the University of Toronto." *Journal of Medical Ethics* 18 (3): 142–47.

Iezzoni, L. I., S. R. Rao, C. M. DesRoches, C. Vogeli, and E. G. Campbell. 2012. "Survey Shows That at Least Some Physicians Are Not Always Open or Honest with Patients." *Health Affairs* 31 (2): 383–91.

Kohn, L. T., J. M. Corrigan, and M. S. Donaldson (eds.). 1999. *To Err Is Human: Building a Safer Health System.* Washington, DC: National Academies Press.

Kraman, S. S., and G. Hamm. 1999. "Risk Management: Extreme Honesty May Be the Best Policy." *Annals of Internal Medicine* 131 (12): 913–67.

Kübler-Ross, E. 1969. *On Death and Dying.* New York: Macmillan Publishing Co.

Makary, M. 2012. *Unaccountable: What Hospitals Won't Tell You and How Transparency Can Revolutionize Health Care.* New York: Bloomsbury Press.

Morreim, E. 2000. "Ethical Imperatives of Medical Errors." *Healthcare Executive* 15 (4): 56–57.

Murphy, E. C. 2013. "Why Do Healthcare Executives Fail?" Murphy Leadership Partners. Accessed May 8. www.murphyleadership.com/on-demand-webinars.

O'Reilly, K. B. 2012a. "Fear of Punitive Response to Hospital Errors Lingers." *American Medical News* February 20. www.amednews.com/article/20120220/profession/302209938/2/.

———. 2012b. "Medicare's No-Pay Rule Sharpens Infection-Control Efforts." *American Medical News* May 14. www.amednews.com/article/20120514/profession/305149943/6/.

———. 2008. "No Pay for 'Never Events' Becoming Standard." *American Medical News* January 7. www.amednews.com/article/20080107/profession/301079966/7/.

Peck, C. 2012. "Better Hospital–Physician Partnerships." *Hospitals & Health Networks Daily* April 5. www.hhnmag.com/hhnmag/HHNDaily/HHNDailyDisplay.dhtml ?id=9270008713.

Pilla, L. 2000. "Clinton Introduces Plan to Reduce Medical Errors." Nurses.com. Published February 22. www.nurses.com/doc/Clinton-Introduces-Plan-to-Reduce-Medical-Err-0001.

Quality Interagency Coordination Task Force. 2000. *Doing What Counts for Patient Safety: Federal Actions to Reduce Medical Errors and Their Impact.* Accessed April 27, 2013. http://archive.ahrq.gov/quic/report/mederr2.htm.

Rice, J., and F. Perry. 2013. *Healthcare Leadership Excellence: Creating a Career of Impact.* Chicago: Health Administration Press.

CHAPTER 4

Conflicting Moral Demands: Qual Plus HMO

FOR TEN YEARS, Jim Goodrich has been the chief operating officer (COO) of Qual *Case* Plus, a successful not-for-profit, staff-model managed care organization (MCO) with *Study* 275,000 members in a major metropolitan area on the West Coast. The organization has been so financially successful, in some measure because of Jim's efforts, that it is about to embark on the construction of a $12 million corporate office complex to house its business activities. As COO, Jim has been responsible for the planning and development of the project, the purchase of the land, and the presentation of the construction proposal to the 12-member board of directors. Following the board's approval, the building and grounds committee of the board will select a general contractor and submit the construction contract to the entire board for its approval.

The committee-established selection criteria for the general contractor included demonstrated quality of work, ability to meet construction deadlines and work within budget, financial solvency of the firm, and competitive costs. Only local firms known to adhere to ethical business practices were asked to bid on the project.

The request for bids indicated that all bids must be sealed and delivered by noon on December 9 to the COO's office. Bids received after this designated time or not in this designated manner would not be considered. The committee was scheduled to meet at 1:00 pm that day to open the bids, review them, and select a general contractor to submit for board approval.

Joe Smith had served on the building and grounds committee for a number of years. Well liked by the other members of the board, he had been appointed to this committee because, as the owner of Smith Masonry, he had expert knowledge of construction and related fields.

At the appointed time, the committee met, opened the bids, and began its review. Of the bids received, three met all criteria. The costs associated with two of the bids were close. The cost of the third bid, offered by Acme Construction, was considerably higher. Joe was visibly shaken. Knowing that Acme subcontracted with Joe's firm for masonry work, Jim assumed Joe would declare a conflict of interest and abstain when it came time for a vote. Jim did not anticipate what happened next.

As the discussion was about to begin, Joe moved that the committee take a ten-minute recess before continuing its deliberations. When the committee reconvened, Joe made a motion that the three contractors who had made the final cut be offered the opportunity to submit a "final" bid in 24 hours. The committee would then reconvene the next day to review these final bids. Jim was astonished at the motion and at its immediate support from the rest of the committee and questioned the rationale, legality, and ethical implications of this action. He was told quite simply that because all three finalists were being given the same opportunity, it should not be considered illegal or improper. As for rationale, the committee believed that Acme Construction, which met all of the other criteria, may have inadvertently made a calculation error that placed its bid so much higher than the other two finalists. Joe indicated that it would, in fact, be unfair and unethical not to allow a final bid from a contractor known to be competitive in pricing and highly regarded in the building community when the difference in the bid was obviously great enough to be a miscalculation. The motion was quickly called, and the vote was unanimous that "final" bids would be sought from the three contractors.

Jim was shocked and angry that the board committee would take action that he believed to be blatantly unethical, if not illegal. Furthermore, as the executive responsible for this project, he was expected to concur with their decision, an expectation that he was uncomfortable with and believed to be in conflict with his responsibility as an administrator. As soon as he was in his office, Jim called the organization's attorney and reviewed the committee action with him. When asked about the legality of this action, the attorney said he believed it to be a bit unusual but not illegal. Jim suspected that the attorney was reluctant to explore the matter more fully because it was individual board members' actions that were being questioned, rather than the action of the board as a whole.

At this point, Jim knew he had to report the events of the afternoon to Brent Williams, his boss. Brent had been CEO of Qual Plus since its inception 15 years ago and had the unfailing support of the board of directors. Jim liked Brent, and his reporting relationship with him had been mutually satisfying. Brent trusted Jim and gave him the latitude to run the operations of the organization. At times Jim felt that Brent might play a little fast and loose with propriety, but the issues were always personal ones that did not really affect Jim or the operations of the organization. Rumors had circulated that Brent's home had been remodeled at no cost to him through Joe's largesse and that his automobiles were provided at no cost to him by another board member. He was also known to vacation often in a luxury condo in the Caribbean owned by yet another board member. More disturbing to Jim, however, was the fact that Brent's administrative assistant took care of all of his personal errands and business and was often gone from the office for extended periods of time.

When Jim told Brent about the committee action, Brent dismissed it with a shrug. "It's a board committee—it's their call," he said. Jim persisted and told Brent that he was not comfortable with the committee's actions, especially because he was the one expected to execute their decision, and that he was going to request an opinion from the Qual Plus ethics committee. Brent appeared agitated at this suggestion and said abruptly, "I would not recommend that, but if you feel you must, go ahead. Just remember, it's your job that's on the line here." He then stood up, indicating that the discussion was over.

Jim was disappointed with Brent's reaction. With a mortgage, twin girls in college, a son in high school, and a wife with professional ties to the community, Jim was not prepared to relocate. He doubted he could match his current salary in another position. Brent and the board had been extremely generous with his compensation package. Jim did not want to jeopardize his position at Qual Plus. On the other hand, he was seriously troubled by his dilemma.

He called the chair of the organization's ethics committee, who said she did not believe this situation fell within the purview of her committee because it was a board action but agreed to poll her committee and get back to Jim with a response by late afternoon. Jim was not surprised when she called back to say that her committee agreed with her earlier assessment. Jim had come to the conclusion that no one at Qual Plus was ready to take on the board members over this issue. Frustrated, Jim knew that he was expected to keep his mouth shut and carry out the board committee's wishes. He also knew that if he did this, he would be violating his personal principles and would make himself vulnerable to future expectations of unethical behavior.

ETHICS ISSUES

Conflict of interest: Do Joe's actions constitute a flagrant conflict of interest? Does Qual Plus have an organizational policy on conflicts of interest that specifically provides guidance and direction for governing board members?

Management's role and responsibility: What is management's role and responsibility in this matter? Specifically, what is the role of the CEO related to actions of governing board members? Have Brent's special relationships with board members compromised his position and authority as CEO? Is management's primary responsibility to the governing board or to the organization?

Use of organizational resources: Is having the administrative assistant perform personal business for the CEO an appropriate use of organizational resources? Is it appropriate for the CEO to accept personal favors of such value as home remodeling, luxury cars, and vacations from board members?

Adherence to the organization's mission statement, ethical standards, and values statement: Are the actions of the Qual Plus board committee consistent with the organization's mission statement, ethical standards, and values statement? What about Jim's reaction and Joe's reaction?

Adherence to professional codes of ethical conduct: Are the actions here consistent with the codes of conduct promulgated by the professional organizations and associations representing healthcare executives, governing board members, and MCOs?

Organizational implications and evaluating the effectiveness of ethics committees: What is the role of the Qual Plus ethics committee in this situation? What does it say about the organizational culture if so many staff and governing board members appear to find the board committee's action to be acceptable? What effects do the actions of the leadership at Qual Plus have on the organizational culture?

Conflicting moral demands: What is the responsibility of a healthcare executive when she is asked to do something that she feels is unethical? What is the responsibility of a healthcare executive when she observes her boss or others acting unethically? How does she reconcile professional and personal ethical demands when they are in conflict with one another?

Legal implications: Does the action of the board committee in this case constitute a violation of the organization's bid process? Is any aspect of the action illegal? What is the responsibility of the organization's attorney in this case? Is the misuse or waste of charitable or community resources a legal concern as well as unethical?

Justice and fairness: Even if it is not illegal, is the board committee's action fair to the other contractors who participated in good faith in the bid process as stated in the written request for bids?

DISCUSSION

Conflict of Interest

What is a conflict of interest? According to the *Encyclopedia of American Law,* the term *conflict of interest* is "used to describe the situation in which a public official or fiduciary who, contrary to the obligation and absolute duty to act for the benefit of thc public or a designated individual, exploits the relationship for personal benefit, typically pecuniary" (Gale Cengage Learning 2010). In healthcare, a conflict of interest typically arises when an individual or group, such as a board of trustees, has been entrusted with the assets of an organization but acts for personal gain rather than in the organization's best interests. A conflict of interest may be present if even the potential for personal gain exists. Conflicts of interest are very real dangers, both to organizations and to careers. Healthcare managers must always be mindful of potential clashes between their professional obligations and personal interests because even the appearance of a conflict of interest can be damaging.

The American College of Healthcare Executives (ACHE) believes that conflicts of interest are significant enough to warrant reference in two of its policy statements. In its "Considerations for Healthcare Executive–Supplier Interactions," ACHE (2011a) states that

> In interacting with current and potential suppliers, healthcare executives must act in ways that merit trust, confidence and respect, while fulfilling their duties to the public, their organizations and the profession. Further, it is important to avoid even the appearance of conflicts of interest that may seem to unduly advantage the healthcare executive, the organization or the supplier. Thus, healthcare executives must demonstrate the utmost integrity and embrace the need for transparency in interactions with suppliers.

In its policy statement "Ethical Decision Making for Healthcare Executives," ACHE (2011b) states that

> Ethical decision making is required when the healthcare executive must address a conflict or uncertainty regarding competing values, such as personal, organizational, professional and societal values. . . . Healthcare organizations should have mechanisms that may include ethics committees, ethics consultation services, and written policies, procedures and guidelines to assist them with the ethics decision-making process. With these organizational mechanisms and guidelines in place, conflicting interests involving patients, families, caregivers, the organization, payors and the community can be thoughtfully and appropriately reviewed.

State licensures for professionals also may include standards of conduct that address conflicts of interest.

Conflicts of interest most often involve money. A conflict of interest becomes an issue when an individual's personal ties could influence his professional judgment or when an individual is in a position to influence the business of the organization in ways that could lead to his personal gain or that of close family or friends. In some cases, individuals may be quick to exercise caution when their own personal gain is at issue but lax toward the gain of others in their realm of family, friends, or, more significantly, those in authority. However, the same principle applies.

Healthcare executives who know they are not doing anything wrong may not consider the appearance of impropriety as seriously as they should. Sometimes, the healthcare executive may be so close to the issue that she cannot see how her actions appear to others and may not realize that her actions are unfair to legitimate stakeholders because her conflict of interest favors other parties. Of particular relevance in the Qual Plus case is this value of fairness and how it relates to the other general contractors who have fulfilled the criteria required by the organization's formal bid process. Corporate policies and procedures should, above all, be fair to all parties concerned.

Conflicts of interest seem to feature in newspaper headlines with increasing regularity amid the ever-changing complexities of the US healthcare system and in American society where some people find it acceptable to stretch the limits of the law and propriety for economic or personal advantage. Legal and ethical implications will continue to multiply as more and more hospitals and physicians contract for services, as employers and insurers contract with hospitals and physician groups, and as issues of third-party payers, corporation-sponsored research, physician investments, mergers, and the like complicate the relationships involved.

Avoiding Conflicts of Interest

Conflicts of interest and the appearance of impropriety are easier to avoid than to explain. Academic health centers and universities in particular are aware of conflicts of interest associated with physicians' entrepreneurial activities and academic research, especially when funded by corporations. Some universities require that individuals, when hired and periodically thereafter, disclose significant financial, personal, and professional relationships that may represent potential conflicts between their academic role and outside interests. Teaching organizations routinely require that faculty refrain from promoting services or products that bring them personal gain—financial or otherwise.

Governing board members of healthcare organizations are typically required to complete and sign an annual conflict-of-interest disclosure form, noting any financial interests or governing responsibilities they may have in businesses or entities that transact with the healthcare organization. Some organizations include conflict-of-interest clauses in senior-level executive contracts. Healthcare executives have a responsibility to abide by these standards even if they are not required to sign any conflict-of-interest agreement, however. They also must remember that the standards apply when close family or friends have a substantial interest in businesses that interact with the healthcare organization.

While formal agreements are effective in preventing conflicts of interest from becoming major problems, informal realities in each organization also have a considerable impact on how business is conducted and what is considered appropriate behavior. Corporate norms, social groups, role modeling, and interpersonal relationships all play a role in determining behaviors. The burden of responsibility for ethical conduct in the organization is placed on the leaders of the organization, who ultimately are accountable for the corporate culture.

Professional codes of conduct usually address conflicts of interest. The ACHE policy statements cited earlier in this chapter address the professional responsibilities of healthcare executives. The "Conflict of Interest Guidelines for Organized Medical Staffs" of the American Medical Association (AMA 2007) address the responsibilities of physicians who represent the organized medical staff of a healthcare organization on boards, committees, and other governing or decision-making bodies, recommending that the physicians complete and sign a disclosure form and statement of compliance regarding any "actual or potential interest that a reasonable person would believe to be a conflict." Failure on the part of a physician to disclose a conflict is addressed by a clause covering "involuntary recusal for conflicts of interest" (AMA 2007).

The Association of Governing Boards (2013) is clear about its three standards of board responsibility:

1. The duty of care requires the full attention to one's duties as a board member, setting aside competing personal or professional interests to protect the assets of the institution. This includes financial assets to be sure, but it also includes the institution's reputation, personnel, and tangible assets as well. The expectation is that a board member acts reasonably, competently, and prudently when making decisions as a steward of the institution.

2. The duty of loyalty requires board members to put the interests of the institution before all others. It prohibits a board member from acting out of self-interest. The board's conflict-of-interest policy provides guidance on how a conflicted board member can avoid putting personal interests first.

3. The duty of obedience refers to the board member's obligation to advance the mission of the [organization]. It also includes an expectation that board members will act in a manner that is consistent with the mission and goals of the institution. Failure of this duty can result in a loss of public confidence in the institution.

Although these standards of responsibility are directed at governing board members of colleges and universities, they are instructive for healthcare managers as well because they address the organization's reputation, personnel, and other assets. Indeed, managers who fail to live up to firm ethical standards of conduct harm the reputation of the organization and the people who are part of it, whether they are personally guilty of unethical conduct or not.

Because it generally falls to senior management to plan and coordinate board orientation and continuing education, ensuring that the board's conflict-of-interest policy is current, well understood, and appropriately implemented is an essential part of that responsibility.

A Formal, Fair Bid Process

Organizational conflict-of-interest policies and procedures should be written to provide guidance for employees and staff and help them define and avoid difficult situations. A formal bid process typically embodies this kind of protection for staff and ensures fair and equal treatment of vendors. The process and the selection criteria should be well publicized, and bids should be solicited from the broadest range of potential providers. The bids should be sealed and kept confidential, and they should be opened and reviewed simultaneously. Under no circumstances should one vendor know another's bid. The perception of wrongdoing must be avoided. Rumors of unethical business practices, even if untrue, may damage the reputation of the organization and cause it to lose future business. Improperly disclosing confidential information of one vendor to another could even be cause for litigation.

To ensure the integrity of the bid process, a blind consideration of all bids on merit, without identifying names, could be undertaken. If any question of conflict of interest remains, the individual involved should recuse himself from any decision making or discussion that may influence others' votes, to avoid the appearance of preferential treatment or bid rigging.

Clearly, policies, procedures, codes of conduct, and the like will help the health-care manager avoid problems associated with conflicts of interest. Equally important is candid, open discussion among coworkers and professional colleagues when questions of conflict of interest arise. This kind of honest dialogue can help substantially to eradicate any perceptions of wrongdoing before they develop.

Management's Role and Responsibility

Generally, executive leaders in healthcare organizations are expected to be "servant leaders"—that is, to serve the needs of their organization and its stakeholders. However, this leadership style may become problematic if the demands of patients, clients, governing board members, or others in the organization conflict with one's personal values. When a board member uses his board appointment to acquire personal financial gain, to obtain confidential information, or to secure favorable treatment for family or friends, it presents an ethical dilemma for the healthcare executive. Strong, capable leadership can handle this situation without compromising personal integrity. Occasions may arise when a healthcare executive must compromise her personal preferences or liking for the good of the organization, but such compromise is different from sacrificing personal values or standards of ethical conduct. A CEO's responsibility to the organization also outweighs her responsibility to any individual board member. Having clearly written and well-understood policies for the conduct of the governing board is one way to preempt unreasonable and sometimes unethical requests from individual board members.

So, what should Brent have done in the case of Qual Plus? An appropriate and ethical approach in this situation may have been for the CEO and the board chair to discuss the situation and then meet privately with the board member in question to review the inappropriateness of his actions related to the bid process. Of course, this approach assumes that the CEO has previously implemented guidelines and codes of conduct for the organization and the board, including signed documents of conflict-of-interest disclosures. This approach also assumes that the CEO has been a visible role model for ethical conduct throughout the organization and the community and has included ethics education as part of the board's orientation and continuing education. Certainly, if these structural mechanisms were in place, questionable ethical practices like the one surrounding the Qual Plus bid process would not have occurred.

Further complicating the situation at Qual Plus and Brent's leadership abilities has been Brent's poor behavior as an effective role model. He dismisses Jim's concerns with little thought. He does not take the situation or Jim's discomfort with it seriously and shows no support or willingness to pursue an analysis of the ethical implications of the board committee's actions.

Use of Organizational Resources

The CEO's cavalier personal use of organizational resources sends a signal to employees and staff that such misuse is acceptable. He uses his administrative assistant as his personal valet, while the organization pays her salary and reaps small benefit from her time "at work." He drives luxury cars and takes frequent Caribbean vacations. He has created the impression of a lavish lifestyle garnered from being an executive of an HMO—and this at a time when the rising costs of healthcare and efforts to reduce those costs loom high on the national agenda and MCOs are touted as an effective solution. The CEO has provided fertile ground for the appearance of impropriety and suspicions that other questionable business practices may just not be visible. MCOs, like other healthcare institutions, are vulnerable to public scrutiny and accountability because they receive public benefits in the form of tax exemptions. Any suggestion that the organization's operations and business practices involve conflicts of interest, profit-making at whatever cost, or unethical practices may threaten its tax status.

Executives with reputations for excess have been in trouble with the law, the government, and the public. The political and corporate worlds provide us with too many examples to list here. Healthcare executives are not exempt from temptation. Prominent, successful leaders can be found in the headlines and across the Internet captured in humiliating, unethical, and sometimes illegal acts. More often than not, their misdeeds involve financial or sexual transgressions that can be traced to hubris—the arrogant belief that they deserve special treatment and perks and that they are above the rules of ordinary men and women. Unfortunately, great leaders sometimes possess major character flaws. In the literature, this has come to be known as "the Clinton phenomenon." Like President Bill Clinton, these leaders may not lose their jobs or go to jail, but their organizations, their relationships, or their reputations may incur irreparable damage when they exhibit questionable behavior (Rice and Perry 2013, 35).

At Qual Plus, the propriety of the gifts and favors Brent receives from board members is also questionable. Gift giving is a reciprocal act, in which the recipient is expected to express gratitude in some way—by a subsequent gift, favor, or special consideration. In this case, what could the board members presenting the gifts to Brent reasonably expect in return? The answer, as any experienced senior-level manager knows, is political considerations and personal favors. Brent is on dangerous ground because he may develop a sense that he is beholden to the gift givers and expected to provide favors that compromise his obligations to the organization and to the other board members. Such a feeling may, in some part, account for Brent's reluctance to challenge the board committee's actions at Qual Plus—a reluctance that is mirrored by that of the ethics committee and the attorney representing Qual Plus. The staff and employees in an organization take their cues from the CEO and the role modeling that she demonstrates on a day-to-day basis. Such is the power of example. The CEO has the responsibility for establishing an ethical culture in the organization, implementing standards of ethical conduct, educating trustees and staff on these standards, and fulfilling the organization's ethical responsibilities to its community. The CEO must conduct her personal and professional life in an ethical manner worthy of emulation. Healthcare leaders must set high standards and then lead by example. Leaders must practice the standards that they expect of their employees and staff, who will follow what is lived rather than what is written. This is true regardless of the scope of a manager's sphere of influence. We have all known pillars of excellence within organizations. Chances are these departments have managers who set and live high ethical standards. While clinicians may bring their own codes of conduct to the workplace, management must set the tone for how business is conducted, how professionals interact, and how patients and clients are served. The culture of the organization quickly teaches newcomers what is acceptable, what is rewarded, and what is frowned on.

Leadership creates the organizational culture, and the culture at Qual Plus appears to be toxic. Why do those in leadership positions sometimes behave in such obviously wrong ways? What impact does leadership behavior have on the organization? Savvy executives never underestimate the far-reaching influence of leadership throughout the organization. Leaders at the top are role models, and those under them will seek to emulate them in an effort to gain favor in the management hierarchy. Wise leaders will consider how to influence managers and informal leaders throughout the organization in positive ways.

Adherence to the Organization's Mission Statement, Ethical Standards, and Values Statement

While an organization must have a code of conduct, clear ethical standards must also be articulated and well understood by all members of the organization. Formal education of staff, trustees, physicians, vendors, and suppliers must ensure that everyone knows the ethical rules governing the organization and that everyone plays by them. Each program decision, resource allocation, personnel practice, corporate policy, and so forth, whether at the board level or below, must be undertaken only after the ethical implications have been examined and found to meet the organization's standards. In an ethical culture, staff are encouraged to question decisions and probe for the ethics issues that may be present. Forums for discussion and mechanisms for consultation contribute to sound ethical decisions.

A major responsibility of the CEO in the development of an ethical culture is educating trustees. Because trustees are typically community members, often in business, the board must have a clear conflict-of-interest policy. The governing board must mandate that each trustee declare conflicts of interest and abstain from voting whenever decisions of the board would bring business advantages to them, either directly or indirectly. Policies related to competitive bidding procedures must be clear and information kept confidential.

Most trustees are aware of their fiduciary responsibilities to the organization. Too often, however, financial decisions may be reached without a full understanding of their ramifications. Trustees have an ethical responsibility to make informed financial decisions and to spend the organization's resources wisely. The healthcare executive must assist trustees in fulfilling this obligation by providing complete information and recommending continuing education when needed.

Information regarding patients, clients, physicians, staff, suppliers, and the organization must be treated as confidential by trustees unless otherwise specified. Frequently, trustees may be asked by friends or family to provide information that must be kept in confidence. A clear confidentiality policy must be in place and well understood. All board members must be educated regarding the Health Insurance Portability and Accountability Act and its requirements.

Only a few of the areas requiring trustee education are mentioned here. These areas were chosen because of their relevance to the case in point. However, some CEOs fail to make board education the priority that they should. Some fear that a strong, effective board may challenge their authority. Experienced executives know that a well-educated board is needed to move an organization forward. As governing boards become increasingly accountable for quality of care, financial oversight, and other important challenges, healthcare executives must take very seriously their responsibility to ensure their organization has an effective board in place.

Adherence to Professional Codes of Ethical Conduct

ACHE (2013) has published an "Ethics Self-Assessment" designed to help healthcare executives evaluate their areas of ethical strength and opportunities for improvement (see Appendix A). Among the assessment's many questions are three that are relevant to the Qual Plus case:

1. I have a routine system in place for board members to make full disclosure and reveal potential conflicts of interest.
2. I personally disclose and expect board members, staff members, and clinicians to disclose any possible conflicts of interest before pursuing or entering into relationships with potential business partners.
3. I advocate ethical decision making by the board, management team, and medical staff.

The "Ethics Self-Assessment" is one of several tools available to help healthcare executives develop an ethical corporate culture and create management strategies and programs that support ethical decision making. The best practices of other healthcare organizations can also provide valuable guidance. In particular, healthcare organizations that focus on performance excellence will not fail to have an ethical culture. Malcolm Baldrige National Quality Award winners share their best practices willingly through both personal contacts and webinars that cover such topics as leadership, quality, and innovation. Henry Ford Health System (HFHS), a 2011 Baldrige Award winner, has a strong and comprehensive code of conduct that leaves no doubt about the values its staff should practice and the importance of complying with its principles: "Violation of the Code of Conduct and related policies may lead to corrective action up to and including termination and criminal prosecution" (HFHS 2013, 8). Significantly, leadership at HFHS does not abdicate its personal or professional responsibility to abide by its code of conduct; a letter from CEO Nancy Schlichting to all HFHS employees that accompanies the code of conduct states that "leadership must serve not only as a model of compliance to the Code, but also must communicate and create a supportive culture for it, teach it and observe closely for violations, correcting these swiftly when detected" (HFHS 2013, 1). Schlichting has also said, "I attend new-employee orientation, give out my e-mail address, and tell the employees to let me know if they have concerns about whether we are meeting our [ethical] standards" (Rice and Perry 2013, 35). Relevant to the Qual Plus case, the HFHS code of conduct contains a comprehensive section on conflicts of interest. Its guidelines address financial interests, vendor relationships, business entertainment, professional discounts, expert testimony, outside employment, board service, donations, gifts, awards, and other potential conflicts (HFHS 2013, 3–4).

Compliance programs provide an opportunity to combine the responsibilities of compliance and ethics management in an organization. While a compliance program may address some ethical issues, separate compliance and ethics programs should be established that complement one another. Conduct that is legal may not be ethical, even though to be ethical an organization must comply with legal mandates.

A paramount responsibility of leadership in an organization, especially in a healthcare organization whose mission is to serve humanity, is to create a corporate culture where sound ethical decisions are a way of life. Healthcare executives must not forget that "the essence of a profession is that its members commit themselves to a set of standards higher than the morals of the marketplace" (Association of Academic Health Centers 1990, 5).

Organizational Implications and Evaluating the Effectiveness of Ethics Committees

Historically, ethics committees and ethics consultants in healthcare organizations were called on to assist in resolving ethical issues related to end of life, access to treatment, and the like. Typically, the majority of committee members were clinicians, and the knotty issues brought to these committees were clinical in nature.

As the "business" of healthcare delivery has become more complicated, the lines between clinical and business ethical issues frequently blur. Healthcare executives are confronted with more ambiguities, potential for ethical dilemmas, and uncharted waters than ever before. Ethics committees can serve as a valuable sounding board to test ideas and explore potential solutions to ethical dilemmas, and they can be especially helpful to CEOs who may be removed from day-to-day operations.

However, to be prepared to deal with such multifaceted issues as managed care contracting, mergers and acquisitions, compliance, physician investment, and the like, ethics committees must regularly review their scope and function as well as their member composition. Expanding ethics committee responsibilities to include addressing organizational issues and providing advice and counsel to healthcare managers is imperative. Healthcare managers familiar with the clinical issues may be inexperienced with the business issues they now encounter. If ethics committees have not expanded their purposes, they may not be used where the greatest need exists.

For a number of reasons, an ethics committee may not be used as effectively as it should be. Staff and employees may not understand what the committee's role and functions are, what issues it deals with, or how to refer questions or concerns to it. They may be uncomfortable suggesting that the organization's actions, contemplated or otherwise, may not be ethical. They may not know the committee's deliberations are confidential. They may believe the committee deals only with clinical issues because membership typically includes physicians and nurses. Management needs to address these issues through staff education and increased visibility of the committee's work.

Ethics committees play an important role in ensuring an organization is meeting its obligations to patients, clients, and the community. If a healthcare organization is to make sound ethical decisions on a daily basis, its ethics committee must be readily accessible to staff and its effectiveness must be regularly evaluated. Chapter 16 offers practical strategies for evaluating the effectiveness of ethics committees and useful insights on committee self-assessment.

Conflicting Moral Demands

Ethical dilemmas in healthcare are seldom one-dimensional and are rarely, if ever, under the control of a single well-meaning manager. By definition, a dilemma implies conflicting choices with different consequences, usually undesirable. The conflicting moral demands of one's boss and one's conscience are a major challenge for the most ethical of healthcare managers. This dilemma lies at the heart of the matter in the Qual Plus case.

The 2011 National Business Ethics Survey, conducted by the Ethics Resource Center (ERC 2012) and titled *Workplace Ethics in Transition,* reported that signs point to an ethics downturn among our nation's public and private institutions. Findings showed that 45 percent of US workers observed misconduct in the workplace; 65 percent of those who witnessed wrongdoing reported it; and of those who reported, 22 percent experienced some form of retaliation—an all-time high. In addition, compared with the previous survey two years before, the percentage of employees who felt pressure to compromise standards to do their job climbed from 8 percent to 13 percent, and the percentage of employees who viewed their supervisor's ethics negatively rose from 24 percent to 34 percent.

Given the impact of organizational culture on ethical conduct, perhaps the most significant finding had to do with organizations' strength of ethics culture, which declined dramatically. Strength of ethics culture was measured by three critical aspects: ethical leadership, supervisor reinforcement, and peer commitment and support. Survey respondents graded their organization's ethics culture as strong, strong leaning, weak leaning, or weak. The percentage of employees who said their organization had a weak ethics culture increased to 42 percent from 35 percent two years before. The survey indicated that where cultures are weaker, misconduct is more prevalent. An organizational culture may condone unethical conduct simply by overlooking it. Sometimes overlooking seemingly small examples of unethical behavior gives a colleague the green light to misbehave in bigger ways. In contrast, questioning the colleague and challenging his actions can alert him to an opportunity for behavior modification.

So what do you do when someone in authority asks you to act unethically? Standing up for what is right is always commendable, but before you do so, you must calculate the costs and the unintended consequences of your actions. Most people cannot afford to stand up for their principles lest they lose their job—especially during an economic recession. As the ERC (2012) survey indicated, of those who reported wrongdoing, 22 percent suffered retaliation of some kind.

Indeed, an employee facing this dilemma is at great personal risk if he refuses to perform unethical acts and if, as in the Qual Plus case, those in authority are the CEO and board members who control his job and, to some extent, his future career. Aside from potentially losing his job, what other considerations must weigh heavily on Jim's decision? What about his family obligations, his children's education, and his wife's ties to the community? Jim believes he would have difficulty matching his current compensation package if he were fired. Is this a valid consideration in his decision making? Are his personal well-being and the well-being of his family separate from morality? How would he explain his termination, if that should occur? What about his references for new employment? Would he be labeled as "not a team player"? Is he the only one who sees anything wrong? Would all of the parties involved deny any wrongdoing if the situation were made public? Does Jim have any personal liability if he acts unethically?

On the other hand, if Jim acquiesces to the board committee's requests and takes action that he deems unethical, what consequences can he expect? Jim knows that he will have difficulty living with himself if he makes that decision. It will be a terrible blow to his self-esteem. He worries that if he complies with the committee's wishes, he will be expected to abandon his principles in future decisions—in essence, be "held hostage" by this action in whatever unethical murky situations lie ahead. Most employees simply give in under this kind of pressure and become "organization people."

A physician who was asked about a similar dilemma responded, "I'm not so narcissistic that I would stand firm in my righteousness while my family starved." Perhaps he was exaggerating, but his comment makes an interesting point: One's moral obligations are complex. There are no simple answers. An experienced senior-level executive in a multinational corporation, when told of the physician's remark, immediately replied, "He's using his family as a rationalization for not doing the difficult thing." He went on to explain that he had been with a company that gave very large bonuses to its top senior executives (himself included) but at the same time told the executives to cut the salaries of all their direct reports. When he complained that this was unfair, he was told the decision had been made. He decided he couldn't live with that and resigned. It took him three months to find another position, but he said he never regretted his decision and his family supported him in it. Although we do not know all of the circumstances in either the physician's or the executive's case, we can appreciate that they both faced challenging dilemmas and that a number of considerations entered into their decisions.

Given all the risks involved, can a senior-level manager defy authority more easily than a secretary or an administrative assistant can? Who has more to lose? Being asked to ignore or participate in ethical misconduct presents challenges at all levels of the organization. Resolution is difficult for any employee, and the difficulty is only intensified by personal circumstances.

The federal government recognizes the difficulty that employees face when they are asked to do something unethical or when they observe unethical conduct on the part of their coworkers. In 1991, Congress passed the Federal Sentencing Guidelines for Organizations (USSC 2012). The guidelines apply to all profit and not-for-profit organizations, associations, corporations, and the like; mandate strict punishment for those convicted of federal crimes; and hold an organization responsible for the wrongful acts of its employees if the employees are acting in their official capacities. The guidelines include fines for the organizations and jail sentences and/or fines both for those involved and for managers and executives, whether they knew about the illegal actions or not. If the company has an effective ethics and compliance program, penalties may be significantly reduced. Criteria for an effective program include

- compliance standards and procedures,
- oversight by high-level personnel,
- due care in delegating authority,
- training programs that communicate ethical standards and ensure compliance,
- internal auditing and reporting systems,
- consistent enforcement of standards through disciplinary measures, and
- measures to prevent recurrence of offenses.

The Federal Sentencing Guidelines expect organizations to train and counsel employees to act lawfully and ethically. The guidelines also require that employees be able to report suspected violations without fear of reprisal. Employees of most organizations are guaranteed further protection against reprisal when they disclose actions that violate federal statutes: Title VII of the Civil Rights Act, the Age Discrimination in Employment Act, and the Occupational Safety and Health Act all contain anti-retaliation protection. Government agencies, such as the Environmental Protection Agency, the Department of Health & Human Services, and the Antitrust Division of the Department of Justice, have developed model compliance programs, programs for self-reporting, and programs for amnesty.

The act of whistle-blowing has become even more complicated with the passage of two federal laws. The False Claims Act of 1986 and the Sarbanes-Oxley Act of 2002 seek to recover government funds from organizations found guilty of misdeeds and to provide financial rewards for whistle-blowers in amounts that can be substantial. The potential rewards have caused some employees to make premature or false claims and have caused others to question the motivation of some whistle-blowers interested more in money than in "doing the right thing" (Friedman 2007).

Friedman (2007) provides some solid advice for those who may consider whistle-blowing:

- Have some basis in fact.
- Don't wait until the evidence is overwhelming.
- Listen to the concerns of people closest to the situation.
- Don't try to cover the situation up; someone will find out.
- Support your colleagues who blow the whistle.
- Make your report to the appropriate individual or entity, starting internally.
- Respect that confidential sources must remain confidential.
- Consider whether the organization's culture provides protection for whistle-blowers.
- Understand the consequences of your decision.
- Decide if whistle-blowing is worth it.

While some protection exists for those who do not wish to participate in unethical or illegal acts or stand by while they observe others participate, risks remain. Healthcare managers who find themselves in a dilemma must carefully weigh both current and future consequences of their actions on themselves personally as well as on family, colleagues, and those for whom they are a role model. We all make choices that we believe we can live with, but rarely does compromising our principles come to a good end.

Knowing the right thing to do is easier than doing the right thing. Some managers may choose simply to remove themselves from a situation that requires them to compromise their principles and their personal value system. Others may decide to "ride it out" and allow freedom and flexibility to work out problems. Sometimes this course of action is an acceptable one. But healthcare managers ought to think carefully through the difficult choices before them and consider both the short- and the long-term consequences of their decisions for their organizations, their families, and their careers.

REFERENCES

American College of Healthcare Executives (ACHE). 2013. "Ethics Self-Assessment." Accessed May 1. www.ache.org/newclub/career/Ethics_self-assessment.pdf.

———. 2011a. "Considerations for Healthcare Executive–Supplier Interactions." Ethical policy statement. Revised November 14. www.ache.org/policy/execsuppliers.cfm.

———. 2011b. "Ethical Decision Making for Healthcare Executives." Ethical policy statement. Revised November 14. www.ache.org/policy/decision.cfm.

American Medical Association (AMA). 2007. "Conflict of Interest Guidelines for Organized Medical Staffs." Revised October. www.ama-assn.org/resources/doc/omss/coiguidelines2007.pdf.

Association of Academic Health Centers. 1990. "Conflicts of Interest in Academic Health Centers." Report of the AHC Task Force on Science Policy. Washington, DC: Association of Academic Health Centers.

Association of Governing Boards. 2013. "Three Standards of Board Responsibility." Accessed May 1. http://agb.org/knowledge-center/briefs/fiduciary-duties.

Ethics Resource Center (ERC). 2012. *Workplace Ethics in Transition*. 2011 National Business Ethics Survey. www.ethics.org/nbes/files/FinalNBES-web.pdf.

Friedman, E. 2007. "Hear That Long, Lonesome Whistle Blow." *Hospitals & Health Networks Daily* October 2.

Gale Cengage Learning. 2010. *Encyclopedia of American Law,* third edition. Volume 14, *Dictionary of Legal Terms*. Farmington Hills, MI: Gale Cengage Learning.

Henry Ford Health System (HFHS). 2013. "Code of Conduct." Accessed June 28. www.henryford.com/documents/Medical%20Education/HFMH%20GME/Rehab%20Internship/HFHS%20Code%20of%20Conduct.pdf.

Rice, J., and F. Perry. 2013. *Healthcare Leadership Excellence: Creating a Career of Impact*. Chicago: Health Administration Press.

US Sentencing Commission (USSC). 2012. "Sentencing of Organizations." Chapter 8 of the USSC *Guidelines Manual*. www.ussc.gov/Guidelines.

CHAPTER 5

Gender Discrimination:
Rolling Meadows Community Hospital

ROLLING MEADOWS COMMUNITY HOSPITAL is a 200-bed acute care facility *Case* located in an affluent suburb of a major metropolitan area in the Midwest. The *Study* hospital is highly regarded in the community, especially for its obstetrics program and innovative birthing center, its ambulatory care program, and its geriatrics center. The hospital is supported by a large group practice of young, well-trained primary care physicians who occupy an adjacent medical office building owned by the hospital. Despite turmoil in healthcare delivery during the past decade, Rolling Meadows has remained financially strong. Indeed, it has prospered in an environment that quickly became dominated by managed care in recent years.

Rolling Meadows was well positioned for such changes. Its financial stability, its strong primary care base, and its modern facilities predicted success. In addition, its location among the rolling meadows for which it is named and its proximity to an exclusive golf course make the hospital a desirable place of employment for professional and nonprofessional staff alike.

John Waverly has been the CEO of Rolling Meadows for five years. The hospital's governing board had conducted a national search and aggressively recruited John, who at 42 years old was an up-and-coming HMO executive on the West Coast. The board still congratulates itself on its foresight and wisdom. John was just what Rolling Meadows needed to make the hospital a major player in the then-emerging managed care market. The hospital has thrived under John's leadership and has compensated him well for his efforts. In addition, John continues to enjoy the favor of a governing board that, although conservative, has remained supportive of his innovative management style. John is the envy of his peers in other, more beleaguered healthcare institutions and, at age 47, he feels good about his professional achievements and status.

In retrospect, his decision to take the CEO position at Rolling Meadows had been a good one. At the time of his recruitment, John had major reservations about relocating to the Midwest, especially to the conservative community surrounding Rolling Meadows. He wasn't sure his wife and children would easily adjust. Indeed, they have never fully embraced this community, a fact that continues to be a source of tension in John's life.

In the beginning, John had also been uneasy about his credentials and unsure about how well his educational background would translate to the delivery side of healthcare. John knew he would have to work especially hard to compensate for his lack of hospital experience.

Six months ago, John hired a bright, ambitious postgraduate fellow from a prestigious university program in hospital administration. At the time, John was about to enter into discussions with two nearby powerful healthcare financing and delivery systems, both of which wanted Rolling Meadows to become a part of their multihospital structure. John knew that these discussions and evaluations of any proposals they submitted would be time consuming and demand a great deal of research and preparation. Having a capable postgraduate fellow on board to perform staff work appeared to be a win–win situation. The arrangement would provide both valuable experience for the fellow and needed manpower for the organization. John especially liked the idea of working with someone who was well schooled in the latest academic trends in healthcare administration.

Over the past six months, the partnership proved to be as fruitful as expected. The CEO and his young protégée worked closely together for long hours and week-ends, and Rolling Meadows benefited greatly from their hard work. John and his protégée found themselves celebrating success after success. It was a most enjoy-able partnership. She admired and respected John; he was flattered by her admira-tion. He found himself seeking out opportunities to spend more and more time with her. She began accompanying him to all of his meetings, even those unrelated to her assigned projects. He looked for educational conferences in attractive loca-tions where the two of them enjoyed fine dining and upscale accommodations.

Now her fellowship was nearing its close, and she approached John about her future career plans. Her performance evaluations had been outstanding, as indeed had been her accomplishments. Rolling Meadows had profited greatly from her efforts, and she fully expected to be awarded a postgraduate fellowship position. After all, many of her peers already had received job offers from their fellowship organizations even though they had no significant accomplishments to report from their fellowship experiences. John had been an outstanding mentor, and her admi-ration and respect for him bordered on hero worship.

John was not unprepared for this discussion. After much thought, he had decided it would not be prudent for him to offer her a position at Rolling Meadows. He candidly explained the situation to her. Her performance was outstanding, many had noted her professionalism, and she was a brilliant strategist. But, he said, he was personally attracted to her and he felt this attraction was reciprocated. He *Study* believed that if they continued to spend time together, this attraction would esca-late to a physical relationship. *Case*

He offered to help her in her job search by providing impeccable references and contacting his colleagues in progressive, innovative organizations where her talents would be showcased. She was astonished and humiliated. In view of her accom-plishments and her close working relationship with John, she assumed a position was a given. She felt used and betrayed. Angry, she said this treatment constituted nothing other than sexual harassment. John believed this remark was an idle threat and that reason would overcome her emotional outburst.

The following day, John received a phone call from a member of the governing board informing him that an executive session of the board had been scheduled to discuss "this appalling situation" and the action that should be taken to avert a lawsuit. He told John to be prepared to respond to the allegations at this meeting, and if they were accurate, he should consider resignation to spare the hospital any adverse publicity.

John was surprised by the call and by the tone of the conversation but felt confident that he had done nothing wrong. In fact, he believed he had honestly appraised the potential dangers of his relationship with the fellow and had avoided any misconduct. He believed his actions had been in the best interests of the orga-nization and that the governing board would agree.

ETHICS ISSUES

Legal implications: Do John's actions in this situation constitute sexual harassment? If so, are John and the hospital both liable for these actions? Could this situation be viewed as a case of gender discrimination? Does it matter?

Adherence to the organization's mission statement, ethical standards, and values statement: Are John's actions in this situation consistent with the hospital's ethical standards and values?

Adherence to professional codes of ethical conduct: Is John's conduct in this situation consistent with the professional codes of ethics as promulgated by the professional organizations representing healthcare executives and hospitals?

Organizational implications: Have organizational resources been used prudently? Has this situation, including John's actions specifically, had any effect on other employees in the organization? Have the image and reputation of the organization been affected by this situation? How significant an impact might this situation have on the operations and success of the organization? Are there financial implications to John's actions?

Leadership responsibilities: Was John's conduct in this situation consistent with the role and responsibility inherent in the position of CEO of a healthcare organization?

Expectations of a mentorship program: What are the role and responsibilities of a mentor? Of a protégé? On completion of a postgraduate fellowship, what can each of the participants expect to have achieved? In this case, has the postgraduate fellowship met or failed its expectations?

Justice and fairness: Has the postgraduate fellow in this case been treated fairly? Is John being treated fairly by the governing board, considering his candor and honesty regarding the situation?

Community values: Has John taken sufficient consideration of community standards and values into account? What about the board, when identifying their expectations of the CEO and the needs of his family? When new staff members are recruited to a community, how important are the standards and expectations that the community may have for its professionals?

DISCUSSION

Legal Implications

The fundamental question in this case may well be: Did John, in fact, do anything wrong? Formal allegations of sexual harassment may be forthcoming. Do John's actions here constitute sexual harassment? John would vehemently deny any explicit or implicit actions or expressions that would suggest sexual harassment. He admits to his attraction to the fellow but insists that the long hours worked together, the meetings, and the out-of-town conferences were work related and that she was never coerced to spend this time with him. Indeed, he would argue that she seemed to be attracted to him and, in fact, to have encouraged his attentions with frequent flattery and expressions of gratitude for the time and effort he was putting into her fellowship experience.

Some might argue that John's superior position as CEO gives him a power advantage that "implies" coercion, overt or not. But if John and his protégée both willingly and actively participated in this relationship, does that not imply acceptable activity between two consenting adults? And as such, would this relationship not be consistent with prevailing societal norms and therefore lack coercion?

If John is not guilty of sexual harassment, then perhaps he is guilty of sexual misconduct. However, John and the fellow did not engage in any sexual or physical activity. In fact, no expression of desire or intimacy was involved. To himself, John would admit flirtation, but nothing more. Is attraction not acted on a form of sexual misconduct—adultery of the heart, so to speak, as admitted publicly by former president Jimmy Carter? Some religious beliefs delineate clearly between desire or intention and action. These beliefs suggest that the action is what is "sinful," and if the "evil" desires are overcome by will and hence not acted on, such behavior may be considered virtuous. In this case, John chose not to take the relationship to the next level—assuming that the choice was his alone to make, that is.

Or is this gender discrimination? Would this postgraduate fellow have been offered a position with the organization if she had been a man? High-performing postgraduate fellows are not guaranteed a position on completion of the fellowship, but offering a position is a common practice among healthcare organizations. An American College of Healthcare Executives (ACHE 2010) study found that 63 percent of postgraduate fellows surveyed were offered a position following their fellowship. However, 90 percent of the postgraduate fellowship group surveyed expected to be offered a position. While healthcare executives will admit that postgraduate fellowships are a great source of new talent for an organization, mentors are wise to clearly state at the outset that there is no guarantee a position with the organization will be offered at the end of the fellowship.

Were there financial improprieties in this situation? Were the out-of-state conferences necessary, or were they merely boondoggles? Is it wrong to consider these conferences in upscale locations as a well-deserved and appropriate reward for high-performing staff who may be putting in long hours in uncompensated or lowly compensated positions, especially when conferences are infrequent and have educational merit?

Is John's conduct in this case simply an example of bad judgment? Were his actions motivated by a sense of power and a belief that his status and accomplishments placed him above the need to avoid any appearance of impropriety? John would argue that his actions were always in the best interests of the organization. He can cite significant accomplishments as a result of this mentor–protégé relationship. According to John, his intentions were always to serve as a diligent preceptor, and he believes the fellowship has been an educationally rewarding experience for the fellow. He is stunned that anyone on the governing board would consider his actions to be anything other than in the best interests of the organization. After all, for the good of the organization he denied a position to this fellow. John believes the only thing he may be guilty of is misplaced honesty, and he greatly regrets admitting his attraction to the postgraduate fellow.

In their upcoming review of this case, the governing board members must, to the extent possible, set aside personal standards of conduct and rely on the hospital's standards and policies and on professional codes of ethics if they are to make a fair and just assessment of this situation. Is it likely they will be able to do so?

Adherence to the Organization's Mission Statement, Ethical Standards, and Values Statement

To resolve the issues of this case, access to the hospital's ethical standards and values would be advantageous. Indeed, assistance in the resolution of ethical questions is ample justification for written standards of ethical practice in an organization. Such written standards also provide valuable guidelines for an organization's day-to-day professional and business operations.

The "Principles of Accountability for Hospitals and Health Care Organizations" of the American Hospital Association (AHA 1999, I) make it clear that the governing board has a responsibility for establishing the ethical standards that guide the organization's operations. Legal and accreditation requirements address this obligation as well.

Emanating from the hospital's mission statement, these ethical standards frequently reflect the mission of the organization in responding to the needs of its community and the prevailing standards of behavior in its community. In this particular case, no such written standards of ethical conduct or values statement are in place, but Rolling Meadows's mission statement does reference "family values" in its stated commitment to serve its community through state-of-the-art programs in family practice, obstetrics and gynecology, and geriatrics. The service area for Rolling Meadows is family oriented, religious, and conservative, and the board members representing this community reflect these same values. Under these circumstances, is it safe to assume that John's behavior will be judged in the same framework as that of his colleagues in other healthcare organizations? If not, is this disparate treatment fair?

When recruiting John to be the CEO of Rolling Meadows, did the board make clear the community's standards and expectations for its professionals? Did the board take into account how important a satisfactory adjustment of one's family is to the positive job performance of the hospital's CEO? If not, is the board acting fairly now?

Typically, healthcare organizations are a vital and visible part of any community. They serve the community's healthcare needs, but they are also a source of employment and an economic force in the community. Accordingly, leaders of healthcare organizations are expected to be pillars of the community. Disregarding community values can be career limiting, or at least embarrassing, for the CEO or other senior-level staff. For example, in one Michigan hospital with a board chair who was a retired plant manager for Chevrolet, a vice president made the mistake of parking his foreign-made automobile in the hospital parking lot and was publicly chastised at the board meeting for disloyalty to the community.

Adherence to Professional Codes of Ethical Conduct

ACHE's *Code of Ethics* provides guidelines for the ethical conduct of healthcare executives (see Appendix B). It identifies standards of ethical behavior for healthcare executives in their professional and personal relationships, especially when their "conduct directly relates to the role and identity of the healthcare executive." The *Code* advises that healthcare executives should serve as "moral advocates" and should "act in ways that will merit the trust, confidence and respect" of all. In doing so, "healthcare executives should lead lives that embody an exemplary system of values and ethics" (ACHE 2011, Preamble). If these standards are to be applied to the Rolling Meadows case, the key word here may be "exemplary."

In the section on the healthcare executive's responsibilities to employees, the *Code* obligates healthcare executives to promote "a healthy work environment which includes freedom from harassment, sexual and other, and coercion of any kind" and "a culture of inclusivity that seeks to prevent discrimination on the basis of race, ethnicity, religion, gender, sexual orientation, age or disability" (ACHE 2011, Section IV, C, D).

Organizational Implications

Are financial improprieties evident in John's actions? The answer to this question must follow a careful review of the hospital's policies related to educational conferences and business travel. Adherence to these policies must be uniform among the staff, including the CEO.

Has this situation, and John's behavior specifically, had any effect on other employees in the organization? Regardless of how discreet the individuals in any "special" relationship may be, the relationship is usually quickly perceived by most of the staff who have contact with the participants—particularly when the CEO is involved, because of his high visibility. Such special relationships are often a frequent topic of office gossip and speculation. They are bound to be an unneeded distraction at best and a threat to the credibility of management at worst. Regardless of what the participants may believe, favoritism, physical attractions, and flirtations are always obvious to outside observers and do affect the functioning of the organization, however negligible in some cases.

If office rumors filter outside the organization into other, more public domains, as they often do, the image of the organization and the effectiveness of the CEO may suffer. These considerations have prompted many organizations to establish policies limiting or prohibiting workplace liaisons. A survey of more than 2,000 working professionals indicated that office life is "erotically charged and occasionally lurid" (Cohen 2012). While this survey may not reflect the typical healthcare environment, it gives one pause. Resisting the temptation of being human is not always easy, but ethical leadership requires self-discipline.

In a recent article about Gloria Allred, the highly sought-after lawyer for sexual harassment and discrimination cases was quoted as saying, "There is an epidemic of sexual harassment and discrimination against women in companies all across

America" (Kolhatkar 2012). The article reported that 28,534 sex discrimination charges were filed with the US Equal Employment Opportunity Commission (EEOC) in 2011, and Allred has been highly successful in prosecuting such cases. She says, "Some very intelligent men can be so successful in business and so stupid in the workplace."

Leadership and Power

Effective leaders have certain characteristics in common: vision, integrity, intelligence, initiative, interpersonal skills, ethics, and flexibility, to name a few. Leaders are expected to serve as positive role models, to motivate staff and employees, to be committed to the organization's mission and goals, to be responsive to the community's needs, to establish ethical standards, and to be of strong moral character.

The higher the leader is in the organization, the more important and visible her moral character becomes. The moral character of the leader can serve as the standard for acceptable behavior, or it can destroy the organization's reputation and effectiveness. At Rolling Meadows, John's preferential treatment of the postgraduate fellow has eroded staff morale, and rumors about the relationship are fraying his credibility. Healthcare executives, especially CEOs, may liberally reward their immediate subordinates for jobs well done, while others in the organization may perform equally well yet go unrewarded. Executives may be oblivious to the effect that this behavior has on the remainder of the staff.

It's lonely at the top. Unfortunately, to be effective, a leader must willingly take on this hardship. Too often, the job is just not that much fun. The leader may enjoy friendship and confidences among professional colleagues in other organizations (noncompetitors, of course) but not in her organization without the risk of compromising her position.

Further complicating the role and responsibilities of leaders is the issue of professional power. When you are the boss and have the power to reward others (or not), do your subordinates always tell you the truth, or do they tell you what they think you want to hear? Some subordinates may want nothing other than to please you (the superior) and be liked by you. Taken to extremes, the subordinate may begin to adopt your manner of dress, appearance, and work habits. If the behavior borders on the obsequious, the subordinate may be ridiculed by other employees and called a "yes man" or even worse. Some subordinates who exhibit this behavior seek career advancement; others simply want to be closer to those in authority.

The behavior of the superior in this dynamic can be interesting as well. While some bosses may feel flattered and enjoy such behavior, others may dismiss it and seek more original thinking and intellectual challenge from their subordinates. As in all circumstances, the boss takes the lead in defining the patterns of behavior that will prevail in an organization.

An additional source of power for executives, whether in healthcare or the corporate world, are the rituals and symbols that define the "executive office" and impart power to those who inhabit it. Berger and Luckmann (1967, 91) posit that all reality is socially constructed by the interactions of the participants. They believe that symbols and rituals structure and influence this interaction and distribute power accordingly. The corner office, the executive furniture, the Mont Blanc pens, the executive attire, and the framed diploma all signify authority and set the executives apart from the less powerful employees. No wonder many executives seek to keep these tokens of power in place.

Executives often underestimate the level of power that they exercise. In fact, it can be dangerous when the powerful are unaware of the power they wield. Equally dangerous, however, is when the powerful become so aware and so seduced by power that they act in arrogant disregard of the norms, laws, and standards intended for everyone in a profession, an organization, or a society. The idea of hubris—excessive pride or self-inflation—and its downfall are often noted in mythology and history. In Greek mythology, the hero aspiring to be like the gods was usually punished by death. In modern times, examples abound of political figures who believed they were above the law and suffered a demolished career and reputation as a result. Less conspicuous but more common in healthcare management is the highly regarded and committed leader who develops a sense of entitlement regarding the "perks" of the position as a result of the long hours and personal sacrifices that she has endured.

Finally, some leaders struggle with a desire to do the right thing in the face of ethical dilemmas and ambiguities. The close scrutiny of their actions in their organization, in the healthcare field, and in the media and the community at large makes them especially vulnerable to questions.

Effective leaders are self-aware. They reflect on their words, actions, and the effect they have on others and on their organizations. These leaders are not always perfect, but they are open to learning new communication styles and leadership strategies. They know that if they want high-performing teams, they must model the behaviors they wish their staff to emulate. Effective leaders are moral leaders who promote morality among subordinates.

A multitude of resources provide ethical guidance, including professional organizations, university programs, publications, educational programs, ethics consultants, networking, and the Internet. However, the best source of guidance remains the organization's mission statement, which should help define the ethical standards of the organization and provide a sense of purpose and direction to staff.

Kramer (2003) offers useful questions that leaders can ask themselves from time to time to determine if they are in danger of reckless behavior:

1. Are you spending most of your time plugging holes and papering over cracks?
2. How do you respond to those annoying dissenting voices in your organization?
3. Whom can you really trust to tell you the emperor has no clothes?
4. Do you have illusions of grandeur?
5. Are you too greedy for your own good?
6. Is this a good time to pause, consider doing something different, or even nothing at all?

The situation at Rolling Meadows points out the very real need for healthcare leaders at all levels to have a trustworthy confidant who can advise and alert them when their actions are questionable and may have untoward consequences. Some managers neglect this advice because their insecurity or naiveté does not invite criticism. But effective leaders must be able to anticipate the consequences of personal and professional actions both on their careers and on their organizations. Wise managers will seek out a respected and trustworthy staff member, colleague, or friend who can offer candid criticism in confidence.

In the Rolling Meadows case, should the fellow be considered blameless in what appears to be an escalating personal relationship? Perhaps not. One would think that having completed a graduate program, the fellow would be mature enough to recognize inappropriate behavior, whether her own or that of others. Nevertheless, university programs should include professionalism and ethical conduct as an important component of coursework. Regardless of the fellow's responsibility, however, the power equation of superior–subordinate tips the balance of blame toward the CEO mentor.

Sex Discrimination and Sexual Harassment

Sex discrimination is against the law and has been since Congress passed the Civil Rights Act of 1964. This law, along with various state and local statutes, prohibits discrimination based on race, sex, religion, age, national origin, and disability. Title VII of the Civil Rights Act of 1964 prohibits discrimination in private employment with respect to compensation and the terms, conditions, and privileges of employment. These include hiring, firing, promotion, transfer, job training, and apprenticeship decisions. The Civil Rights Act of 1991 awarded to victims of such discrimination the right to jury trials and compensatory and punitive damages (EEOC 2013). The EEOC is the federal agency established to administer the law.

In 2009, President Barack Obama signed the Lilly Ledbetter Fair Pay Act, a law named for an Alabama woman who, at the end of her 19-year career as a supervisor at Goodyear Tire and Rubber, discovered that she had been paid less than men in the same position. Her claim was originally denied by the US Supreme Court, which said she should have filed her suit within 180 days of the date that Goodyear first paid her less. This new law resets the six-month statute of limitations every time the worker receives a paycheck.

Sex discrimination was not part of the Civil Rights Act of 1964 as it was originally written. Gender was added at the last minute by conservative southern opponents of the bill who thought that something as "ludicrous" as equality of the sexes would surely cause the bill to founder. The bill passed and became law, but the EEOC took no action against sex discrimination in employment for several years until pressure from the women's movement made it an issue. A case was subsequently made that sexual harassment is, in fact, a form of sex discrimination. In 1980, the EEOC defined sexual harassment as a form of sex discrimination prohibited by the Civil Rights Act, and in 1986, the Supreme Court held that sexual harassment on the job was a form of sex discrimination (Lazar and Volberg 2013).

In the case of Rolling Meadows Community Hospital, an examination of the possibility of disparate treatment because of gender may be in order. If an employee was treated less favorably because of gender, or if he was treated both differently and less favorably, disparate treatment and discrimination may be involved. The complainant must show that the employer intended to discriminate because of gender. That is, the employee must show that he was qualified and applied for a job or promotion that the employer was seeking to fill, that he was denied, and that the employer continued to seek applications. The employer does not need to prove a lack of discrimination. Employers are given a great deal of latitude in this area and can disguise questionable employment practices as business decisions. The complainant, on the other hand, must show direct evidence, such as derogatory statements by the employer; comparative evidence, such as similar situations where others were treated more favorably; or evidence that the employer acted contrary to its own policies (Lazar and Volberg 2013; Outten, Rabin, and Lipman 1994).

While sexual harassment is a form of sex discrimination, it is not always as easy to define. Typically, the legal issues focus on whether the conduct in question is sexual in nature, unreasonable, severe, and unwelcome. Title VII of the Civil Rights Act considers sexual harassment as unwelcome sexual conduct of two types: (1) quid pro quo, or sexual favors for job benefits, and (2) hostile work environment, where the employee is forced to endure unpleasant conduct because of gender. In quid pro quo situations, the harasser must be one who has authority over the victim's job and benefits. In hostile work environments, any conduct of a sexual nature that interferes with an employee's work is considered hostile (Lazar and Volberg 2013; Outten, Rabin, and Lipman 1994).

Most experts agree that a key determinant of sexual harassment is whether the conduct is unwelcome, but this perception is not always readily apparent. The EEOC (2010) has stated that "because sexual attraction may often play a role in the day-to-day social exchange between employees, the distinction between invited, uninvited but welcome, offensive but tolerated, and flatly rejected advances may well be difficult to discern." Italie (2013) asks, "Are workplace compliments focused on looks or other personal details like dress ever OK? When do such remarks rise to actionable harassment or become worthy of a friendly rebuff or a trip to HR?" In the opinion of compliance experts, human resources managers, and labor lawyers, "tone, context, and a pattern of behavior are everything when it comes to unwanted remarks" (Italie 2013). Some compliments mean nothing; others aim to change the power dynamic between two individuals.

Office romances are an inevitable fact of life. Some people attribute them to the greater number of women now in the workforce; others point to the fact that many workers are putting in longer hours. A recent CareerBuilders survey found that almost 39 percent of workers have dated a coworker, and of those, nearly 17 percent have dated a coworker at least twice. Despite the prevalence of office affairs, a Society for Human Resource Management survey found that only 13 percent of companies have a policy on workplace romance, perhaps because many human resources managers believe a formal policy would intrude too much on employees' personal lives (Singh 2013).

Workplace romances, real or imagined, have an impact on the work environment. They change the dynamics and chemistry between workers. The perception of favoritism can erode productivity and morale. When a breakup occurs, negative fallout brings unwanted tension.

Affairs between managers and subordinates are the most dangerous liaisons. The manager undermines his authority, jeopardizes his working relationships with other reports, and is often seen as having a conflict of interest. Despite a perception of favoritism, the subordinate may, in fact, be treated less favorably in an attempt to cover up the relationship. Coworkers may view her as an informant and avoid her. She may not have access to the information or teamwork she needs to do her job effectively. Charges of sexual harassment against someone in authority are often scrutinized more closely than others because of the possible abuse of power.

Although other managers may not be so fortunate, many CEOs have survived office affairs and not been fired for sexual misconduct. Governing boards appear to be more interested in financial performance than in their CEO's sexual escapades. Still, in a widely publicized scandal, the CEO of Beth Israel Deaconess Medical Center in Boston was fined $50,000 by the hospital's board for his "lapses in judgment" in a personal relationship with a female employee (Kowalczyk 2010b, 2010c). This action followed an investigation of an anonymous complaint letter to the board alleging inappropriate hiring practices and sexual relationships involving the CEO and hospital employees. In spite of this "punitive" fine and the board's public "expression of their disappointment" in their CEO, the board expressed "unanimous continued confidence" in his leadership of the medical center. The board cited his "exemplary record . . . , the current performance of the hospital, [and] his role as the chief architect of the hospital's leading position in quality and safety" in a public statement concerning its actions.

These public statements notwithstanding, some dissension among board members regarding its decision was reported, and the board subsequently asked the Massachusetts attorney general's office to review its decision and determine if it had appropriately fulfilled its responsibility in its handling of the matter. In September 2010, the attorney general found "no evidence of misuse or abuse of charitable funds" in the hiring or compensation of the employee with whom the CEO admitted to having a personal relationship (Massachusetts Office of the Attorney General 2010).

However, the report of the attorney general continued:

The predictable and unfortunate result of combining personal and professional relationships within a workplace environment means decisions made regarding the employee's hiring, transfer, pay, bonuses, and performance reviews will always be subject to the perception they may have been influenced as much by the personal relationship . . . as by her own professional performance. . . . The outstanding reputation of an organization and its CEO are valuable assets of any charitable organization. The personal relationship between the CEO and the employee, which continued throughout her tenure despite repeated expressions of concern by senior staff and certain board members, clearly damaged his reputation, and of greater concern, endangered the reputation of the institution and its management.

The attorney general's review further concluded that the hospital board had acted appropriately in its investigation and deliberations but indicated that the board should have taken earlier disciplinary action given the CEO's continued personal relationship after repeated expressions of concern by senior staff and some board members. The attorney general subsequently urged the board of Beth Israel Deaconess Medical Center to do "some soul searching" about the CEO's ability to continue leading the hospital (Kowalczyk 2010a). The CEO stayed on for a few months and then announced his retirement in January 2011, claiming his resignation was unrelated to the controversy of the previous year.

Much can be learned from this unfortunate incident. Personal relationships, especially those of a sexual nature, will not go unnoticed by hospital staff and employees, and the perception of favoritism and unlimited access to the boss will have negative consequences. In this incident, the anonymous complaint letter was signed "concerned employees of BIDMC." The fallout from a tarnished institutional image, although not immediately apparent, may negatively affect future donor support or recruitment of professional and clinical talent. The energy and resources committed to investigation of the allegations and management of the public relations related to this incident may have been diverted from more pressing, patient-centered activities.

Like John at Rolling Meadows, the CEO of Beth Israel Deaconess Medical Center had served as a mentor to the employee in question, who, like the fellow at Rolling Meadows, was by all accounts a competent healthcare manager with positive performance reviews. A close mentoring relationship requires that the mentor wisely establish boundaries that keep the relationship at a professional level; neither CEO in these scenarios was attentive to boundaries. Finally, wise healthcare executives pay attention when colleagues tell them their behaviors are being perceived as inappropriate and potentially harmful to the organization.

Sexual misconduct, and especially charges of sexual harassment, can be costly to an organization. Employers are almost always responsible for the actions of a superior when a subordinate files such charges. The average cost of defense against a sexual harassment claim is $150,000, and the average settlement is $350,000 (Becker 2010). In 1998, Mitsubishi Motor Manufacturing of America settled what was at the time probably the most globally publicized claim of sexual harassment ever for $34 million. In 2011, a St. Louis woman was awarded $95 million in a sexual harassment suit against Aaron's Inc., a rent-to-own furniture store. This jury award is believed to be the largest payout in a sexual harassment suit to date (Patrick 2011).

Just as the dollar amounts for settlements have increased, so has the number of sexual harassment claims filed by men. From 1990 to 2009, the percentage of claims filed by men doubled from 8 percent to 16 percent (Becker 2010). Although some charges allege harassment by women supervisors or coworkers, most charges involve men harassing other men.

The less tangible—but perhaps even more detrimental—effects of sexual harassment claims are distrust of management, high turnover, loss of productivity, and damage to the organization's public image. Questions, such as the following, also remain as to how far the costs of sexual harassment claims extend beyond the individual companies directly involved.

- Does the publicity surrounding settlements foster complaints in other organizations?

- Are more false claims filed because the complainant despises the boss, was rejected by a superior, was humiliated or made to feel inferior, hates the company, or is just seeking financial gain?
- Is the government overregulating the workplace?
- Are sexual harassment claims making our society more litigious—and driving up healthcare costs?

All of these questions should be part of the discussion. But regardless, sexual harassment is against the law, and the employer is responsible for establishing strong policies that prohibit it in the workplace, effective investigative procedures, and comprehensive training programs for all employees, managers, and governing board members.

Sexual harassment is not a simple issue, and its complexities make it a major ethical challenge for organizations. Smart organizations will meet this challenge and commit the necessary resources to create a working environment free from harassment because they know it is costly not to do so.

Mentoring

Corporate leaders often rank mentoring second only to education as a significant factor in their success. In interviews with 21 nationally prominent healthcare executives, a respected mentor was often credited with early guidance and instilling a sense of purpose in them (Rice and Perry 2013, 57). The executives interviewed indicated that they, in turn, have cultivated their effectiveness as mentors by intentionally developing leadership teams and by sharing relevant career experiences with their direct reports. They believe in the power of mentoring and expect that those whom they mentor will mentor others in turn.

The mentor's protégé is often a postgraduate fellow. A postgraduate fellowship is "a structured, preceptor-directed, planned program of development that consists of a learning and working experience in a healthcare facility . . . after the conferring of the academic degree" (ACHE 2006). A fellowship provides an opportunity for the protégé or fellow to gain real-world experience in his professional field, to refine skills, to test academic concepts, and to learn about the dynamics and politics of organizations.

The preceptor or mentor is typically a senior-level executive who is interested in teaching and sharing experiences, insights, and knowledge with young professionals embarking on their careers. Some view mentoring as a mechanism whereby executives can contribute to their field and assist in the professional development of future colleagues.

To be effective, the mentor must be an emotionally secure individual who possesses high ethical standards and values and behaves in a rational, consistent manner. These traits are important because the mentor serves as a role model and teaches by example. Protégés often adopt the behaviors and value systems of their mentors and retain this learned work philosophy throughout their careers. Early careerists may pattern their professional lives after that of their mentors. Seen in this light, mentoring provides the executive with considerable responsibility as well as an opportunity to prepare healthcare leaders of the future.

Because of position and experience, the mentor can provide the direction and guidance that the protégé needs to achieve career goals. The mentor serves as a teacher and protector and provides learning opportunities. The mentor makes it safe for the protégé to make mistakes but intervenes when circumstances become difficult or complex. Effective mentors are good teachers, enjoy a favorable professional reputation and network of colleagues, and commit the necessary time to the relationship. Time is a precious commodity in the life of an executive, and mentoring takes time. Minimally, the mentor must plan the fellowship experience, assign meaningful projects, confer at least weekly with the protégé to assess progress, and provide honest evaluation. Most important, the protégé must have access to the mentor.

Having access to the boss sometimes creates problems among other employees, who may feel that the protégé enjoys special privileges. The perception of favoritism is just one of the pitfalls of mentoring. Mentors must also avoid teaching only what they believe to be true. They must encourage their protégés to be critical thinkers and to challenge their ideas and methods. Mentors who teach thoughtful questioning and tactful disagreement will provide their protégé with valuable interpersonal skills. Collaborating closely, sharing thoughts, and spending a lot of time together can predispose the principal participants in a fellowship to a romantic attraction. This possibility could be one reason some male executives may be reluctant to mentor women.

Given that most CEOs are men, gender could be a potential barrier to desirable mentorship situations for women. Further limiting mentorship opportunities for women is the unfortunate reality that women executives who rise to the top are often reluctant to mentor other women (Tahmincioglu 2010). Women face other barriers as well: Male managers may have more access than do female managers to informal executive networks, which tend to be the dominant organizational coalitions that provide access to mentors. It is no myth that a great deal of business is conducted on the golf course and other predominantly male social venues. The prevalence of this dynamic makes it especially important for women to interact with senior-level executives through fellowships, membership in professional societies such as ACHE, service on local or state healthcare committees, and the like.

The absence of such executive interaction diminishes a woman's ability to develop the network needed for career advancement.

Executive-level interaction and mentorship that crosses gender lines does carry risk for inappropriate sexual behavior on the part of one or both of the participants. Recognizing this risk, the American Medical Association (AMA 2013) has published guidelines for preventing sexual harassment that include a code of behavior for teacher–learner relationships in medical education. This code of behavior notes that "the teacher–learner relationship should be based on mutual trust, respect and responsibility. This relationship should be carried out in a professional manner, in a learning environment that places strong focus on education, high quality patient care and ethical conduct." The teacher is expected to provide instruction, guidance, inspiration, and leadership. The learner is expected to make the effort to acquire the necessary knowledge and skill to become an effective professional. In addition to defining and prohibiting sexual harassment, the AMA (1994) specifically addresses consensual amorous relationships between teacher and student, noting that the fundamental power imbalance between the two partners and the possibility of biased evaluations, either positively or negatively, make these relationships unethical.

Despite the time, energy, and resources needed to establish and participate in mentoring younger, less experienced healthcare managers, valuable benefits accrue to the mentor and to the organization from mentoring. Mentoring requires mentors to objectively analyze their way of addressing an issue, examine their choice of actions more closely, and stay current with best practices in the field (Perry 2012).

Clayton M. Christensen (2010), an influential management expert, asked the Harvard Business School class of 2010, "How will you measure your life?" His own answer to this question was:

> Management is the most noble of professions if it's practiced well. No other occupation offers as many ways to help others learn and grow, take responsibility and be recognized for achievement, and contribute to the success of a team. More and more MBA students come to school thinking that a career in business means buying, selling, and investing in companies. That's unfortunate. Doing deals doesn't yield the deep rewards that come from building up people. . . . I've concluded that the metric by which God will assess my life isn't dollars but the individual lives I've touched. . . . Don't worry about the level of individual prominence you have achieved; worry about the individuals you have helped become better people.

REFERENCES

American College of Healthcare Executives (ACHE). 2011. *Code of Ethics*. Updated November 14. www.ache.org/abt_ache/code.cfm#patients.

———. 2010. "Administrative Residencies and Postgraduate Fellowships in Healthcare Administration." Summary report prepared by Strategic Communications on May 12. www.ache.org/postgrad/SummaryReport.pdf.

———. 2006. "A Comparison of the Career Attainments of Men and Women Healthcare Executives." Published December. www.ache.org/pubs/research/gender_study_full_report.pdf.

American Hospital Association (AHA). 1999. "Principles of Accountability for Hospitals and Health Care Organizations." Approved November 11–12. www.aha.org/content/00-10/AHAPrinciplesAccountability.pdf.

American Medical Association (AMA). 2013. "Teacher–Learner Relationship in Medical Education." AMA Policy H-295.955. Accessed July 3. www.ama-assn.org/resources/doc/PolicyFinder/policyfiles/HnE/H-295.955.HTM.

———. 1994. "Sexual Harassment and Exploitation Between Medical Supervisors and Trainees." Opinion 3.08 of the AMA *Code of Medical Ethics*. Updated June. www.ama-assn.org/ama/pub/physician-resources/medical-ethics/code-medical-ethics/opinion308.page.

Becker, A. 2010. "Sexual Harassment: Stati[sti]cs, Facts and Impact It Could Have on Your Organization." Career Management Associates. Posted August 13. www.cmacareer.com/for-organizations/2010/08/sexual-harassment-statics-facts-and-impact-it-could-have-on-your-organization.

Berger, P. L., and T. Luckmann. 1967. *The Social Construction of Reality*. Garden City, NY: Anchor Books, Doubleday and Co.

Christensen, C. M. 2010. "How Will You Measure Your Life?" *Harvard Business Review* July. http://hbr.org/2010/07/how-will-you-measure-your-life/ar/pr.

Cohen, A. 2012. "Sex and the Workplace." *Bloomberg Businessweek* May 10. http://images.businessweek.com/slideshows/2012-05-10/sex-and-the-workplace.

Italie, L. 2013. "Sexism Walks a Fine Line." *The Albuquerque Journal* May 12, H2.

Kolhatkar, S. 2012. "Why They All Want Gloria Allred." *Bloomberg Businessweek* July 19. www.businessweek.com/articles/2012-07-19/gloria-allred-is-on-a-very-public-crusade.

Kowalczyk, L. 2010a. "AG Urges Beth Israel to Rethink CEO's Fitness." *Boston Globe* September 2.

———. 2010b. "Hospital Chief Sorry for 'Poor Judgment.'" *Boston Globe* April 27.

———. 2010c. "Levy Is Fined $50,000 for Lapses in Judgment." *Boston Globe* May 4.

Kramer, R. M. 2003. "The Harder They Fall." *Harvard Business Review* 81: 58–66.

Lazar, W. S., and D. I. Volberg. 2013. "Sexual Harassment in the Workplace." Outten & Golden. Accessed July 2. www.outtengolden.com/sites/default/files/sexual_harassment_in_the_workplace.pdf.

Massachusetts Office of the Attorney General. 2010. "Letter from Assistant Attorney General Jed M. Nosal to Chairman Stephen Kai, Beth Israel Deaconess Medical Center." Accessed May 3, 2013. www.mass.gov/ago/docs/nonprofit/findings-and-recommendations/beth-israel-hosptial-review-090110.pdf.

Outten, W. N., R. J. Rabin, and L. R. Lipman. 1994. *The Basic ACLU Guide to the Rights of Employees and Union Members*, second edition. Carbondale, IL: Southern Illinois University Press.

Patrick, R. 2011. "Jury Awards $95 Million in Fairview Heights Sex Harassment Suit." *St. Louis Post-Dispatch* June 10.

Perry, F. 2012. *Healthcare Leadership That Makes a Difference: Creating Your Legacy*. Self-study course. Chicago: Health Administration Press.

Rice, J., and F. Perry. 2013. *Healthcare Leadership Excellence: Creating a Career of Impact*. Chicago: Health Administration Press.

Singh, R. 2013. "HR—the Third Umpire in Office Romance." People Matters. Accessed August 5. www.peoplematters.in/articles/learning-curve/hr-the-third-umpire-in-office-romance.

Tahmincioglu, E. 2010. "Women Still Reluctant to Help Each Other." NBC News. Updated July 6. www.nbcnews.com/id/38060072/ns/business-careers/t/women-still-reluctant-help-each-other/.

US Equal Employment Opportunity Commission (EEOC). 2013. "The Civil Rights Act of 1991." Accessed July 2. www.eeoc.gov/eeoc/history/35th/1990s/civilrights.html.

———. 2010. "Enforcement Guidance: Policy Guidance on Current Issues of Sexual Harassment." Reformatted June 28. www.eeoc.gov/eeoc/publications/upload/currentissues.pdf.

Physician Impairment: University Hospital

UNIVERSITY HOSPITAL HAS long been designated as the Level I trauma center serv- *Case* ing a tri-county area of a northwestern state. It enjoys a favorable reputation among *Study* healthcare professionals and the public it serves. Its teaching, research, and patient care programs are of the highest caliber. Its trauma center is nationally known for its excellent medical staff, and the resident physicians who train there are in demand across the country when they graduate from the program.

Jan Adams has been the second-shift operating room (OR) supervisor for ten years. She knows her job and is well liked and highly respected by staff and physicians alike. She makes certain that the surgeons follow protocol and never get out of hand. She probably knows more about the skill levels of the surgical staff than most of the surgeons themselves.

Jan likes working second shift and likes working with trauma patients. She receives a great deal of satisfaction from the life-saving immediacy so visible with trauma patients.

Friday nights have always been the busiest of the week for trauma, and this Friday was no exception. The helicopter was on its way in with a 42-year-old who had been in an automobile accident, struck head-on by a drunk driver going the wrong way on the interstate.

The resident, Dr. Truman, was already scrubbing, as were the two other house staff who would be assisting. The scrub nurse and circulating nurse had the room set up and were waiting. Dr. Spalding, the trauma surgeon on call, was on his way to the hospital, and the anesthesiologist was setting up when the patient arrived. Things looked grim—lots of bleeding, vitals fading. Dr. Truman quickly prepped and draped the unconscious patient and readied to make his incision. Although Dr. Spalding had not yet arrived, Dr. Truman knew he had to proceed if the patient was going to make it.

Jan was concerned that Dr. Spalding had not yet arrived. As the trauma surgeon on call, he was responsible for being in attendance when a resident performed surgery. Jan tried calling him several more times but received no response. She considered calling the surgeon on second call but was reluctant to cause any problems for Dr. Spalding. She checked to see how the surgery was going and waited. The patient's ruptured spleen had been removed, and his lacerated liver was being repaired. He was still losing blood, and the residents were looking for additional sources of the bleeding.

Almost three hours had elapsed when Dr. Spalding finally arrived. As Jan began to brief him on the patient's status, she noticed the unmistakable odor of alcohol. This was not the first time Dr. Spalding had arrived in the OR smelling of alcohol while on call. He was known to have a drink or two, but no one had ever questioned his operating skill. In fact, Jan had said that if it were she or one of her family members on that operating table, there was no surgeon she'd rather have operating than Dr. Spalding. He was a superb teacher as well; the residents consistently voted him "Faculty of the Year." He was well liked, confident but never arrogant, and always considerate of the staff. The scrub nurses would volunteer to work overtime if it meant the opportunity to scrub for him.

This Friday night was different. His speech was slurred, and Jan knew he was drunk. She suggested they talk in the doctors' lounge, and once there, she gave him coffee and told him she thought it best if he stayed in the lounge instead of scrubbing in. When she went back into the OR, they were closing and the patient was stable. Jan breathed a sigh of relief, believing a crisis had been averted.

On Saturday morning, she received a call at home from the vice president of nursing, who had been contacted by a reporter from the local newspaper. He said the reporter had information that emergency surgery had been performed last night on a critical patient by a physician in training because the surgeon showed up drunk. He was giving University Hospital an opportunity to comment before he contacted the patient's family. The story would appear in that afternoon's newspaper.

ETHICS ISSUES

Patient safety: What is the hospital's responsibility for the safety of the patients entrusted to its care? Of the licensed professionals administering that care?

Impaired healthcare professionals: When caring for patients, what is the responsibility of healthcare professionals related to impairment—their own and that of others?

Adherence to professional codes of ethical conduct: Were the actions in this case consistent with the professional codes of conduct for physicians? For nurses? For resident physicians?

Adherence to the organization's mission statement, ethical standards, and values statement: Were Jan's actions consistent with the organization's mission statement, ethical standards, and values statement? Were Dr. Spalding's?

Management's role and responsibility: As the OR supervisor, what is Jan's role and responsibility in this situation? What is senior management's responsibility following this incident?

Failure to apply hospital policies in a fair and equitable manner: Could the way Jan treated Dr. Spalding in this case be perceived as favoritism? What are the repercussions of favoritism on staff morale? On staff performance? On management credibility? On the culture of the OR?

Legal implications: What is the hospital's liability for allowing a resident to perform surgery without the supervision of an attending physician? What is Jan's liability? What are the legal implications of failing to follow hospital policies and protocols consistently? How will this surgery be billed?

Organizational implications: How will this incident be perceived by the public? What will its effect on the organization be? What effect will Jan's actions have on the staff and culture of the OR? Does this incident involve issues related to compliance with regulatory or accrediting agencies? What will the patient or his family be told about his surgery?

Implications for graduate medical education: What are the implications of this incident for the surgical residency program? Should the program director for surgery education have been notified?

DISCUSSION

Patient Safety

Patient safety must be the primary concern and focus in this case. It can never be trumped by personal or organizational loyalties. The mission, values, and code of ethical conduct of this and all healthcare organizations must clearly identify patient safety as the institution's primary goal, ahead of all other goals and activities. "Do no harm" is clear in both the Hippocratic oath and the professional codes of conduct of other professional healthcare disciplines. Hospital policies need to be clear and specific about this point and absolutely must focus on patient care and safety to merit the public's trust.

Impaired Healthcare Professionals

In addition to drugs and alcohol, causes of impairment among healthcare professionals may include mental or emotional instability, cognitive dysfunction, physical limitations, and the mental or physical effects of aging. Aging may become more of a problem as an increasing proportion of the population, which includes many brilliant and capable physicians, grows older. Although the University Hospital case deals with an impaired physician, impairment can occur at all levels of the clinical staff and throughout the organization.

Drug and alcohol abuse is a national issue that has significant social, financial, and ethical implications. Substance abuse crosses all socioeconomic lines, but the problem is particularly serious in healthcare because healthcare professionals are responsible for the health, well-being, and safety of patients and can ill afford to have their competence and judgment compromised by addiction. Healthcare professionals are also looked up to as role models of healthy lifestyles and behaviors, and they must take this role seriously. Professional impairment has both direct consequences (harm to patients) and indirect ones (erosion of public trust and confidence in the profession). Therefore, the ethical obligations of organizations—and everyone who works in them—in matters of substance abuse and those affected by it are considerable. Research suggests that at some point during their careers, 10 to 15 percent of healthcare professionals will misuse drugs or alcohol (Angres, Bologeorges, and Chou 2013).

Some reasons for this marked propensity include opportunity and availability of substances, knowledge about drugs and their effects, the perception that this knowledge provides immunity from addiction, and enhanced genetic predisposition among the helping professions (Bissonnette and Doerr 2010). Although some may dispute this prevalence of substance abuse, no one can deny the dangers of substance abuse among healthcare professionals who have been entrusted with the lives of patients in their care. Admitting to substance abuse and seeking treatment may be problematic for healthcare professionals, whose livelihood, like that of airline pilots, depends on the trust of the public. Healthcare professionals who abuse substances often suffer in isolation that is enabled by the silence of coworkers, who fear that reporting a colleague may cause him to lose his professional credibility or license to practice.

Having organizational policies and programs in place that provide help and access to treatment for impaired individuals is therefore all the more important. Early detection, reporting, and treatment will not only protect the impaired individual from embarrassment but will also safeguard patients from undue harm. A solid, trusting relationship with a surgery department chair, residency program director, or chief of staff can be valuable to an administrator who, confidentially and for the good of the individual physician as well as the hospital, could ask that an investigation be undertaken to determine if a problem exists and if early intervention is needed.

Although healthcare is an extremely rewarding occupation, it is also a very stressful one, especially for those on the front lines of patient care who often must work long hours and cope with the sadness associated with death and dying patients. A recent survey presented the following statistics (Physician Wellness Services and Cejka Search 2011):

- Almost 87 percent of physicians report feeling "moderately to severely stressed and burned out on an average day."
- Nearly two-thirds of the survey's respondents said that their stress levels had increased moderately to dramatically over the past three years.
- 14 percent said that they left their practice because of stress.
- The top four causes of work-related stress were administrative demands of the job, long hours, on-call requirements, and worry about malpractice lawsuits.
- Only 15 percent of those surveyed said their organization helps them cope with stress or burnout.

Further complicating matters, physicians may view alcohol and drugs as a way to reduce stress and fatigue.

Physician stress has implications for the entire organization and the patients treated there. It can result in disruptive behaviors, lower productivity, increased turnover, and—most alarming—patient safety and quality issues (Best and Rosenstein 2012). For good reason, therefore, healthcare leaders need to pay attention to physician stress and provide programs that address this growing problem. Wise healthcare managers recognize that healthy clinicians must care for patients and will seek solutions that are compatible with physicians' availability and that have the support and sanction of the medical staff. Dealing with physician stress is much easier than dealing with alcohol and substance abuse. Time and money are better spent addressing the causes of physician stress and impairment than managing the consequences.

Adherence to Professional Codes of Ethical Conduct

Most healthcare organizations, professional societies, and associations have addressed the issue of drug and alcohol abuse and impaired healthcare professionals in ethical policy statements, codes of conduct, human resources policies, and the like. The ethical policy statement "Impaired Healthcare Executives" of the American College of Healthcare Executives (ACHE 2012; see Appendix C) reminds us that impairment results in more than just personal damage to the abuser and her family. Impairment affects her organization, colleagues, patients, clients, profession, community, and society as a whole. Impairment typically leads to misconduct, incompetence, unsafe or unprofessional behavior, errors in judgment, and the like. The organization may suffer from a loss of public confidence and support. The ACHE policy statement defines the ethical obligations of the healthcare executive, which include

- behaving in a personal and professional manner that is free of impairment,
- urging impaired colleagues to seek treatment,
- reporting those colleagues to the appropriate authorities if they do not, and
- recommending or providing resources for treatment within the organization and community.

The current opinion of the American Medical Association (AMA 2004) on the reporting of impaired colleagues says that "physicians have an ethical obligation to report impaired . . . colleagues in accordance with the legal requirements in each state." The opinion states that "physicians' responsibilities . . . include timely intervention to ensure that these colleagues cease practicing and receive appropriate assistance from a physician health program. . . . Ethically and legally, it may be necessary to report an impaired physician who continues to practice despite reasonable offers of assistance and referral to a hospital or state physician health program." If the physician does not enter an impairment program, then he should be reported directly to the state licensing authority.

Both the ACHE and the AMA policies emphasize treatment as the first solution but clearly say that impaired professionals must be reported to the appropriate authorities if they do not enter treatment programs or if they continue to demonstrate impairment in professional activities. Given the medical staff "chain of command" in the hospital setting, in the case of University Hospital Jan could have appropriately reported Dr. Spalding to the chief of the department of surgery, and Dr. Truman should have reported him to the program director for the surgery residency.

The *Code of Ethics for Nurses* of the American Nurses Association (ANA 2001) is clear on nurses' responsibility to "promote, advocate for, and strive to protect the health, safety and rights of the patient." The nurse's highest duty is always to the patient. The ANA position on impairment is grounded in this provision of its code of ethics: "In a situation where a nurse suspects another's practice may be impaired, the nurse's duty is to take action designed both to protect patients and to assure that the impaired individual receives assistance in regaining optimal function" (ANA 2001).

Management's Role and Responsibility

The healthcare organization's mission statement and ethical standards almost certainly address the hospital's responsibility for the safety of patients and the delivery of quality healthcare. The mission statement and standards mandate that management address the issue of impairment in the workplace with programs that protect the patient and ensure a work environment that is conducive to effective patient care.

Progressive discipline for substance abuse is the norm in most healthcare organizations today, and many organizations have employee assistance programs (EAPs). But EAPs are not always the answer. They still carry some stigma, and some employees fear that entering such a program will damage their career. Even though EAPs ensure confidentiality, many employees avoid them for fear that their problem will become public. In addition, insurance does not always cover the costs of an EAP program, so employees may have to pay out-of-pocket.

For impaired professionals who want more anonymity than their hospital's treatment program provides, some states have recovery programs that promise confidentiality. For example, the Michigan legislature has established the Health Professional Recovery Program to offer healthcare professionals a confidential, non-disciplinary approach to support recovery from substance abuse, chemical addiction, and mental illness.

An effective substance abuse program must have clear policies, developed through a collaborative process, that clearly identify why drug and alcohol use is unacceptable in the organization and what actions need to be taken when it occurs. The collaboration should include representatives of human resources, legal counsel, safety departments, medical staff, and employees. If the organization is unionized, a union representative should be included as well. The program that is implemented must fit the organization, its culture and philosophy, and its business activity.

The program should include easy access to a reporting system that may function more effectively if it is anonymous. As in the case at University Hospital, coworkers may be reluctant to report an impaired colleague, especially one whom they like and respect. They may not want to get him into trouble or hamper his career. They may be reluctant to report him for fear he may have his privileges suspended, lose his licensure, or be reported to the National Practitioner Data Bank. Concerned coworkers do not have many options when dealing with an impaired colleague. They may urge the individual to seek treatment or ask someone close to him to intervene. But if the impaired healthcare professional does not refrain from professional activity, he must be reported to protect the patients receiving care from the organization. Colleagues and coworkers must recognize that although reporting an impaired professional is difficult, early intervention will protect the individual from doing harm to himself and others.

Having effective programs and policies in place is never enough. Management must make certain that those policies and procedures are well known and followed by staff. The most common workplace drug—alcohol—is especially dangerous because it is not illegal, it is socially acceptable, and supervisors and coworkers tend to overlook its abuse. Coworkers may even rationalize a colleague's misconduct by saying to themselves, "he was drunk at the time." But being drunk never justifies unethical, incompetent, or erratic behavior. Employees must be made well aware of the dangers that being under the influence of alcohol poses for patients.

As the second-shift OR supervisor, Jan is the manager in this case and has responsibility for reporting incidents beyond her remedy or control to the next in command—administratively, medically, or both. Nurses are expected to be reliable in assuming this responsibility. Some time ago, a surgeon was overheard saying that physicians rely on nurses to report unethical conduct because "nurses have a more highly developed conscience than physicians." Whether or not this statement is true, physicians are not relieved of their burden of responsibility for the safety of patients or their compassion for colleagues in need. Some physicians may believe that their scope of responsibility is limited to their own patients; others may simply wish to avoid conflict. This attitude is not surprising—most physicians, even those employed by the hospital, view themselves as independent practitioners and strongly believe in personal accountability. Bujak (2008) tells us, "Physicians define quality as 'the way I take care of (my) patients.'" In a sense, this implies that others in the organization can take care of other matters. However, the AMA (2004) makes it clear that physicians have an ethical obligation to report impaired colleagues to the appropriate bodies.

Physicians are apparently not the only ones who rank nurses high on the ethical scale. A recent Gallup poll found that nurses were the professionals whom Americans consider most honest and ethical. They were ranked ahead of pharmacists, doctors, engineers, and all others (Lewis 2012). Licensed nurses have sworn to uphold a code of ethics that, for most, means "they have a nonnegotiable set of moral standards that govern the way they interact with patients, patient's families and other medical professionals" (Lyder 2011). Healthcare executives should take advantage of this perception of ethical superiority and consider nurses among their most valuable advocates when developing an ethical organizational culture.

Failure to Apply Hospital Policies in a Fair and Equitable Manner

Applying the same standards of behavior and discipline to high-performing staff as to moderate-performing staff may be difficult, especially in the case of a staff member who is well liked. However, the consequences of inconsistency can be far reaching. The OR staff who witnessed Jan's accommodating treatment of Dr. Spalding may perceive her actions as favoritism, because she likes Dr. Spalding so much. What effect may Jan's actions have on the morale and culture of the OR and on the behavior and performance of other physicians and OR staff? Could their performance suffer, taking a back seat to efforts at making sure that Jan "likes" them? What kind of role modeling does this case involve? The adverse effects of favoritism on staff morale, productivity, and teamwork are predictable, and favoritism lowers the bar for everyone as far as standards of conduct are concerned.

Legal Implications

As the legal analysis of this case in Chapter 12 observes, failure to follow existing hospital policies or to consistently apply hospital policies can be difficult to defend in a court of law. In this case, two policies were ignored: the policy regarding on-call surgeons and the one related to impaired professionals. Jan may also have exposed the organization to future litigation, if different standards and disciplinary actions are applied in future incidents involving other staff members or physicians. Leadership actions always have broader implications than may at first appear to be the case.

Graduate Medical Education

The high quality of patient care for which teaching hospitals are known can erode if those hospitals do not conform to the highest ethical standards. Public trust in teaching hospitals can give way to fear and uncertainty if healthcare professionals are unknown to the patient. The public has been educated to believe that (1) physicians in training are closely supervised by practicing physician specialists and subspecialists who are board certified in their particular fields and (2) patient care is delivered in an environment of intellectual inquiry that fosters the state-of-the-art practice of medicine.

If a physician in training performs unsupervised surgery, the action invites mistrust of the institution and its healthcare professionals. It also threatens the certification of the residency program by the Accreditation Council for Graduate Medical Education (ACGME), which can have financial implications for the teaching hospital. A new ACGME rule now requires that residents and faculty in training programs inform patients about a resident's role in the patient's surgery (Hill 2011). A faculty physician who arrives in surgery intoxicated only compounds this mistrust, further erodes the integrity of the program, and compromises the credibility of the institution that would allow such misconduct. Because teaching hospitals receive public benefits—such as tax exemptions, training support, and research grants—they must do their utmost to preserve the public's trust and confidence.

Organizational Implications

Reisor (1994, 28) suggests that "institutions have ethical lives and characters just as their individual members do." He cautions that the day-to-day interactions in a healthcare organization must reflect the values that it professes. To illustrate his point, he examines some of the contradictions often seen in academic health centers. For example, faculty may lecture medical students on the need to treat indigent patients the same as the insured but then turn the care of indigents over to residents; hospitals may build special facilities for the wealthy and ignore the poor in the neighborhood; faculty may instruct medical students to treat people with dignity but then treat those medical students as nonpersons; and administrators may call for cooperation while undermining competitors. Reisor (1994, 28–29) says that contradictions between what institutions say and what they do breed cynicism among employees and staff as well as public mistrust of the institution.

In the case of University Hospital, Jan's tolerance of Dr. Spalding's intoxication while on call has not gone unnoticed by the OR staff. Her failure to report him or to call the surgeon on second call has surely cost her the respect of her staff.

What about Dr. Truman and his responsibility as the resident in this case? Dr. Truman may be in a more precarious situation because resident physicians rely on teaching physicians for their evaluations. Many residents also stay where they train and rely on faculty physicians there for references and referrals. Reisor (1994, 30) reminds us that teachers and students are "bound together as family and subject to the ties that interdependence brings" and that the regard for each other's needs should set the tone for them to follow ethical standards in their other healthcare relationships. This kind of teacher–student relationship would make Dr. Truman vulnerable to compromising situations. That vulnerability is one of the reasons graduate medical education has policies to guide and protect physicians in training in such situations (Reisor 1994, 32). The accreditation bodies that review residency programs are interested in the policies and procedures that ensure sound educational practices, and accreditation decisions affect the funding of residency programs. Dr. Spalding's behavior is not just a personal matter; it is a program matter as well. As a teacher, Dr. Spalding has a responsibility to serve as an ethical role model. In this case, he is teaching that unsafe patient care is acceptable.

Dr. Truman and Jan demonstrate misplaced loyalty in this case. As healthcare professionals, their primary loyalty should be to the patient. The codes of conduct for the professions of both medicine and nursing are clear on this point. But both Jan and Dr. Truman like and respect Dr. Spalding's skill as a surgeon. Their respect for him has muddied their decision and also raises the question of fairness. Would Jan and Dr. Truman be as reluctant to report a surgeon whom they did not like or respect? Probably not. Is this fair? Reisor (1994, 32) tells us that fairness has a special significance in healthcare organizations, which cannot promote the equal valuing of all people and simultaneously condone discriminatory practices. When we like someone, we tend to favor that person, sometimes overlooking foibles that we would not overlook in others or allowing her outstanding attributes to eclipse her flaws. Dr. Spalding may have a drinking problem, but his contributions to the hospital and the teaching program are significant. This kind of rationalization can be dangerous; it is reminiscent of the declaration in George Orwell's *Animal Farm* that "all are equal, but some are more equal than others."

The elitist culture of the OR is a contributing factor in this case. The OR is a restricted area where professionals, especially surgeons and nurses, bond with one another, work closely together, and depend on one another. They are isolated from the rest of the hospital, its rules, and its bureaucracy, and they enjoy a less formal atmosphere. (As someone once remarked, "What do you expect? They work in pajamas.") This isolation and elitist attitude can pose a challenge for administrators, who need to be visible and also ensure that OR staff are made to feel a part of the larger organization and accountable to the same policies and standards of behavior.

Much can be learned from identifying and investigating "near miss" situations like the one at University Hospital—incidents that caused no harm, but could have.

REFERENCES

American College of Healthcare Executives (ACHE). 2012. "Impaired Healthcare Executives." Ethical policy statement. Revised November 12. www.ache.org/policy/impaired.cfm.

American Medical Association (AMA). 2004. "Reporting Impaired, Incompetent, or Unethical Colleagues." Opinion 9.031 of the AMA *Code of Medical Ethics.* Updated June. www.ama-assn.org/ama/pub/physician-resources/medical-ethics/code-medical-ethics/opinion9031.page.

American Nurses Association (ANA). 2001. *Code of Ethics for Nurses with Interpretive Statements.* Silver Spring, MD: American Nurses Association.

Angres, D., S. Bologeorges, and J. Chou. 2013. "A Two Year Longitudinal Outcome Study of Addicted Health Care Professionals: An Investigation of the Role of Personality Variables." *Substance Abuse: Research and Treatment* 7: 49–60.

Best, M., and A. Rosenstein. 2012. "Combating Physician Stress." *Hospitals & Health Networks Daily* April 12. www.hhnmag.com/hhnmag/HHNDaily/HHNDailyDisplay.dhtml?id=1560003741.

Bissonnette, T., and J. Doerr. 2010. "Impaired Nursing Practice and the Law in Michigan." *Michigan Nurse* 83 (5): 1–8.

Bujak, J. S. 2008. *Inside the Physician Mind: Finding Common Ground with Doctors.* Chicago: Health Administration Press.

Hill, R. 2011. "Informing Patients About Residents' Role." *Hospitals & Health Networks Daily* December 5. www.hhnmag.com/hhnmag/HHNDaily/HHNDailyDisplay .dhtml?id=8230006534.

Lewis, A. 2012. "Who Do You Trust?" *The Wall Street Journal* December 9. http:// online.wsj.com/article/SB10001424127887324001104578163722945904396.html.

Lyder, C. H. 2011. "Nurses at the Forefront of Change." *Hospitals & Health Networks Daily* November 7. www.hhnmag.com/hhnmag/HHNDaily/HHNDailyDisplay .dhtml?id=3820003826.

Physician Wellness Services and Cejka Search. 2011. "Physician Stress and Burnout Survey." Published November. www.cejkasearch.com/wp-content/uploads/ physician-stress-burnout-survey.pdf.

Reisor, S. J. 1994. "The Ethical Life of Healthcare Organizations." *Hastings Center Report* 24 (6): 28–35.

CHAPTER 7

Workforce Reduction:
Hillside County Medical Center

Glenn A. Fosdick

HILLSIDE COUNTY MEDICAL CENTER is a 475-bed public teaching hospital located *Case* in an urban setting in the Midwest. It serves a city of approximately 250,000 people *Study* in a county whose total population is 500,000. Its primary local competition consists of two regional hospital systems, both not-for-profit. Because of its urban location and its historical status as the county hospital, Hillside provides a significant portion (approximately 70 percent) of the uncompensated care for the community. Nevertheless, it receives no financial subsidies from the city or the county.

For many years, Hillside has been the primary tertiary center providing specialized care in high-risk obstetrics, a Level III neonatal intensive care program, and pediatric intensive and specialized care including pediatric oncology. In addition, Hillside is the regional provider for kidney transplants, burn services, and emergency medicine, experiencing close to 80,000 emergency department (ED) visits per year. Hillside's services have been augmented over the last four years by the development of the region's first American College of Surgeons–verified trauma program. Hillside is affiliated with a major university medical school, with residencies in internal medicine, pediatrics, med/peds, and obstetrics, and has a shared program with other hospitals in radiology and orthopedics. In addition, it has recently added an emergency medicine residency program.

Because Hillside is a public hospital, its board is strongly committed to the community and the hospital's mission. A number of programs have been developed that have increased patient access and the hospital's ability to meet its community health needs, including a large clinic providing primary and urgent care services in the community's most underserved area. Unfortunately, because of the

low reimbursement from outpatient Medicaid and the high percentage of uninsured who are served, the clinic experiences significant financial losses.

Like most hospitals, Hillside prospered until the mid-1990s when changes in reimbursement and increasing competition began to affect it. Hillside is also heavily unionized; nine unions represent 86 percent of its employees. This situation has resulted in higher-than-average benefit and pension costs. After multiple strikes and work actions during the late 1990s, Hillside lost market share to its competitors. As its competitors grew stronger, Hillside started to face significant financial challenges, which culminated in 2000 in a financial loss of close to $7 million. Through the recruitment of new leadership, enhanced strategic planning, and marketing, the organization was able to correct itself and make significant progress. However, in the past several years, it has again faced increasing financial concerns. The dilemma Hillside now faces reflects the variety of problems that are common to most hospitals. These problems result from a number of specific issues, such as decreasing reimbursement, uncompensated care, increasing competition, rising personnel costs, and a depressed economy.

The largest unknown facing Hillside is the exact impact the Patient Protection and Affordable Care Act (ACA) will have on the hospital. Although many ACA provisions are still unclear, all healthcare providers will obviously experience decreased reimbursement and increased vulnerability to financial penalties for quality, satisfaction, and performance issues. In addition, the replacement of inpatient care with ambulatory services will doubtless continue to escalate.

The ACA could also affect Hillside's reimbursement from Medicaid, which represents approximately 25 percent of the hospital's business. Because Hillside serves a high percentage of uninsured and Medicaid patients, it is eligible for Disproportionate Share Hospital (DSH) payments. The ACA could clearly place an increasingly high percentage of Medicaid care into competitive regional and statewide Medicaid contracts if the state decides to participate in this program, which would significantly expand Medicaid eligibility. DSH payments to Hillside could accordingly decrease.

Healthcare providers face unique challenges, unknown in any other industry, that may be further complicated by insurance exchanges and other adaptations associated with the ACA. Although the ACA will decrease the number of uninsured, it is unclear which states will participate and when the impact of this change will be felt. Paralleling national indicators, the amount of uncompensated care that Hillside provides has increased over the past three years. Strategic analysis by the hospital suggests that, at least locally, this is partly the result of the US economy: The instability of the job market has resulted in a higher percentage of jobs that do not provide health insurance benefits.

Hillside also faces the difficulty, common to all healthcare providers, of actually collecting the payment due for services provided. The financial pressures that insurers face appear to encourage them to find ways to make billing more difficult, to find justification for disqualifying bills, and in many circumstances to engineer significant delays in providing reimbursement for services that are properly billed.

Furthermore, Hillside faces increasing challenges from non-hospital competitors in diagnostic and treatment areas that historically have been financially advantageous to the hospital. These areas include ambulatory, surgical, and diagnostic centers, such as MRI facilities and dialysis centers owned and operated on a proprietary basis.

Like most hospitals, Hillside faces the challenge of keeping its patient census as high as it has been in the past. Reductions in reimbursement for patients who stay longer than the appropriate time, expanded competition both regionally and nationally, and increasing use of ambulatory services to treat patients in such areas as chemotherapy, surgery, and diagnostic scenarios all complicate Hillside's ability to maintain its average daily census.

At the same time, hospitals and other healthcare providers are experiencing dramatic increases in the costs associated with providing care. Drug expenditures continue to rise, and medical, surgical, and other supplies continue to experience inflationary increases that exceed annual reimbursement adjustments.

Additional concerns are government mandates and accreditation standards, which require staff for non–patient care requirements. For example, the implementation of the federal APC (ambulatory patient classification) outpatient billing system has necessitated the hiring of additional coders to comply with increased mandates for medical record requirements.

Hospitals also face an intensely competitive environment for the recruitment and retention of healthcare personnel. Perhaps the most significant concern is the future availability of registered professional nurses. The average age of nurses nationally is 45 years. Although the American Association of Colleges of Nursing reported a 5.1 percent increase in enrollment in entry-level baccalaureate programs in 2011 (AACN 2012), this increase may not be sufficient to meet the projected demand for nursing services.

This nursing crisis has been neutralized somewhat by the lethargic economy, which has temporarily discouraged employees from retiring. However, when the economy improves, the turnover rate will be higher than average and nursing resources will be depleted. As pressure for financial control and clinical improvement mounts, fewer qualified personnel are interested in addressing these issues. Other shortages can include, but are not limited to, ultrasound technicians, pharmacists, and radiation therapy personnel. These shortages require that Hillside reexamine its pay and benefit package on a consistent basis to ensure that, while not excessive, it is competitive and capable of attracting the right kind of personnel.

Another concern is the increasing number of professional nursing staff who work for nurse staffing agencies. These agencies allow nurses more control and independence concerning when and how many hours they work, including on weekends and holidays, usually at the expense of benefits and pension plans. This situation contributes to a shortage of staff available to work these unattractive hours, and the higher hourly rates result in additional costs to hospitals that use agency nurses.

These difficulties in recruiting nurses and the financial requirements of tight staffing have increased the need for overtime and mandatory overtime. Not only does overtime mean higher costs, but concerns about the strain on staff and the effect of excessive overtime on the quality of clinical care have also prompted state legislatures to develop controls regarding the use of overtime. Increased overtime also stimulates reaction from unions, which can result in strikes and other work actions.

These combined pressures have resulted in the difficulties that Hillside currently faces. The CEO and management staff have examined their situation and realized that unless significant changes are made quickly, Hillside's financial viability will be compromised. The CEO also recognizes that these issues are more important today than previously. His board, like many, has increasingly identified the hospital's operating margin and financial performance as the primary indicator of the management team's effectiveness.

In addition, the size and complexity of healthcare capital expenses today result in an increasing dependence on the bond market, which puts great significance on bond ratings from recognized financial assessment organizations. A credit rating has a direct, measurable influence on the interest rate required by investors and hence on the firm's cost of debt capital (Gapenski and Pink 2011, 180). Hillside's CFO has noted that whereas 31 not-for-profit hospital bond issues were downgraded in 2007 and 40 were upgraded, 53 issues were downgraded and only 27 were upgraded in 2008 (Gapenski and Pink 2011, 182).

Recognizing the critical importance of swiftly and properly addressing these financial concerns, the CEO has called his senior management team together. He has decided that, to ensure the best results, this issue needs to be addressed from a corporate-wide standpoint and all senior management personnel must be involved.

Because of the matter's financial significance, the CFO takes the initiative. She notes that, as in most healthcare organizations, the highest portion of expense is associated with staff. For example, under the present salary and benefits package, the average employee costs Hillside approximately $61,000 per year. Even with the costs of unemployment liabilities and potential severance programs, she argues, reductions in the workforce are the safest and best-known method of reducing financial deficiencies.

The vice president for human resources reminds the group that in most union contracts and many state labor codes, seniority is a key determinant in workforce reductions. At Hillside, for example, the present contracts with key unions, such as nursing, stipulate that seniority is determined on a hospital-wide basis. She notes that the least senior nursing staff may be located in critical areas, such as the ED and operating rooms, where their services are essential for continuing financial productivity. She also points out that many unions closely monitor the comparative numbers affected from each union and the ratios of reduction to management personnel, which could have implications for labor stability.

The vice president for nursing and the vice president for medical affairs collectively announce that patient care cannot be compromised and that inappropriate reductions in these areas could have a critical effect on the organization's clinical capability and reputation. The vice president for operations questions the effect on community projects, such as the clinic, and asks whether other approaches might be taken. The CEO ponders these questions as he contemplates the right approach to address Hillside's situation successfully.

The CEO tries to identify the dynamics of the healthcare industry that distinguish it from other industries. While other industries have faced the need for employee reductions, these environments do not incorporate the multifaceted responsibilities of the healthcare institution. Certainly, financial performance, while important, is not the only criterion that must be measured. The CEO knows that Hillside must ensure that proper care is provided and available to those who seek it. In no other business does a person receive a service before identifying how payment for that service will be provided. In fact, mandates from the federal government prohibit assessment of financial status prior to providing emergency medical care.

Hillside's mission clearly defines its responsibilities to improve the health of the community. Because the vast majority of hospitals in the United States, like Hillside, have either not-for-profit or public tax status, they are required to provide services in some cases that do not conform to the usual business standards. Unfortunately, too often the public perception is that this requirement is not being met.

The CEO reminds himself that most people do not believe that the quality of care has improved. A recent study found that 40 percent of Americans said the quality of care has declined over the past five years (Bleich 2005, 9). The CEO feels strongly that Hillside must live up to its mission, and he knows that as a public hospital Hillside would be under close scrutiny to see that it did.

ETHICS ISSUES

Organizational implications: What is the most appropriate and ethical method of addressing the organization's potential financial shortcomings? To whom should the CEO listen as he determines the appropriate course of action? Should he include others beyond senior management? If so, whom?

Adherence to the organization's mission statement, ethical standards, and values statement: Does the best approach reflect and adhere to the responsibilities of the organization's mission? How does the CEO prioritize financial viability as compared with clinical quality, organizational mission, and community responsibilities?

Management's role and responsibility: Is rightsizing the only answer or even the best answer to addressing financial difficulties? Does rightsizing ensure that all levels and groups in the organization share the effect of and exposure to these difficulties? Can rightsizing successfully address financial deficiencies without compromising clinical needs? Should the CEO examine other options to address the organization's financial concerns? Does the approach ensure that the effect of the decision does not create even bigger difficulties in the long run?

Clinical quality: Should the decision to cut back be determined from a clinical viewpoint or a business viewpoint?

DISCUSSION

Participation in Problem Resolution

A fundamental question is: Who should participate in the resolution of this problem? Is it enough that the CEO has sought input from the key members of his senior management staff?

A hospital is unique in that the stakeholders involved in and influenced by its actions are very important. With a problem of this magnitude, should the stakeholders be involved and, just as important, can they help? To determine the answer to this question, one must first identify who the stakeholders are, how they may be affected, and what the potential positive and negative ramifications of their involvement may be.

Medical Staff

Because the medical staff have a dominant role in the hospital as a customer, provider of care, leader, and political force, the discussion should begin with them. Any change in clinical staffing or services will directly influence the care provided to their patients, so concerns regarding these issues are to be expected and understood.

In addition, the medical staff have evolved as an informal (and sometimes formal) representative for hospital staff; they will likely hear all the rumors (accurate or not), know the staff's fears, and, in many cases, attempt to defend and protect the staff. Such attempts may include discussion with board members or use of the formal medical staff structure to react to any considered changes or reductions. Because rightsizing is difficult to do without affecting services, in some circumstances their concerns may be legitimate. More important, the medical staff can be valuable when determining how to address this problem.

The CEO must understand that the medical staff will be affected and should be a part of the process in some way. The medical staff can be defensive and disruptive, or they can be collaborative. Because financial problems are unfortunately common in healthcare, members of the medical staff no longer think of staff reductions as inconceivable. Accordingly, the CEO may identify this challenge as one that requires the combined efforts of both the medical staff and management. The CEO should start by educating and sharing his concerns with the medical staff in a variety of settings. Using the formal structure, beginning with the medical executive committee, is beneficial. However, informal discussions at departmental meetings or with key individual physicians are essential.

The medical staff can contribute greatly to the resolution of this problem. Reductions in length of stay, selection and use of medical and surgical supplies, and increases in admissions are possible and may be preferable alternatives to losing popular staff or important services. Finally, involvement in these tough decisions may enhance the medical staff's appreciation that, after thorough analysis, the chosen approach is the most feasible one.

Governing Board Members

The board will be involved in the formal approval stages of the process, but they may provide value in the decision phase as well. Because rightsizing is increasingly common in other industries, some board members may have experience in this area. The CEO must be willing to use all available expertise to accomplish staff reductions with the least negative effect. The more involved the board is, the more support this matter will receive and the better prepared board members will be when responding to any personal inquiries they may receive regarding actions taken.

Unions

Although historically unions are more common in public hospitals, they are active throughout healthcare. In 2010, healthcare unions held 264 elections and won 71 percent of them (Carlson 2011). Although the number of union members in general industry decreased in 2009 and 2010, mostly as a result of the recession and a decrease in government jobs, the number of unions and union members in healthcare increased (Hananel 2012). The increasing involvement of unions has required senior managers to develop new skills to work successfully in a union environment.

Although the most common approach taken by US managers when planning rightsizing is to notify unions of the plan for reductions, the CEO should strongly consider involving union leadership at an earlier stage of the process. Sharing the problem and identifying it as an issue common to all parties may direct negative feelings away from the hospital and management and focus attention on the external forces that are causing the financial problems. In addition, union leadership may have valuable input.

The CEO of Hillside recalls hearing about one organization in similar circumstances that spent more than 30 hours in one week with key union leaders examining the entire operating budget and seeking feedback on each line item. From this process, the organization was able to implement a number of sound ideas for reducing costs that it might not have conceived on its own. Just as important, involving union leadership in solving the problem demonstrated the difficulty that management was facing and its desire to reduce costs in the best and fairest manner possible.

Essential to the success of this approach with union leadership and employees are the following actions:

- The first cuts must be made at the level of vice president, associate administrator, or senior departmental director.
- No particular department or segment of the organization should be exempt from rightsizing, unless this exemption is completely justifiable.
- If possible, the same percentage of managers as of employees should be dismissed.
- Managers should exhibit and communicate to their employees the sacrifices they are making as a result of the rightsizing. For example, managers should indicate the lack of available resources in the financial budget, increased demands on remaining personnel, or other detrimental conditions caused by the rightsizing so that employees understand rightsizing has an equal effect on managers and employees (Lombardi 1997, 42).

These actions will allow union leaders to return to their respective constituents with a strong appreciation of the challenge involved and the intent of management to address it fairly. This appreciation could also be important considering how union leadership may respond to the media. In many cases, a hospital's ability to provide adequate and safe care may be criticized after a reduction in workforce. Such criticism may cause a further reduction in volume and the need for additional cost and staff reductions. However, if union leadership has participated in the process and is comfortable that the actions taken were required, that the actions were fair and consistently executed, and that the focus of the institution remains on the patient, a supportive response from union leadership is possible.

Employees

Progressive and beneficial feedback from employees is also desirable. Giving employees the opportunity to identify cost-saving options, educating them about what will happen if costs cannot be reduced, and incorporating them into the process where possible all have the potential to identify new approaches and to avoid mistrust of management. Communication with employees is critical as the issue develops. Rumors, misinformation, and anger toward management are not beneficial and are traditionally disruptive and counterproductive.

The CEO is responsible for defining guidelines that ensure all staff resources are incorporated into the process, even over the recommendations of members of management who prefer to make these decisions the "easy way." Fear of politically affecting the process and delaying needed reductions is common, and while such caution has merit, this is not the time for management to be autocratic.

When properly managed, rightsizing can lay the foundation for a new, vibrant organization. When poorly managed, it can become the single most dangerous threat to organizational survival and a major cause of employee turnover and low organizational morale. At its worst, rightsizing can cause the demise of a previously successful healthcare organization (Lombardi 1997, 53).

Exploring Other Options

A critical aspect of rightsizing is determining that it is the right or only approach to address the organization's financial difficulties. A common premise is that the desired goal is reducing costs. That premise is not accurate. The primary goal is to improve overall financial viability. The organization is measured on its financial viability, which is essential to its long-term success. The CEO should remember that if cutting costs were the only goal, then closing all the nursing units would do the trick—a large percentage of costs would be eliminated. However, the corresponding loss of revenue obviously precludes that approach. Financial viability can be improved via two avenues: reducing costs and increasing revenues. All too frequently, the focus in healthcare has been on cost reduction.

Although the overall high costs of the healthcare industry certainly support cost reduction, it is not always the best direction for the organization and the community it serves. The CFO often makes cost reduction a primary strategy for several good reasons:

- It is clearly the fastest method of addressing financial concerns.
- It is the most reliable and measurable method in the short run. As the CFO pointed out, even when the unemployment insurance and severance costs are incorporated, the savings from rightsizing are well defined and expedient.
- In healthcare today, the costs of care often exceed reimbursement.

However, the CEO's duty is to consider cost reduction as only one option and ensure that all possibilities are explored for the long-term success of the organization.

In the case of Hillside, one such possibility may be a review of its public status. Although transforming a public hospital to a not-for-profit one may be difficult and expensive, the option is not uncommon. A move of this type has some distinct financial advantages and some potential disadvantages. For example, public hospitals in many states are constrained in their ability to invest cash reserves, which during a highly productive financial market can result in significant limitations on potential returns from investments. In addition, eliminating the public hospital status may increase the hospital's ability to refine its benefit or pension status to a more competitive one that is parallel to those of not-for-profit hospitals. On the negative side, losing its public status could reduce Hillside's access to certain DSH payments and other benefits that have been identified for public hospitals. In sum, Hillside should examine all aspects to determine the value and potential impact of this transformation.

The organization should also examine the potential for reducing or eliminating clinical programs in the hospital itself. Although historically the strategic approach has been to provide as many different services as possible, maintaining programs with decreasing volume and expensive qualifications and support needs may not be beneficial. Collaboration with other providers does not require the closing of services or clinical loss to the community.

Collaborative efforts between organizations may allow agreements that result in one service being reduced at one facility in return for another service being dropped at another. Both facilities may thereby expand their volume and potentially increase their profit margin. The CEO and senior management must not be limited by historical protocol. The fact that other hospitals have "always provided" certain services does not mean they cannot change. A progressive and well-planned effort to reduce duplication of services and commit to their delivery by one provider may be well received by insurers, local industry leaders, and the community. While the physicians and staff currently providing these services may voice some concerns, these concerns may be minimal compared with those caused by the continued reduction of an organization's overall capability.

Revenue Enhancement

In today's competitive healthcare environment, identifying additional opportunities to expand revenue has become increasingly challenging. Efforts should revolve around several key areas:

1. Ensure that payment is received on a timely basis and at the highest amount for services rendered. Opportunities in this area include reviewing the present billing system to identify departmental performance. This assessment includes the following at minimum:
   a. **Days in receivables (compared with state and national averages).** Changes in performance over the last 24 months may reflect problems that have grown or emerged in the recent past.
   b. **Charge rates.** An external review of charge rates may identify possible areas of improvement, particularly in areas such as operating rooms and ambulatory facilities.
   c. **Analysis of individual insurance agreements.** Analysis of insurance agreements may result in renegotiation of certain contracts or consideration of separation from others.
   d. **Internal analysis of charging programs.** Analysis of charging programs will ensure that charges are developed on a timely basis for all services rendered.
2. Review patient volume to ensure that the highest volume of patients is obtained for each service rendered.
   a. An in-depth inspection of admission rates by physician and service, combined with a yearly analysis of market share data, will identify changes or opportunities in volume. It will also give the CEO information to discuss with the medical staff when identifying strategic priorities for the recruitment or placement of new physicians. The CEO should also examine the ages of the medical staff to identify needs for future recruitment.
   b. An analysis of patient satisfaction scores is important because it may reveal factors affecting patient volume. Recognizing the competitive environment requires a clear assessment of the present facilities and a commitment on the part of staff to enhance customer service.
   c. New or additional service opportunities are explored in depth to identify all available revenue sources. The CEO should examine each of these areas in detail with the appropriate staff. Because of the competitive nature of healthcare, finding new revenue-producing programs is not easy. The proverbial low-hanging fruit has probably been picked, and new programs may require significant investment or a time delay before

profits are realized. However, revenue generation is a key responsibility of the CEO to move the organization forward.

To make investments of this type at this time requires the confidence of the board and medical staff and may be criticized by union leaders or other employees. The CEO is responsible for keeping these important stakeholders focused on the vision of the organization's long-term success and for ensuring that other stakeholders appreciate that the actions being taken do not reflect a short-range crisis but rather an industry direction.

Clinical Quality

One challenge facing Hillside's CEO is determining if any contemplated rightsizings will affect the quality of the organization's clinical care. The board, CEO, and senior management must appreciate the need for high quality and understand that quality issues do not allow much room for flexibility.

The 1999 Institute of Medicine report *To Err Is Human* noted that "at least 44,000 people, and perhaps as many as 98,000 people, die in hospitals each year as a result of medical errors" and that medication errors are costly: "2 of every 100 admissions experienced a preventable, adverse drug event resulting in increased hospital costs of $4,700 per admission" (Kohn, Corrigan, and Donaldson 1999). A follow-up review five years later suggested that errors remain high and that many issues around substandard care persist (Bleich 2005, 9).

These efforts require the CEO to analyze every move in a rightsizing effort to ensure that the organization's clinical quality is not compromised. The challenges associated with the expanding demands of clinical capability and decreasing reimbursement do not excuse the organization from performing at a consistent and standard level of quality. A new level of understanding and use of information is required, along with a collaborative working relationship with the medical staff, nursing leadership, and senior management. A series of reactive decisions may compromise the organization's ability to maintain an acceptable level of care.

Community Health

The organization's commitment to community health programs must be given priority. Assessments should take into account both the potential for improved health and efficiencies as well as the possibility of a reduction in programs. The CEO at Hillside must, for example, carefully examine the clinic providing care to the underserved population. At a time when the organization's overall future viability is at stake, programs of this type may be deemed unaffordable. On the other hand, such programs may incur front-end financial losses but also entail significant admissions and laboratory and diagnostic tests that add financial value to the organization. The entire financial contribution of this type of program must be examined to determine its true bottom-line impact on the organization. Identifying what will happen if this program is not in operation is also valuable. Eliminating the program may have a real potential cost if, for example, patients use the ED instead, which results in increased overcrowding and delays in admissions and care for more emergent patients.

Finally, other options for retaining a valuable program should be examined. Is it possible, for example, to share the costs of the program with other healthcare providers? Are grants or governmental funds available that may provide support for a program that contributes to the overall health of the community? Could an existing, federally funded health clinic in the community take over the operation of the Hillside clinic and make it eligible for financial support?

Closing a program of this type may also have a political cost. Underserved communities have become extremely sensitized through ongoing experiences of having services reduced or eliminated, and they may criticize the closure in the media, to community leaders, or in other ways, such as picketing. These concerns must be considered when measuring the true cost of reducing such services.

Collaboration

Financial challenges provide an opportunity for organizations like Hillside to examine the possibility of increased collaboration with competitors. Because the financial difficulties experienced by healthcare organizations are almost universal, competing hospitals are likely facing these challenges as well. In these circumstances, opportunities may exist for the organizations to work collectively and merge certain services to avoid duplication, reduce costs, and enhance the overall quality of programs provided. Opportunities may include programs such as jointly run MRI or other radiological test centers, centralized laboratory systems, and support services such as laundry, freestanding security, and ambulance services. In addition, a strategic assessment may be made of programs that are offered at multiple hospitals and possible collaborations explored.

A joint operating agreement, which allows both institutions to work together and share the savings achieved by avoiding duplication, could formalize this collaboration. For example, an agreement between Hillside and Behavioral Medicine Services resulted in the closure of a freestanding outpatient behavioral center at one facility and the closure of the inpatient pediatric adolescent unit at the other. The end result was significant savings and improved utilization by both parties.

Leadership

The financial problems experienced by Hillside are common in the healthcare industry. Decreases in revenue, increases in cost, and reductions in inpatient volume have required institutions such as Hillside to deal with significant threats to their financial viability, in many cases necessitating immediate action and tough decisions. To some degree, the climate has moved the healthcare industry closer in parallel to other industries in the United States. No longer is the healthcare system a stable industry that does not experience layoffs and workforce reductions. Rather, the dramatic pressures coming from the government, insurance companies, and industry have made it one of the most complicated and uncertain industries in our society.

These challenges require healthcare executives to become better leaders and more sophisticated managers capable of making tough decisions. Financial challenges combined with the expansion of healthcare unions, managed care, and increasing pressure on and from physicians now demand that healthcare executives develop the skills necessary to work collaboratively with medical staff, union leaders, and employees. Healthcare managers must enhance their ability to lead the institution in the strategic planning process, take the strategic vision that evolves, sell it to the primary stakeholders, and make it work. Once key services are defined, executives must be able to monitor and measure these programs to determine if and when they need enhancements or reductions. Recognizing their obligation to community service, leaders must ensure that financially successful programs can pay for those that are not self-sustaining.

As changes take place and outside influences affect the industry, healthcare executives must lead their institutions in the right direction. Too often, actions of external decision makers have had an unforeseen effect on organizations. For example, as government has encouraged the closure of hospital beds and services, they have ignored the impact on the hospital's ED services. Because of the reduction of reimbursement for home and long-term healthcare, more than 25 percent of the home health agencies in the United States have closed over the last several years, and many long-term care providers are facing significant financial problems. These fiscal challenges are magnified as states prolong the approval process for qualifying Medicaid applicants for nursing home services, delaying the discharge process and lengthening hospital lengths of stay. The CEO is responsible for addressing these challenges successfully and ethically without compromising the clinical care his institution provides.

Although many parallels to other industries can be made, the expectations for providers of healthcare are significantly different. Moving a hospital to another community to reduce costs is not an option. Turning away patients who require emergency care because of their financial status is unethical, ill advised, and illegal. Healthcare executives must deal with these challenges in a more compassionate way than would other industry leaders. The willingness of large corporations to cut tens of thousands of jobs to enhance the profit margins of their stockholders is only too well known. To deal with financial concerns, healthcare executives must start by asking themselves whether they have done everything possible to effectively reduce costs, improve financial performance, and enhance the product to make it more attractive to consumers. If they cannot convince themselves of this, they must not take the easy way out and cut staff. The ability to deal with these issues well will separate the successful and ethical executive from the rest of the pack.

REFERENCES

American Association of Colleges of Nursing (AACN). 2012. "New AACN Data Show an Enrollment Surge in Baccalaureate and Graduate Programs Amid Calls for More Highly Educated Nurses." Press release issued March 22. www.aacn.nche .edu/news/articles/2012/enrollment-data.

Bleich, S. 2005. "Medical Errors: Five Years After the IOM Report." *Commonwealth Fund Issue Brief* 830: 1–15.

Carlson, J. 2011. "Power Boost for Labor: Landscape Shift Likely to Trigger New Wave of Organizing in Healthcare." ModernHealthcare.com. Posted September 5. www.modernhealthcare.com/article/20110905/MAGAZINE/309059995.

Gapenski, L. C., and G. H. Pink. 2011. *Understanding Healthcare Financial Management,* sixth edition. Chicago: Health Administration Press.

Hananel, S. 2012. "Union Membership Up Slightly." *USA Today* January 27.

Kohn, L. T., J. M. Corrigan, and M. S. Donaldson (eds.). 1999. *To Err Is Human: Building a Safer Health System.* Washington, DC: National Academies Press.

Lombardi, D. N. 1997. *Reorganization and Renewal: Strategies for Healthcare Leaders.* Chicago: Health Administration Press.

CHAPTER 8

Nurse Shortage:
Metropolitan Community Hospital

METROPOLITAN COMMUNITY HOSPITAL (MCH) was in trouble. The nurse short- *Case*
age, a problem throughout the country, had reached epidemic proportions at MCH. *Study*
While all four of the other hospitals in town were experiencing nurse shortages as
well, none of the competing hospitals was facing the crisis that confronted MCH.
For the first time in her 12-year tenure at MCH, Jane MacArthur, MCH's chief nursing officer, was beginning to feel a little insecure about her position. In fact, she was
updating her resume and had begun to consider new opportunities.

MCH is a 250-bed, privately owned, not-for-profit hospital located in the heart
of a midsize city on the East Coast. The four other hospitals in town range from
200 to 400 beds and include an investor-owned hospital (part of a national chain),
a county hospital, a Catholic hospital (part of a regional network), and another privately owned community hospital. All of these facilities had been aggressively competing for the limited number of nurses in the geographic area, and no matter what
strategies it employed or how many resources it committed to the task, MCH was
clearly losing to the competition. In the past two years, the five area hospitals had
engaged in a bidding war in terms of salaries, sign-on bonuses, and benefits such
as relocation expenses, tuition reimbursement, and domestic partner healthcare
coverage. MCH simply could not match the deep pockets of some of its competitors. The nurse turnover rate at MCH had reached 25 percent as nurses left MCH
to take more lucrative positions at competing hospitals.

MCH's geographic location was an additional recruiting obstacle. Its urban
neighborhood was believed to be a high-crime area, and although statistics dis-
proved this notion, the perception remained among the predominantly young
female nurse population. Jane was aware of this perception, but because it was not
supported in fact, she dismissed it as not needing her attention.

As more and more foreign-born nurses were recruited to MCH and as an increasingly higher percentage of agency staff were used, the budget overrun for nurse staffing had reached record proportions. The board had become impatient with Jane's
attempts at justifying this cost overrun. The board chairman declared, "We can no
longer tolerate explanations for the problem. We need solutions."

The problem had become more significant than just cost overruns. The nurse-
to-patient ratio on the medical/surgical units at MCH was 1 to 12, an unacceptable
level by any standard for both patient safety and quality of care. Patient and family
complaints had increased dramatically over the past year. Adverse events had also
increased, and John Fairfield, the hospital's legal counsel, who had never been one
of Jane's supporters, was quick to remind the CEO and the MCH board that the
source of these potential litigations was failure to remedy the nurse shortage.

Two years earlier, when Eugene Wellborn was hired as CEO at MCH, the nurse
shortage was identified as a problem but did not rank high on the board's list of
priorities for Eugene to tackle. In fact, the board chairman had assured Eugene that
Jane was unquestionably competent and could be relied on to resolve the issue
satisfactorily. The message was clear that nursing took care of itself and that Jane
had the board's full confidence. In retrospect, Eugene wished he had not hesitated
in dealing with the issue. The nurse shortage occupied a huge proportion of his
daily schedule and usurped time and energy he could be spending on the hospital's
other pressing agenda items. Hardly a day passed that Eugene did not have to deal
with an irate patient, family member, or physician.

The nurse shortage at MCH had been the primary topic of discussion at last
month's general medical staff meeting and had been accompanied by threats
of diverting patient admissions to competing hospitals if the situation did not
improve immediately. Jane was quick to point out that physicians were a major
part of the problem and one of the reasons she was having difficulty recruiting and
retaining nurses.

The medical staff enjoyed strong political clout and expected others to defer
to them on questions of authority, facility planning, and patient care. Past administrations had abdicated many of their responsibilities related to patient care and
seemed indifferent to issues other than the financial viability of the institution
and its public image in the community. Attracting physicians had been a priority
in the recent past, and Eugene's predecessor had spent every Wednesday afternoon on the golf course with prominent members of the executive medical staff
committee.

Eugene left this kind of relationship building to Carter Sims, MCH's young,
ambitious chief operating officer. For his part, Eugene believed his role and responsibility as CEO was to focus on the external environment. He needed to develop collaborative relationships and coalitions throughout the community if MCH were to

survive into the future. This was his strong belief and the mandate he had received from the board.

Nevertheless, Eugene was troubled by the powerful position of the medical staff and agreed with Jane that the behavior of some of the physicians contributed to the exodus of nurses. He had been reluctant to confront the medical staff leadership on this issue, believing that he needed to develop a stronger relationship with the physicians before taking on such an adversarial role.

To the nursing staff at MCH, this administrative posture suggested that nurses were not valued and were only supposed to follow the physicians' orders. In this environment, the physicians had become accustomed to behaving in an autocratic and sometimes disrespectful manner toward the nurses. The hospital's legal counsel John Fairfield had on more than one occasion cautioned Eugene about the legal implications of actions that he believed bordered on harassment. These incidents had fueled hostile outbursts between Jane and the chief of the medical staff, who she believed turned a blind eye to the physicians' inappropriate behavior.

In some ways, Jane's management style mirrored the autocratic, disrespectful approach to the nursing staff favored by some physicians. Jane, on the other hand, saw herself as a benevolent dictator, always ready to do battle in defense of her team. The nursing staff resented both of these higher authorities. Behind Jane's back, they referred to her as "the general," and they had even more derogatory nicknames for some of the physicians. The nurses believed that they did all of the work and received none of the rewards. They had no authority or control over their work and no participation in the decision making about patient care. They received no recognition or respect for the physically and emotionally stressful work they were expected to perform without regard to personal or professional preferences. Their work schedules were frequently modified, overtime was often required, and they were arbitrarily pulled from their work units to float in an unfamiliar, understaffed area of the hospital.

The informal leaders among the nursing staff had begun to talk about organizing. Some of them had complained to Carter Sims, the COO, but it seemed that the administration's answer to the nurses' complaints was to throw money at the problem. In fact, Carter Sims was overheard to say, "If we pay them enough, they'll be happy." That did seem to be the case with the foreign-born nurses that MCH recruited. They seemed willing to tolerate the unpleasant working conditions if the pay was good. This difference of opinion created resentment among the US-born nurses, who believed the foreign-born nurses were encouraging unfair treatment by allowing themselves to be exploited. This resentment spawned a lack of cooperation and tension among the nurses that patients observed. Eugene knew it was just a matter of time before news of the disruptive environment at MCH reached the community and he heard about it at the Rotary Club.

The only patient care units in MCH that were peaceful and operated efficiently were the emergency room, the operating room, and the intensive care unit. The physician–nursing coalitions in those patient care units made them untouchable. Both Jane and the attending physicians knew better than to antagonize the skilled, experienced, and confident nurses whom the medical directors of those units considered irreplaceable. Indeed, the nurses were considered more competent and more valuable than some of the attending physicians whose patients were treated there.

As Eugene pondered the situation at MCH, he knew he must take action, and he knew it was not going to be pleasant.

Case originally published in a slightly different format in Mistakes in Healthcare Management: Identification, Correction and Prevention, *edited by Paul B. Hofmann and Frankie Perry. Copyright © 2005 Cambridge University Press. Reprinted with permission.*

ETHICS ISSUES

Patient safety: Has the shortage of nurses responsible for direct patient care threatened patient safety at MCH? If the nurse shortage continues to go unaddressed, will patient safety be further compromised? What effect does the nurse shortage have on the public image of the institution and the willingness of patients to seek care there? What effect does the nurse shortage have on future recruitment and retention of nurses? Do nurse-to-patient staffing ratios have implications for hospital licensure or accreditation?

Adherence to the organization's mission statement, ethical standards, and values statement: Are the actions of the senior executive team at MCH consistent with the organization's mission, code of ethics, and values?

Management's role and responsibility: What is the ethical responsibility of the management of a healthcare organization to focus on mission, to model ethical conduct, and to support patient-centered care?

Ethical responsibilities to employees: What is the ethical responsibility of healthcare executives in the provision of a safe working environment that is free from harassment and discrimination?

Disruptive physician behaviors: What effect has the disruptive behavior of physicians had on recruitment and retention of nurses? On patient care? On the culture of the organization?

Legal implications: What is the hospital's liability for failing to address safe patient care? For failing to address a hostile work environment?

DISCUSSION

Patient Safety

Patient safety must always be the primary focus and concern of any healthcare organization. The presence of an adequate number of direct caregivers with appropriate skills is critical to the safety of patients. Nurses are often the sole professional staff attending to patients 24 hours a day, 7 days a week in the hospital setting. As such, the nurse serves as a clinical coordinator of patient care, addressing vital patient needs and ensuring that other healthcare professionals, including physicians, are contacted and informed of patient requirements and medical status in a timely manner. The nurse is also the monitor of the safety and well-being of the assigned patients and serves as a conduit for communication and interactions with patients and family members. A shortage of these key caregivers requires serious attention.

Because nurses play highly visible roles, a shortage of nurses can be alarming to the public and contribute to negative perceptions of an organization. Such perceptions may impede the recruitment and retention of nurses and deter patients from seeking care at that institution.

In addition, depending on the state in which the institution is located, nurse-to-patient staffing ratios may have a significant effect on licensure. In 2004, California was the first state to implement minimum nurse-to-patient ratios in acute care hospitals. A report released by the Agency for Healthcare Research and Quality of the US Department of Health & Human Services documenting the California experience found that "state-mandated nurse staffing levels alleviate workloads leading to lower patient mortality and higher nurse satisfaction" (AHRQ 2012). In 2010, The Joint Commission announced its interim staffing effectiveness standards. Although those standards do not include staff-to-patient ratios, such ratios remain under examination. As of 2011, 15 states had enacted regulations related to nurse staffing levels, and 17 states had introduced legislation mandating minimum ratios. Staffing effectiveness is on the radar at the national level as more and more stories about patient safety and the costs associated with medical errors and hospital accidents flood the media.

Adherence to the Organization's Mission Statement, Ethical Standards, and Values Statement

In this case, the senior managers at MCH seem to have completely lost sight of the organization's mission and its responsibility to the community it serves. Focus on the mission of the hospital, which should be paramount, has been replaced by focus on self-interests. Eugene, the CEO, has blindly taken his marching orders from the governing board and concentrated all his energies on the external environment, leaving the internal operations of the organization to flounder. Was he more concerned about obliging the board than fulfilling his obligation to the organization? While the CEO may serve at the pleasure of the board, both the CEO and the governing board must be committed to the best interests of the organization they serve. Eugene's failure to conduct a thorough assessment of the organization's operations and senior staff, identify areas in need of attention, and set priorities is a failure of leadership. When leaders focus on mission, they must also pay attention to the people they need to carry out that mission, and Eugene failed to do both.

Management's Role and Responsibility

The most pressing issue at MCH is the nurse shortage, and yet the organization's failure to conduct an in-depth analysis of the crisis is evident. A thorough analysis would have revealed the need to address the factors that underlie the problem, such as disruptive behaviors among physicians, autocratic nursing leadership, lack of inclusiveness and respect, a negative work environment, cultural differences among nurses, and the perception that MCH is located in a high-crime area.

Equally pressing is the need for a careful evaluation of senior management to determine if they are capable of functioning as a team to tackle the organization's problems and carry out its mission of patient care. The senior staff have established beneficial relationships with people who would champion them and their positions—the COO with the medical staff, the CNO with influential board members, and the CEO with the board and community leaders. Those alliances promote individual interests at the expense of the organization's mission. Leadership must create a culture that encourages teamwork and integrates the efforts of staff to achieve organizational goals.

People drive an organization and contribute to its success or failure. "The biggest mistake managers consistently make is to recognize that they have the wrong person in a key position and fail to do something about it" (Russell and Greenspan 2005, 86). Replacing a staff person who is unable to do the job is difficult—especially if the person has been in the position for a long time or has friends on the board or the medical staff. If you have personally hired the person, the situation can also be problematic, especially if you provided a premium hiring package because you were impressed with the person's credentials, experience, or potential. You must admit that you made a mistake. That situation is examined in the Heartland Healthcare System case in Chapter 9.

Decisions about people always seem to be the most difficult but are especially crucial to the success of the organization. Consider Collins's (2001, 41) observation: "The executives who ignited the transformations from good to great [companies] did not first figure out where to drive the bus and then get people to take it there. No, they first got the right people on the bus (and the wrong people off the bus) and then figured out where to drive it."

Ethical Responsibilities to Employees

Healthcare managers, regardless of their areas of responsibility, often find the management of people to be the most challenging part of their jobs. Mastering skills in finance, planning, marketing, information technology, and the like is less difficult for most managers than dealing with the people-related problems and conflicts that arise in the work environment. Adding to the complexity is the diversity of today's workforce and the various values, ethics, and cultural perspectives that influence how each employee sees the world. The healthcare manager must be sensitive to those differences and clearly establish the ethical principles and behaviors that are acceptable when dealing with patients, clients, and coworkers. Then, perhaps even more important, the healthcare manager must actually practice those principles and behaviors when dealing with employees. Healthcare managers are usually acutely aware of their ethical responsibilities to patients, clients, the organization, and the community. Too often, however, they overlook their ethical responsibilities to the people they manage.

The leadership of an organization establishes the ethical culture in which work will be performed and patient care provided. In healthcare, the clinical staff administer patient care, but management is responsible for creating an environment in which top-quality, effective patient care is delivered. Eugene has failed miserably in fulfilling this responsibility. He has focused on the external environment and allowed the internal culture to lapse into a muddle of adversarial relationships, negativity, and distrust. Such a culture will produce patient complaints and staff shortages. Working in such an environment holds little reward. The *Code of Ethics* of the American College of Healthcare Executives (ACHE 2011, IV) is clear about the ethical responsibilities of healthcare executives in this regard:

> Healthcare executives have ethical and professional obligations to the employees they manage that encompass but are not limited to:
> A. Creating a work environment that promotes ethical conduct;
> B. Providing a work environment that encourages a free expression of ethical concerns and provides mechanisms for discussing and addressing such concerns;
> C. Promoting a healthy work environment which includes freedom from harassment, sexual and other, and coercion of any kind, especially to perform illegal or unethical acts;
> D. Promoting a culture of inclusivity that seeks to prevent discrimination on the basis of race, ethnicity, religion, gender, sexual orientation, age or disability;

E. Providing a work environment that promotes the proper use of employees' knowledge and skills; and

F. Providing a safe and healthy work environment.

The management at MCH has also failed to address the perception that the hospital is located in a high-crime neighborhood. Although this perception is not based in fact, "reality is what it is perceived to be" (Berger and Luckmann 1967), and left unchallenged, perceptions can become accepted as truth. Management has a responsibility to address this issue with facts and to make high-profile changes to ensure that patients, visitors, and staff feel safe and secure in the hospital and the surrounding area.

As mentioned, management neglected to complete a comprehensive analysis of the factors leading to nurses' dissatisfaction and resignations. Valuable information could have been gained from exit interviews. A competitive market analysis of salaries and benefits would have been helpful. Focus groups and similar efforts could have shed light on the problem and potential solutions.

If MCH wishes to ensure its viability as a healthcare provider, it should model its approach to nursing on the Magnet Recognition Program, which was developed by the American Nurses Association in response to the nurse shortage of the 1980s. The American Nurses Credentialing Center (ANCC 2008) believes that Magnet organizations are "essential to the continued development of the nursing profession and to quality outcomes in patient care." The program incentivizes healthcare organizations to improve nurse recruitment and retention by means of the 14 Forces of Magnetism, organized under five Magnet Model Components, that differentiate Magnet-recognized hospitals from other hospitals:

1. Transformational leadership
   - **Quality of nursing leadership.** Are they strong, knowledgeable advocates for the staff?
   - **Management style.** Do the leaders invite participation and feedback?
2. Structural empowerment
   - **Organizational structure.** Is it decentralized with strong representation for nurses?
   - **Personnel policies and programs.** Are salaries competitive? Are flexible schedules offered?
   - **Community and the hospital.** Does the hospital have a strong presence in the community?
   - **Image of nursing.** Do other members of the healthcare team view the work of nursing as essential?
   - **Professional development.** Is significant emphasis placed on in-service education, continuing education, and career development?

3. Exemplary professional practice
   - **Professional models of care.** Are nurses given responsibility and authority?
   - **Consultation and resources.** Are there adequate human resources?
   - **Autonomy.** Are nurses allowed independent judgment?
   - **Nurses as teachers.** Are nurses permitted and expected to incorporate teaching in all aspects of practice?
   - **Interdisciplinary relationships.** Is a sense of mutual respect exhibited among all disciplines?
4. New knowledge, innovation, and improvements
   - **Quality improvement.** Are nurses involved?
5. Empirical quality results
   - **Quality of care.** Is it an organizational priority?

Pursuing Magnet recognition has merit. Premier hospitals throughout the nation "vie to meet a rigorous set of requirements and earn this designation, which has become an important element in *U.S. News & World Report* magazine's annual Best Hospitals list" (Lyder 2011). One such hospital is Northern Michigan Regional Hospital, which achieved Magnet recognition in 2011 and is "a paragon of progressive nursing management" (Greene 2012). Such was not always the case—the hospital made headlines some time ago for having the longest nursing strike on record in the United States. Now, with strong nursing representation at the top of the organization and in the boardroom, it is reaping benefits in quality improvement and patient and staff satisfaction.

Nurses are the largest, most visible segment of a hospital's workforce and are widely recognized as the most crucial. According to Bogue (2012), "As payments soon will be tied to quality, building a strong nursing staff will lead to better outcomes—and payment."

Disruptive Physician Behaviors

Disruptive and unprofessional physician behavior is more common than one might think. A national survey by the American College of Physician Executives (ACPE) reported that "more than 2 in 3 US doctors witness other physicians disrupting patient care or collegial relationships at least once a month; more than 1 in 10 say they see it every day." An ACPE representative said, "Our profession is still plagued by doctors acting in a way that is disrespectful, unprofessional and toxic to the workplace" (Knox 2011). Another study found that 80 percent of hospital workers, including doctors and nurses, said they had seen "yelling," "abusive language," "condescension," and "berating of colleagues"—and a quarter of those surveyed said they saw such behavior weekly (Scheinbaum 2012).

The consequences of inappropriate behaviors are many and severe. They result in dysfunctional teams, reduced quality of patient care and medical outcomes, medical errors, poor nurse retention, and increased risk of litigation (Swiggart et al. 2009).

Contributing causes of inappropriate and damaging behavior are thought to be stress, long hours, red tape, and shrinking physician compensation. As a result of their socialization in medical school, physicians expect to be in control of situations, always be right, and never have their orders questioned. In recent years, however, they have lost more and more control over their practices, compensation, and way of life. In addition, stress is intrinsic to their profession, which requires them to deal with life-and-death situations and the ever-present threat of malpractice. However, many physicians fail to develop the social relationships and good physical habits that might serve as stress relievers (Scheinbaum 2012).

Swiggart and colleagues (2009) found that failure to address physicians' disruptive behavior and a lack of consequences reinforce inappropriate conduct. Management may choose to ignore such behavior for many reasons. Perhaps the offender is a high admitter or the only practitioner of a desirable subspecialty. Perhaps administrators fear antagonizing the offender's colleagues or simply wish to avoid conflict. Under those circumstances, the disruptive behaviors are likely to continue and may even escalate. Finally, a physician's inappropriate behavior may be a symptom of a deeper underlying problem, such as addiction or physical or mental illness. Every instance of troublesome conduct requires early intervention to determine its causes.

The American Medical Association (AMA 2001) places responsibility on physicians to "report physicians deficient in character or competence." Physicians, on the other hand, may expect management to handle sensitive situations, especially if the offending physician is well connected politically and professionally. The Joint Commission (2008) is clear on this issue: "To assure quality and promote a culture of safety, health care organizations must address the problem of behaviors that threaten the performance of the health care team." The Joint Commission standard requires hospitals to incorporate codes of conduct into medical staff bylaws and medical agreements that declare zero tolerance for disruptive behavior and provide protections for those who report it (DerGurahian 2008).

So how do healthcare executives go about addressing this often difficult issue? Hickson and colleagues (2007) list the means needed to remedy disruptive and unprofessional behaviors:

- Leadership commitment
- Supportive institutional policies
- Surveillance tools to capture patient and staff allegations
- A model to guide graduated interventions

- A process for reviewing allegations
- Multilevel professional and leadership training
- Resources to help disruptive colleagues
- Resources to help disruptive staff and patients

When dealing with medical staff issues that require behavioral correction, disciplinary action, or cooperation, organizational leaders should collaborate closely with medical leaders and seek their help in pursuing change. Healthcare executives must clearly communicate the effects of disruptive physician behaviors, especially on patient care and staff retention, so that physicians understand how their patients will benefit from explicit methods of dealing with unprofessional conduct. All members of the medical staff must be familiar with policies and procedures pertaining to disruptive behaviors, reporting guidelines, and responsibilities of medical staff officers. Clear definitions of terms such as *discrimination, harassment,* and *disruptive behaviors* are especially important to ensure that staff recognize inappropriate conduct and know that it must be dealt with. Investigations of alleged inappropriate behaviors must be confidential and documented and must allow the physician in question to respond (Hofmann 2010). Interventions and corrective actions must follow allegations proven to be true.

To create a more productive, professional environment, some healthcare organizations have found it helpful to engage the services of an anger management consultant to help physicians learn to control their anger and modify their behavior. One such consultant has created a workbook, *The Practice of Control,* especially for physicians. It teaches that anger, which is often preliminary to disruptive behavior, is as personally harmful as smoking a pack of cigarettes a day (Scheinbaum 2012).

Hofmann (2010) has found that the following management actions promote and support a productive, professional work environment:

1. Provide education and training about inappropriate conduct.
2. Survey staff about the work environment.
3. Enforce compliance with codes of conduct and policies regarding disruptive behavior.
4. Ensure a means for reporting concerns.
5. Promptly investigate allegations.
6. Give timely feedback about complaints.
7. Offer support services for physicians who behave improperly.

All such actions require a commitment from management to provide the necessary time and staff, but healthcare managers with foresight will recognize that the return on investment will be invaluable.

Legal Implications

At MCH, staff shortages, disruptive physician behaviors, conflicts, and poor communication among nurses of different cultures have created a negative work environment and an adversarial climate. Such conditions often lead to medical errors, patient dissatisfaction, and adverse patient events such as falls, surgical complications, hospital-acquired infections, and medication errors. Staff shortages and poor communication among caregivers threaten patient safety and set the stage for malpractice litigation. And nurses are reluctant to question a volatile physician's order, even when doing so might prevent an adverse patient event.

The toxic work environment at MCH invites claims of discrimination and hostile working conditions. Sooner or later, disgruntled employees, patients, or families will decide that management is ignoring their complaints and will seek recourse. The resulting legal, political, and public relations damage will threaten MCH's very existence.

REFERENCES

Agency for Healthcare Research and Quality (AHRQ). 2012. "State-Mandated Nurse Staffing Levels Alleviate Workloads, Leading to Lower Patient Mortality and Higher Nurse Satisfaction." AHRQ Innovations Exchange. Updated October 10. http://innovations.ahrq.gov/content.aspx?id=3708.

American College of Healthcare Executives (ACHE). 2011. *Code of Ethics.* Updated November 14. www.ache.org/abt_ache/code.cfm#patients.

American Medical Association (AMA). 2001. "Principles of Medical Ethics." Preamble of the AMA *Code of Medical Ethics.* Revised June. www.ama-assn.org/ama/pub/physician-resources/medical-ethics/code-medical-ethics/principles-medical-ethics.page.

American Nurses Credentialing Center (ANCC). 2008. "Announcing a New Model for ANCC's Magnet Recognition Program." Accessed August 5, 2013. www.nursecredentialing.org/MagnetModel.aspx.

Berger, P. L., and T. Luckmann. 1967. *The Social Construction of Reality.* Garden City, NY: Anchor Books, Doubleday and Co.

Bogue, R. J. 2012. "Nurses: Key to Making or Breaking Your Future Margin." *Hospitals & Health Networks Daily* May 29. www.hhnmag.com/hhnmag/HHNDaily/HHNDailyDisplay.dhtml?id=5390002938.

Collins, J. 2001. *Good to Great.* New York: HarperCollins.

DerGurahian, J. 2008. "Behavioral Watchdogs: Joint Commission Standard Targets Unruly Staff." *Modern Healthcare* 38 (28): 8–9.

Greene, J. 2012. "A New Voice at the Table." *Trustee* 65 (3): 8–12.

Hickson, G. B., W. Pickert, L. E. Webb, and S. G. Gabbe. 2007. "A Complementary Approach to Promoting Professionalism: Identifying, Measuring, and Addressing Unprofessional Behaviors." *Academic Medicine* 82 (11): 1040–48.

Hofmann, P. B. 2010. "Fulfilling Disruptive-Behavior Policy Objectives: Leaders Must Promptly Address Improper Clinician Behavior." *Healthcare Executive* 25 (3): 62–63.

Joint Commission, The. 2010. "Nurse Staffing Effectiveness in 2010: The Interim Standards." *Briefings on The Joint Commission* March 2010.

———. 2008. "Behaviors That Undermine a Culture of Safety." *Sentinel Event Alert* Issue 40, July 9. www.jointcommission.org/assets/1/18/SEA_40.pdf.

Knox, R. 2011. "Doctors Behaving Badly? They Say It Happens All the Time." *NPR* May 25. www.npr.org/blogs/health/2011/05/28/136648516/doctors-behaving-badly-they-say-it-happens-all-the-time.

Lyder, C. H. 2011. "Nurses at the Forefront of Change." *Hospitals & Health Networks Daily* November 17. www.hhnmag.com/hhnmag/HHNDaily/HHNDailyDisplay.dhtml?id=3820003826.

Russell, J. A., and B. Greenspan. 2005. "Correcting and Preventing Management Mistakes." In *Management Mistakes in Healthcare: Identification, Correction and Prevention,* edited by P. B. Hofmann and F. Perry, 84–102. New York: Cambridge University Press.

Scheinbaum, C. 2012. "Doctors Without Boundaries: An Anger Management Pioneer Tries to Defuse Rageaholic Physicians." *Bloomberg Businessweek* August 6–12.

Swiggart, W. H., C. M. Dewey, G. B. Hickson, A. J. R. Finlayson, and W. A. Spickard, Jr. 2009. "A Plan for Identification, Treatment, and Remediation of Disruptive Behaviors in Physicians." *Frontiers of Health Services Management* 25 (4): 3–11.

CHAPTER 9

Information Technology Setback: Heartland Healthcare System

JACK MOORE HAD been frustrated throughout most of his career. Information *Case* technology (IT) was breaking new ground in the medical and corporate worlds, *Study* yet Jack found himself continually compromised by unimaginative bosses and organizations crippled by a lack of resources. But it looked as though things were about to change. Jack had recently been hired as the chief information officer (CIO) of Heartland Healthcare System, a successful multihospital system. It was his dream position.

The flagship 500-bed hospital is located in the major metropolitan area of a predominantly rural state in the Great Plains region. Heartland's five smaller hospitals of 50 or fewer beds are scattered throughout the rural regions of the state within a 100-mile radius of the flagship hospital. In addition, three specialty hospitals (heart, pediatrics, and orthopedics) thrive in the metropolitan area along with a very busy outpatient surgical center. The hospitals that make up the Heartland system are connected by a sophisticated helicopter transport system that quickly transports patients in need to the flagship hospital. The hospital system employs more than 5,000 staff members and 300 physicians, mostly subspecialists. An additional 900 private-practice physicians have privileges at Heartland. Heartland's staff includes a sizeable number of nurse practitioners, who play a significant role in caring for the state's rural population and who staff a number of the primary healthcare clinics located in the metropolitan area as well.

When Jack was hired as CIO at Heartland, he was charged with two major responsibilities: (1) ensure access and interconnectivity of medical information among all of the system's hospitals, urgent care centers, primary care clinics, and private physician offices; and (2) install computerized physician order entry (CPOE). To make his job easier, he would report directly to the CEO.

Richard Smith had been the CEO of Heartland for more than 15 years and was largely responsible for the success of the system. His one disappointment had been his inability to enhance the IT at Heartland. His failure to do so was in some measure attributable to John Forbes, the previous CIO, who was retiring after more than 20 years at Heartland and who was thought to be out-of-date with the current available technology. Richard had often berated himself for not investing more in IT and for not forcing early retirement on John to better achieve this goal.

Richard was pleased with his recruitment of Jack, who had very impressive IT credentials, although not in healthcare, and seemed competent and eager to move Heartland into the next generation of IT. Richard assured Jack that the needed resources had been budgeted and approved to achieve rapid progress, based on an earlier feasibility study by a reputable IT consulting firm. Heartland had engaged the firm to conduct the study, and both Richard and the Heartland board had been pleased with the firm's work. The IT consultants had indicated in their study that the existing XYZ system at Heartland could be upgraded to the new CPOE system for a cost of $3 million. An upgrade seemed like a reasonable solution to the immediate problem, but Jack felt it was a myopic strategy if Heartland were to move into future cutting-edge technologies necessary to maintain its command of the market. The plan certainly did not mesh with his personal ambition to build an IT system at Heartland that would be the envy of healthcare organizations across the Midwest. Eager to bring Heartland's system up-to-date as quickly as possible, Richard did not need much convincing of the wisdom inherent in Jack's strategy. Subsequently, a three-vendor search and formal bid process yielded a $10 million contract with MedCor to implement a new IT system with promises of the desired interconnectivity throughout Heartland, electronic medical records, and CPOE—in short, state-of-the-art healthcare delivery system technology.

As the project progressed, Jack hired Les Atkins, a local independent contractor, to manage the hardware conversion. This conversion was a much more complex undertaking than Jack's previous experience had prepared him for, but he felt that with Les's help, the project would move forward. As work progressed, Jack found himself relying more and more on Les and his advice on managing the project. Les began contracting for more and more staff time from his firm to work on the implementation, even though using Heartland IT staff would have been less expensive and certainly better for Heartland staff morale. The staff were beginning to grumble that they were being left out of the loop and did not know what was going on. The sense of being left out of the decision making on the implementation began to escalate as the accounting staff responsible for patient billing and the nursing staff responsible for patient care were ignored. The nursing staff became especially vocal in their chagrin at not being consulted as decisions were made that affected their patient care activities. The vice president (VP) for nursing wasted no time in making her concerns known to the CEO, but they were largely unheeded. Richard thought this was yet another example of the VP's marginal cooperation with other departments in the organization, a problem he had raised during her last annual performance review.

To the hospital staff, Jack and Les seemed to be making decisions in isolation with the unflinching support of the CEO. To Richard, the hospital staff, especially nursing, were being resistant to change as usual and were attempting to thwart the forward progress necessary to bring Heartland's IT into the twenty-first century.

As staff morale plummeted, speculation among the staff began to focus on the appropriateness of Les's firm's business transactions with Heartland. The purchasing staff let it be known that Heartland had purchased 40 keyboards and mice from Les's firm without a formal bid process.

Then the unthinkable happened. Two years into the contract and $8 million into the $10 million project, MedCor was sold to another company, which dropped the patient billing system product that was an integral part of the project. Nothing in the contract protected Heartland from this eventuality. In an effort to minimize the financial loss, Jack went back to XYZ, which said that with the remaining budget of $2 million, they could upgrade to the new CPOE system.

Richard was dumbfounded. Jack had recommended MedCor so strongly and was so confident that it was the perfect fit for Heartland. Following the initial shock of the disclosure, however, Jack was able to convince Richard that this unfortunate turn of events could not have been foreseen. As Jack put it, it was a minor setback that would not prevent Heartland from moving into the technology future they both desired.

In the aftermath of the MedCor debacle, Heartland hired Les as its full-time manager of hardware support. Jack was shaken by the MedCor departure and believed that he needed Les even more. It was common knowledge among the Heartland IT staff that Les had no formal degree. Not only had Heartland waived the position's requirements for Les, but it had also not posted the position.

Today, Richard still has high hopes that Heartland can acquire state-of-the-art technology like that of hardware system giants in the corporate world. Although he has less confidence in Jack and suspects that Jack is more interested in building his own personal technology empire, he does not necessarily see their goals as being mutually exclusive.

The hospital's IT staff clearly lack confidence in Jack's leadership ability. They see a firewall between the employees doing application support and IT management. The nursing staff believe that Jack has no concept of the hospital's mission of patient care and no interest in involving patient care staff in technology planning and implementation. The accounting staff are convinced that Jack has no business savvy and does not adequately focus on business applications. In fact, one employee was recently overheard to say, "Jack is more intent on being a cutting-edge IT think tank than being an integral part of a hospital system whose job is to serve patients."

Case originally published in a slightly different format in Mistakes in Healthcare Management: Identification, Correction and Prevention, *edited by Paul B. Hofmann and Frankie Perry. Copyright © 2005 Cambridge University Press. Reprinted with permission.*

ETHICS ISSUES

Management's role and responsibility: What are Richard's role and responsibility in this case? What are Jack's? How does Richard's and Jack's treatment of the other senior staff inform the situation? Were project goals established with metrics to measure progress? Was appropriate accountability and oversight established for a project of this magnitude? Were contracting, purchasing, and human resources practices judicious and ethical?

Organizational implications: Given the fiduciary obligation of administrators to their organization, how could the CEO and CIO have avoided, or at least minimized, the possible damage if their IT plan ran into difficulty? Who is more accountable—Jack, for convincing Richard to change plans, or Richard, for allowing himself to be swayed without conducting more due diligence? What is the board's role? What are the implications of this situation for quality improvement at Heartland? How will reimbursements be affected? Staff satisfaction? Patient satisfaction? What effect will this failed project have on future staff collaboration and productivity? On staff's trust of management?

Adherence to the organization's mission statement, ethical standards, and values statement: Are the actions in this case consistent with the organization's mission statement, ethical standards, and values statement? Was Jack unethical in his management of the IT project? Did Richard behave ethically in his obligations as CEO? Have personal goals and ambitions trumped the organization's mission and responsibility to the community?

Conflict of interest: What are the conflicts of interest in this case? Did Jack truly believe that the solution he proposed would provide greater benefit to Heartland and its patients? How might the situation have been different if Richard had examined the interests of all parties (including his own) in an objective way?

Use of consultants: What factors should be considered when hiring a consultant? What steps should be taken during the hiring process? Did Jack use his consultant effectively and appropriately? What could Jack have done to improve the situation?

Justice and fairness: How do issues of justice and fairness enter into this case? Did Jack manage personnel and other resources fairly? What role did bias play in the situation and its outcome? Did the relationship between Richard and Jack support or inhibit fair and just relationships with others? How did Jack's relationship with Les affect members of the IT staff? How might the situation at Heartland have been different if Jack and Les had listened to and engaged other leaders and staff?

DISCUSSION

by Pete Shelkin and Melissa Cole

This case tells the story of a CIO who lands his dream job and is looking forward to making his mark by raising his employer's IT infrastructure to a level that will be the envy of other hospital systems. Such opportunities can be great motivators because they challenge people to prove their abilities. However, this case also demonstrates that it takes more than desire and motivation to ensure success and that straying from the path to success can be easy once the first missteps are taken. Along the way, ethical challenges arise that people can increasingly succumb to as pressures mount.

The following discussion addresses the pitfalls of confusing one's own goals with those of an organization and the consequences of not knowing when to ask for or properly use help.

Management's Role and Responsibility

Before dealing with ethics, we need to discuss roles and responsibilities. In Richard's case, the board would consider his CEO responsibilities to include setting clear direction, creating the management organization chart, staffing the executive team, ensuring that budgets are set and met, and making sure that decisions are well made and executed (White and Griffith 2010, 56–57). Richard has further responsibilities to his management team that include giving clear direction, assessing performance, and providing coaching and guidance when necessary (Morrison 2011). In addition, in his role as Heartland's CEO, Richard has a responsibility to all Heartland staff to ensure just treatment and to all patients and the community to ensure that patient trust is not violated and that patients can expect to be satisfied by the services that they receive (Morrison 2011).

As a member of the senior executive team, Jack is responsible for achieving the goals that the CEO sets for him and to do so in ways that will ensure the best results. Those results are typically measured in terms of quality, costs, benefits, and the like. As the CIO, Jack is also responsible for working closely with clinical leaders to ensure that he understands their needs and to prepare strategic and operational plans that take those needs into account. More important, in executing his plans he is expected to meet the clinicians' needs as closely as possible. Given unlimited wants and limited budgets, meeting these needs can be a difficult task, but the expectation is legitimate. Established models and practices show that this responsibility can be successfully fulfilled (White and Griffith 2010, 428, 433). Finally, Jack is responsible for setting clear direction in the IT department and ensuring just treatment of his staff (AMIA 2007).

The financial management function projects future needs, arranges to meet them, and manages the organization's assets and liabilities in ways that increase its profitability (White and Griffith 2010, 434). Executives have a fiduciary responsibility to protect the resources of their institution. The loss of $8 million and two years of effort opens the door to charges that Heartland's administrators, particularly the CIO and CEO, have failed to uphold their fiduciary responsibility. The board may even ask questions about managerial malpractice and negligence when they learn that the contract with MedCor had no provisions protecting Heartland in the event that MedCor was sold. Although the CEO and the legal counsel may share in the blame, the CIO has primary responsibility to ensure that relatively common issues with IT vendors are identified and addressed in such an important IT contract.

Even if we lay the blame for the troubled IT project at the feet of the CIO, we must still ask what the CEO could have (or should have) done to minimize or even avoid the damage. Healthcare administrators are ethically bound to ensure that staff who work at their institutions are competent (Morrison 2011). This obligation is most clear in the areas of direct care delivery, where many staff are required to be licensed or certified and to stay up-to-date through continuing education. Although healthcare executives are not required to be licensed or certified, they are expected to be highly competent in their respective fields, and their managers are expected to validate that competency on a regular basis. The Joint Commission (2012) standard requiring that all staff, not just line staff, receive performance evaluations reinforces that expectation.

In this context, we must ask why the CIO is able to persuade the CEO to ignore the $3 million budget that the board previously approved and to pursue a much more expensive strategy. And then, after the sale of MedCor, why is the CEO willing to believe that the debacle is only a minor setback? Finally, after the VP for nursing voices her concerns about being left out of decision making, how can Richard continue to avoid questioning Jack's ability to handle the job of CIO?

While we may forgive Richard for seeing Jack in only his best light during the hiring process, ethical questions begin to arise in regard to Richard's response—or rather his lack of response—to warning signs about Jack's ability to take direction and his competency in general. At what point between the initial honeymoon period granted to a new hire and the catastrophic failure of the IT project did the CEO fail in his duty to ensure that Heartland had a competent CIO? Could following a schedule of required formal performance assessments that included gathering feedback from others at key intervals have helped the CEO keep the CIO on a course to success?

Organizational Implications

Clearly, the loss of $8 million and two years of effort will have a significant impact on Heartland. Not only have the goals of installing CPOE and ensuring interconnectivity been delayed, but the benefits that could have been gained by spending that $8 million on other capital projects have also been forfeited. Even without further details about Heartland's financials, we have enough information about the size of the system and its operations to make some reasonable assumptions. For example, the Healthcare Information and Management Systems Society Analytics Database (HIMSS 2013) shows that midwestern hospitals with 500 to 600 beds have average total annual operating revenues of $496 million and average total capital expenses of $19.6 million. Most hospitals also set a goal of maintaining a 2.7 percent operating margin to achieve an A credit rating.

Assuming that Heartland is like other midwestern hospital systems of its size, its $8 million loss would have amounted to 20 percent of its annual capital budget during each of the last two years. The lack of corresponding assets on the balance sheet will drive down Heartland's margin and have an adverse effect on its financial and operating ratios. As substantial as the damage appears to be when the HIMSS averages are used as a basis, the picture would be even worse if Heartland's financial performance were below average to begin with. The damage is sufficiently great that the CFO and the board's finance committee will have to make some tough decisions as they watch Heartland's ratios decline and risk losing its A rating.

The effect on Heartland will likely go beyond the damage to its financial statements and operating ratios and may extend to staff and patients alike. Questions that the CEO should anticipate hearing from the board include the following: What quality improvement initiatives were initially postponed to fund the IT projects, and will they now be postponed even further? Are quality metrics stagnating, or worse yet, declining, while improvement efforts await funding? If so, how will reimbursements be affected now that reimbursements are being tied to outcomes? The board may also want to know if staff satisfaction is being affected by delays in improvements or if patient satisfaction is being affected by quality issues, deterioration of the physical plant, or perceptions of outdated equipment.

The losses resulting from Jack's actions have implications that reach far beyond the IT department.

Given the ethical obligation of administrators to serve in a fiduciary role, how might the CEO and CIO have avoided, or at least minimized, any negative consequences? Why has the original consulting report been discounted? The report was provided by a reputable firm, and the board is pleased with it. Heartland is planning to act on the report's recommendations until Jack arrives and convinces Richard to think bigger. In his enthusiasm to move Heartland into a cutting-edge IT future, Richard fails to exercise due diligence, such as having the consulting firm review Jack's new proposal and compare it with its earlier recommendation. If the consulting firm is truly reputable, and if Jack's plan has merit and is backed by facts, the firm could easily modify its recommendation in light of the new information and Jack's leadership. Given the effect of the change in plans, who is more accountable? What is the board's role? Have they approved the change in plans without asking questions of their own? As tends to be the case when leaders look back at massive failures, they may see many missed opportunities that might have ensured accountability and prudent corrections.

Questions also remain about how MedCor has been selected and how the project is managed within the organization. Whether the selection committee includes representatives of all stakeholders is unknown; however, Jack's exclusion of key stakeholders from decision making during the new system's implementation suggests that he also does not consider stakeholder input during the selection process. Ignoring stakeholder input is a primary cause of failure for IT projects (Glaser 2009). Given that Jack fails to use stakeholder input as the basis of his planning and decision processes, the project would likely run into serious trouble even if MedCor had not been sold.

Adherence to the Organization's Mission Statement, Ethical Standards, and Values Statement

Although we do not have access to Heartland's mission statement and strategic goals, we do know that Jack has two major responsibilities: achieving interconnectivity and implementing CPOE. Jack's primary goals are probably tied directly to Heartland's strategic plan, which is—by definition and necessity—intended to support Heartland's mission and vision.

Jack clearly has not met the goals that he was responsible for. However, is failure unethical? One could easily argue that failing to meet a business goal is not in and of itself an ethical failure. To determine the existence of an ethical breach, we need to understand why a failure occurred. For instance, a failure might occur because an unethical person misrepresented his skills or experience to get a job. An obvious example of this in healthcare is someone who impersonates a physician and harms patients by giving bad advice and bungling procedures (ABC News 2010; Janes 2012). However, Jack appeared to have impressive IT credentials when Heartland hired him and so does not seem guilty of outright fraud. Later we learn that Heartland's project was "a much more complex undertaking than Jack's previous experience had prepared him for." Nonetheless, Jack's willingness to take on such a difficult project would not necessarily be an ethical breach because eagerness to tackle ever greater challenges is often encouraged and admired in successful leaders.

What distinguishes an ethical failure from an unethical one is the motive involved (Collis 1998). Jack certainly wanted to make Heartland a successful show-case of technology, but he may have been motivated more by his ambitions than by a desire to support Heartland's mission. According to the opening paragraph, Jack had been frustrated throughout most of his career and felt that he had been continually compromised by unimaginative bosses. Jack's personal ambition was "to build an IT system at Heartland that would be the envy of healthcare organizations across the Midwest." Jack's ambition raises questions about his adherence to Heartland's mission, which focuses on serving patients and, we can assume, makes no mention of causing competitors to be envious. In light of such information, Jack's motives might be questioned, as might the ethics of his priorities and actions.

Conflict of Interest

Conflict is not necessarily bad or unethical. In fact, many innovations have come about because people's perspectives conflicted with the status quo, and their interest in providing a more valuable product or service drove them to challenge accepted assumptions or previous decisions. Some people also discover that they are working for an unethical organization and seek to expose the unprincipled activities. Although such whistle-blowers are motivated by the conflict between their personal interests and their responsibilities to their employers, they are usually regarded as acting ethically. In the end, the determining factor is the whistle-blower's motivation: Is the individual focused primarily on personal gain or on benefiting the organization?

In the case under consideration, the goals of the CIO, the CEO, and Heartland initially appear to be aligned: They all share the goal of using technology to move the health system into a productive and efficient future where quality rises and cost per unit of service declines. Conflict comes into play almost immediately, however, when the CIO decides that the board-approved solution is myopic and lobbies successfully to pursue an alternative strategy at a much higher cost. Where do the CIO's interests lie when he persuades the CEO, and presumably the board, to change direction? Does he believe that his solution will result in greater benefit to Heartland and its patients? Perhaps he does; however, we are told that a primary reason the CIO believes that the approved solution is shortsighted is that it does not mesh with his personal ambitions. When that is considered along with the statement in the opening paragraph that throughout his career the CIO had felt "continually compromised by unimaginative bosses," we get a sense that while the parties' goals may be aligned, their motives may not be. The term *conflict of interest* is commonly used to describe such situations; perhaps the term *conflict of motive* can be thought of as the key to identifying a conflict of interest that is unethical.

In the Heartland case, other interests besides those of the CEO and CIO are at play as well. For example, the CIO's interests seem to conflict with those of the VP for nursing and her nursing staff, the accounting staff, and the IT staff. While mounting evidence suggests that the CIO's selfish motives are at the root of those conflicts, each interest should be examined on its own merits. All too often a mob mentality can take over when a crisis reaches critical mass and people rally to find a scapegoat. To guard against a situation such as that at Heartland, people must avoid accepting the easy conclusion and falling into an ethical trap. The CEO's actions are evidence of this tendency: Instead of fully investigating the situation, Richard quickly dismisses the VP for nursing's objections because he sees them as proof of her marginal cooperation. In fact, as the project gets deeper and deeper into trouble, the more others complain and the more they are ignored. How might the situation have been different if the CEO examined all parties' interests and assessed the validity of each perspective?

Use of Consultants

Healthcare leaders must frequently decide whether to use outside expertise or internal talent. Large IT projects are especially likely to call for such decisions because the needed skills and the duration of those needs usually differ greatly from the needs of day-to-day operations.

Ideally, when organizations hire consultants for temporary support and enhancement of their own staff, the staff gain valuable new knowledge and abilities. Laying the foundation for a successful collaboration requires input from the project's stakeholders to clearly define the scope of work to be accomplished as well as thorough research by the in-house project manager to locate a consultant with the right skills, experience, and credentials. A contract is then negotiated that documents the scope, the deliverables (which should include knowledge transfer), and a clear timeline that includes project benchmarks. (Of course, use of consultants for open-ended operational activities would not require such a strict plan.)

At Heartland, the CIO seems not to have taken any of those steps when hiring his consultant. He instead hires a consultant who can make up for his own lack of experience: "This conversion was a much more complex undertaking than Jack's previous experience had prepared him for, but he felt that with Les's help, the project would move forward." In short, Jack creates a situation that discourages the consultant from transferring the knowledge needed to sustain the new system, because, from the consultant's perspective, doing so would bring an end to what has turned out to be an open-ended, lucrative project. In addition, the consultant's lack of credentials, compounded by his inability to connect with the VP for nursing and other leadership, leaves him open to criticism and takes a toll on staff morale. Clinical, accounting, and IT staff all feel left out of the decision making and therefore have no buy-in to the project or its success.

The "Code of Professional Ethical Conduct" of the American Medical Informatics Association (AMIA 2007) states:

> Disclose to colleagues any personal biases, prejudices, technical shortcomings, or other constraints that may hinder your ability to discharge your professional responsibilities.

Has Jack followed the AMIA's code and admitted his technical shortcomings? On the surface, his choice to use a consultant implies that he recognizes the gap in his abilities. However, instead of expanding his own abilities or those of his staff, he appears to use company resources to keep his shortcomings covered up.

By failing to define the roles of his consultant and his IT staff, the CIO also opens the door for dissension and frustration: He does not engage his staff in the knowledge-building process, and his actions create a wedge as opposed to a bridge. Although he is ethically bound to ensure that the goals and activities of his department are aligned with Heartland's mission and vision, Jack's pursuit of his personal goals creates an environment that is counterproductive and distracting for his team. The CIO has painted himself into a corner and feels forced to convert what should have been a defined consulting project for Les into a permanent job. By ensuring that Les reports directly to him, Jack ultimately removes the need to improve on his own skills.

Justice and Fairness

Richard and Jack certainly have focused goals: move forward with CPOE, create a legacy of supporting patient safety, and provide a state-of-the-art IT system for use by staff across the enterprise. Their vision is clear, and the resources they need seem readily available. But when they begin working toward achieving those goals, they are unwilling to listen to stakeholders, especially those with differing views, and thus fail to find common ground.

All people have biases, and if pressed, most will admit to them. Fair and just leaders know how to identify potentially damaging biases and keep them in check. They also know that openly disclosing affiliations and financial ties helps clear blind spots, reduces liability, and increases the trust of staff and colleagues.

Consider why people develop a bias toward a favorite source of input. Is it because that person helps them come to the best conclusion and grow in the process? Or because that person fills a gap that they have and helps them avoid detection? Which reason best explains the relationship that the Heartland CIO has with the IT consultant? How may the CIO's waiving of Heartland's hiring criteria for the hardware manager position be viewed by the IT staff, particularly those who may actually have qualifications for the position that the consultant lacks?

Managers may naturally gravitate toward one or two staff members when they are seeking advice. We all seek advice from people who have the skills and experience to help us. The way managers respond to input from people other than trusted advisers can raise ethical questions, however, especially when that input conflicts with the managers' point of view. To be fair, managers should listen to all opinions with an open mind. Clearly, Heartland's CIO has not done so. By failing to listen to those he viewed as critics and adversaries, he has failed to include information that may have helped him create the most serviceable IT system for all users.

Heartland's CIO and CEO have allowed their biases to influence whom they listen to. Would a strong focus on fair and equitable treatment have helped them avoid the compromising situation that they now find themselves in? Imagine if the CEO had listened without bias to nursing and accounting staff and put them in leadership roles on the project. Consider how working conditions might have changed in the IT department if the CIO had listened to his team as much as he listened to his consultant. In a fair and just organizational culture, the IT project would have turned out quite differently than the project at Heartland, where the CIO and CEO gave in to their biases.

Fairness does not imply consensus seeking or weakness; nor does it mean compromising on goals or outcomes. Ethical and just leaders do not choose sides—they maintain their vision of success for all. They bring dissenting voices together via shared goals. People often have differing opinions about "how." The true, ethical leader reminds them of "why."

Lessons Learned

The *Code of Ethics* of the American College of Healthcare Executives (ACHE 2011) states,

The fundamental objectives of the healthcare management profession are to maintain or enhance the overall quality of life, dignity and well-being of every individual needing healthcare service and to create a more equitable, accessible, effective and efficient healthcare system. Healthcare executives have an obligation to act in ways that will merit the trust, confidence, and respect of healthcare professionals and the general public.

It also enjoins us to "use this *Code* to further the interests of the profession and not for selfish reasons." These passages provide a good ethical framework for examining the case of Heartland Healthcare System.

In the Heartland case, the CEO and CIO are very shortsighted as they move forward with CPOE and system integration. Despite many setbacks, the CEO remains satisfied with the CIO's performance and seems unable to respond to feedback from others to the contrary. While he has "an obligation to act in ways that will merit the trust, confidence, and respect" (ACHE 2011) of his executive team, he does not listen to his VP for nursing and thus erodes her trust. Healthcare leaders must provide everyone a place to be heard, even when the motivation behind dissenting voices might be in question. In a highly engaged team, all ideas are not necessarily supported, but all voices are heard. Ensuring that level of engagement is the responsibility of every leader, especially the CEO.

At Heartland, the CIO becomes increasingly dependent on the consultant, and in doing so he allows the balance of power to shift away from his team and to an outsider. This dependence causes growing concern among others in the organization, concern that is compounded by the CIO's failure to consider their input. Leaders must communicate when their abilities are stretched. Asking for help is indeed a challenge. People all strive to appear competent, and many worry that by asking for assistance or admitting they do not have all the answers, they risk exposure—or worse, repercussions. Successful leaders understand their shortcomings and use help in targeted ways to get specific results. Less successful leaders sometimes use help as a cover, hoping that the helper will solve all the problems before they fully manifest themselves and derail a project.

Following are steps to take when help is needed:

1. **Learn to recognize an error.** First, assess if an error has been made. If so, immediately confer with an executive stakeholder who can assist with any course corrections. Ethical leaders monitor themselves, recognize errors, and model to staff how best to respond to mistakes.
2. **Be willing to seek specific help.** Identify personal strengths and weaknesses, and recognize when help is needed. Be specific about the help needed by clearly defining the tasks, roles, and outcomes sought. Be clear about what you know, what you need from others, and what you expect moving

forward. By defining the need and the expectations, you make the distinction between using help and being helpless.

3. **Engage others.** Connect with others early and often to gather relevant information and develop strong employee involvement. This can be the most valuable time you invest in a project because collaboration improves outcomes. By engaging others from the beginning, you may be able to prevent an error or avoid the need to ask for help later. If you recognize the need for a course correction, promptly acknowledge any error and then ask for help. Demonstrating humility and acknowledging what others can contribute will earn the trust needed to move forward.

4. **Request feedback.** Seek counsel from peers, stakeholders, and supervisors. Reach out to a mentor, ideally someone outside the organization, who has succeeded with similar projects. After making (and admitting to) an error, engage people of influence to ensure a turnaround and success.

5. **Remain open.** Keep firmly in mind that the concerns voiced by people you may perceive as resistant could have some validity. Get past your preconceptions and hear the true message. Do not alienate people whose support and guidance you may need in the future.

6. **Focus on the solution.** Once an error or misstep has been acknowledged, gather your team and begin working to correct it. Recognize that even individuals who have resisted your plans likely share your goal: to make the organization more successful. Focusing on the solution overcomes any unpleasantness caused by disagreement. Also, giving detractors a role in planning the solution ensures their buy-in, which will be critical not only for the success of the project but also for sustained operational success.

Healthcare IT is evolving at a rapid rate, and no one person can have expertise in every area. Acknowledge when additional expertise is needed and engage stakeholders to ensure adoption of proposals and their cost-effective implementation.

Perhaps the most significant ethical lapse by Heartland's CIO is to disregard his responsibility to identify when the project's demands exceeded his technical ability or to draw on appropriate resources and stakeholders to ensure the project's success. By not engaging key stakeholders or asking for feedback, and by attempting to do everything on his own (helped only by Les), Jack has alienated all of the team members he needs to successfully define and implement his project.

Ultimately, the ACHE *Code of Ethics* identifies healthcare leaders' responsibilities in five key areas (ACHE 2011):

1. The profession of healthcare management
2. Patients or others served

3. The organization
4. Employees
5. Community and society

When healthcare executives lose sight of their mission or lose their ethical grounding, they have a tendency to make poor decisions. Poor decisions will result in criticism, and if they fail to respond properly to justifiable criticism, they lose the trust of those they lead or serve. As Greer (2012) has observed, "in the absence of trust, we try for control," and the Heartland case illustrates that trust cannot be won back simply through the exercise of control.

Ideally, we all have an ingrained set of ethics—an internal compass that helps us differentiate between right and wrong. When we find ourselves confronted by an ethical dilemma at work, we can reach into our professional toolbox, which includes our mentors, our colleagues, and our professional code of ethics. Our code of ethics is the foundation of all our activities, decisions, and behaviors; by broadening our perspective, it enables us to see beyond our personal interests and pursue higher goals.

The leaders in this case had wonderful intentions. When their project became too difficult for them, however, they reacted by trying to hold onto control instead of admitting that they needed help. Had they behaved ethically when problems arose instead of becoming entrenched in a battle for control, the outcome probably would have been much different.

REFERENCES

ABC News. 2010. "Man Charged with Impersonating Doctor." Posted November 23. http://abclocal.go.com/wtvd/story?section=news/local&id=7805604.

American College of Healthcare Executives (ACHE). 2011. *Code of Ethics*. Updated November 14. www.ache.org/abt_ache/code.cfm#preamble.

American Medical Informatics Association (AMIA). 2007. "A Code of Professional Ethical Conduct for AMIA." White paper. *Journal of the American Medical Informatics Association* 14 (5): 686.

Collis, J. W. 1998. *The Seven Fatal Management Sins: Understanding and Avoiding Managerial Malpractice*. Boca Raton, FL: St. Lucie Press.

Glaser, J. 2009. "Implementing Electronic Health Records: 10 Factors for Success." *Healthcare Financial Management* 63 (1): 50–52, 54.

Greer, T. 2012. "Physician Hospital Integration in the 21st Century." Panel discussion held at the 5th Annual New Mexico Healthcare Managers Forum, Albuquerque, October 19.

Healthcare Information and Management Systems Society (HIMSS). 2013. "HIMSS Analytics Database." Accessed April 11. www.himssanalytics.org/data/HADB.aspx.

Janes, P. 2012. "Lincoln Man Sentenced for Impersonating Doctor, Prescribing Drugs." *ABC News 10.* Posted March 28. http://rocklinloomis.news10.net/news/crime/95823-lincoln-man-sentenced-impersonating-doctor-prescribing-drugs.

Joint Commission, The. 2012. "Standards and Elements of Performance (EPs) Applicable to the Proposed Long Term Care Core: Human Resources Chapter." Accessed April 11. www.jointcommission.org/assets/1/6/LTC_Core_HR.pdf.

Morrison, E. E. 2011. *Ethics in Health Administration: A Practical Approach for Decision Makers,* second edition. Sudbury, MA: Jones and Bartlett Publishers.

White, K. R., and J. R. Griffith. 2010. *The Well-Managed Healthcare Organization,* seventh edition. Chicago: Health Administration Press.

CHAPTER 10

Failed Hospital Merger: Richland River Valley Healthcare System

THE SCENIC RICHLAND RIVER meanders through historically prosperous Clay County. In the heart of this fertile valley lies the charming and picturesque city of Richland. The suburban area surrounding Richland, with its rolling hills and abundance of natural beauty, has attracted developers and now boasts elite resorts and retirement communities for the wealthy. The population of Clay County, including the city of Richland, is just under 500,000. *Case Study*

Clay County is proud of its healthcare services and touts them in its promotions to attract new industry to the area. The county has six hospitals, four in the city of Richland and two in the outlying suburban areas. Suburban Medical Center is a 150-bed general acute care hospital, and Community Behavioral Health Center is a 50-bed residential center with an innovative and highly regarded outpatient treatment center. In the city of Richland, the main healthcare providers are Trinity Medical Center and Sutton Memorial Hospital. The other two general acute care hospitals in the city of Richland, both with fewer than 200 beds, are not considered major players in the healthcare arena of Clay County. On the other hand, both Trinity and Sutton Memorial are the providers of choice for the vast majority of the population of Clay County.

While both of these organizations are well-respected providers of high-quality healthcare, they are very different in mission and structure. Trinity Medical Center is a faith-based organization that is part of a larger, regional religious system. Its mission is to care for those in need regardless of their ability to pay, and as a result, Trinity provides the vast majority of indigent care in Clay County. Its programs have been developed in response to the needs of the younger population it tends to serve. Enormous resources have been committed to its high-risk obstetrics program, neonatal intensive care unit, and pediatrics program with its attendant pediatrics intensive care unit. Trinity is also the designated Level I trauma center for the county and has committed considerable resources to its critical care programs, which include a surgical and medical intensive care unit and renal dialysis and burn units. In addition to its general medical/surgical units, it operates oncology, cardiology, and orthopedics programs, all supported by active outpatient clinics and rehabilitation programs. The professional personnel at Trinity, especially the nurses, are exceptionally loyal to the hospital and are highly skilled, competent, and compassionate. They are also unionized, but Trinity has implemented strong, effective management–employee programs, and the unions are committed to the continued success of the Trinity organization.

The J. Blair Sutton Memorial Hospital is a privately owned, richly endowed healthcare organization whose namesake was the founder of Sutton Manufacturing and Construction Inc., a company that brought great wealth to its founder and employment to many of the residents of Richland. The Sutton family is "old money" and originally acquired their wealth from sawmills along the Richland River. J. Blair Sutton was quick to respond to modern technologies, and when the time was right, he diversified his holdings and entered commercial construction and the manufacturing of doors, windows, and lumber products. That was in the 1940s, and now the Sutton name and its products are known nationwide. To manage the family money, the Sutton progeny moved from Richland to New York City, but the Sutton name still graces the streets of Richland on schools, avenues, plazas, and prominent buildings throughout the community.

J. Blair Sutton Memorial Hospital is one such legacy. The 275-bed acute care hospital is renowned throughout the state for its cardiology services, including a respected and successful open heart surgery program, an orthopedic surgery program specializing in hip replacements, and a cancer care program that has attracted nationally recognized oncologists and cancer surgeons. In addition to those "pillars of excellence," Sutton Memorial offers general medical/surgical, obstetrics, and pediatrics services, but these programs command fewer resources because the hospital's mission is to serve the healthcare needs of the "older families" of Clay County. The governing board of Sutton Memorial has no problem supporting this mission. After all, Trinity very capably and compassionately cares for the indigent in Clay County. Sutton Memorial's mission is to provide healthcare to those who continue to commit their personal wealth to enrich the Richland community. This philosophy is in keeping with J. Blair Sutton's personal philosophy, deeply rooted in American capitalism and the right of the individual to reap the rewards and privileges of his hard work. His philosophy did not abide government intervention of any manner, and accordingly, the Sutton Memorial board did all that it could for as long as it could to legally avoid caring for Medicare and Medicaid patients. The hospital operated on a cash basis until the recent past. This system was very appealing to the members of the Sutton Memorial board, the majority of whom are corporate executives with companies of international stature who were recruited to the board by the influential Sutton family.

In contrast, the Trinity governing board comprises representatives of the community, the religious order, and local bank and corporate executives. These two governing boards, very different in philosophy, have little reason to interact. They do not travel in the same social circles, and the Sutton Memorial board members are most often out of town running their corporations in other states. The Sutton Memorial board meets quarterly, while the Trinity board, with its local members, meets monthly. The administrations of the two organizations seemed content with maintaining the status quo. After all, both organizations were operating well. Strong governing boards at both hospitals made it clear to their respective CEOs that their jobs were to manage operations. In spite of their differences, the two organizations amicably coexisted in the city of Richland, each successful in its own right.

All of this was about to change as national for-profit hospital corporations were emerging as a force in healthcare. Indeed, one of these corporations, Continental Healthcare, began purchasing private, not-for-profit hospitals in Clay County. Continental had already purchased one of the smaller hospitals in the city of Richland and had also entered into negotiations with Suburban Medical Center. Both Trinity and Sutton Memorial were alarmed and fearful of losing their positions of prominence in Clay County. After much separate discussion, the governing board at each hospital arrived at the same conclusion: The hospital needed to partner with another organization to shore up its position in the community. As each organization sought an appropriate partner, it became clear that all they had was each other.

The governing boards of the two organizations took the lead in exploring the merger of Trinity and Sutton Memorial. The administrations of the two organizations were only minimally involved and, for the most part, remained focused on daily operations. Each governing board engaged the services of a consultant to explore the feasibility of the merger. Following the consultants' reports, both Trinity and Sutton Memorial decided a merger into a system was in the best interests of their respective organization. At this point the two governing boards met for their first face-to-face discussion, during which they decided to jointly engage the services of a nationally known consulting firm with experience in successfully implementing the mergers of healthcare organizations. The consulting firm's report clearly laid out enormous benefits, both present and future, that would accrue to both organizations once the merger was fully implemented. This report evolved into the only strategic plan used by the newly merged system and showed savings of millions of dollars from merging business operations and sharing expensive medical technology. The report also promised that the merger would increase bargaining power with health plans.

An initial step in the process was to determine the asset value of each organization. Trinity's assets were valued at $25 million more than those of Sutton Memo-
rial. For the two organizations to enter into the merger as equal partners, Trinity
placed $25 million into a newly created foundation for the merged system, named
Richland River Valley Healthcare System (RRVHS), to use for healthcare programs
in Clay County. Although it agreed to this resolution, the Sutton Memorial board
was visibly annoyed with the results of the asset valuation. Its members were unac-
customed to being second best at anything.

As the implementation of the merger moved forward, both sides agreed that
the RRVHS governing board would have 25 members: 12 from Trinity, 12 from Sutton Memorial, and the new RRVHS CEO. The RRVHS board would be responsible
for strategic planning and financial oversight of the system. Sutton Memorial would
appoint the board chair for a two-year term. Trinity would then appoint the succeed-
ing board chair for a two-year term, and so on. As it turned out, the most powerful,
influential members of each hospital board were appointed to the system board,
and the hospital boards retained the less powerful members. The hospital governing boards would now be responsible for operations, credentialing, and facilities
management at their respective organizations. The powerful RRVHS board decided
that the hospital governing boards would no longer receive operating budgets or
routine financial reports. The RRVHS board would provide financial oversight of
both hospitals and would control the flow of financial information. Friction soon
developed between the system board and the hospital boards, whose members
became so frustrated at one point that the two hospital boards considered joint
legal action against the system board.

The RRVHS board further decided that neither of the current hospital CEOs
was capable of assuming the position of system CEO and hired an executive search
firm to recruit an experienced system CEO. The RRVHS board, with powerful representatives from both hospitals, could not agree on an acceptable candidate to lead
the newly merged entity. This dissension resulted in a lengthy and combative CEO
search that left the new entity adrift with no management leadership for over a year.

Curtis Tower was finally hired as system CEO. During the recruitment process,
Tower made it clear that the board needed to leave the management of the new
system to him, and the search committee agreed to this condition. Soon after Tower
assumed leadership responsibilities, however, he realized the board was either unwilling or unable to stay out of the management of the new system. The RRVHS board
directed Tower to fire all of the senior administrators at both hospitals and conduct
a national search to replace them. By following this directive, Tower lost vital corporate memory at a time when it may have been needed most. The corporate cultures
of both organizations were visibly shaken by this massive administrative turnover.

Organizational values were questioned by the staffs of both hospitals, who became increasingly anxious in this uncertain environment.

Amid all of this uncertainty, physicians in Clay County became a major influential force. Throughout the merger process, the hospitals' two medical staffs had been relegated to the sidelines. But a new opportunity presented itself in Richland: Physicians Partners, Inc., a proprietary corporation that purchases and operates physician practices, began buying physician practices in Richland. Now the RRVHS board and the two hospital boards had a common worry: What if their admitting physicians decided to admit elsewhere? A group of ten physicians who controlled most of the admissions, referrals, and outpatient ancillary services at both Trinity and Sutton Memorial began approaching board members at social gatherings with an idea. These physicians had lost their ability to leverage one hospital against the other with the creation of RRVHS. Now with Physician Partners, Inc., rolling into town, the physicians had bargaining power once more. They suggested that RRVHS purchase their practices and asserted that through their personal connections to a renowned East Coast medical school, they could arrange for the establishment of an affiliated major medical clinic in Richland that would attract national and international patients. Such a clinic would secure the success of the new merger.

RRVHS entered into what proved to be a very lucrative arrangement for the physicians involved, and news of the agreement and the planned medical school–affiliated clinic disseminated rapidly throughout the medical community. Questions about who would control the clinic and, more important, who would be allowed to practice there were put to the RRVHS board. Dissension among the medical staff was palpable. Those physicians who continued to practice independently gave the RRVHS board an ultimatum: If plans for the clinic went forward, they would boycott both hospitals. The RRVHS board rejected the proposed affiliated clinic. The contract physicians became angry and resentful. The independent physicians remained distrustful and hostile. Throughout these discussions, negotiations, and agreements, the administrations of both hospitals had been absent.

Two years into the merger, RRVHS has yet to consolidate clinical services as recommended by the consultant's plan guiding implementation. The hospitals, four miles apart, are still duplicating all but business operations.

Equally troubling is the lack of medical staff consolidation. The differences in medical staff organization and structure at the two hospitals have proven to be significant barriers. Medical staff officers at Trinity are elected by the general medical staff, while medical staff officers at Sutton Memorial are appointed by the Sutton Memorial board. After much political maneuvering, it is agreed that consolidated medical staff officers will be elected, but the decision is just one more contentious issue between the two hospitals.

Case Study The administrative offices for the system are constructed in available space at Sutton Memorial, which further increases ill will between the hospitals. The members of the two hospital governing boards do not like each other, and more significant, their counterparts on the RRVHS board do not like each other either. The governing styles of the two hospitals are in conflict. Sutton Memorial operates with a corporate approach to healthcare delivery: be innovative, operate efficiently, practice good business management. Social status is important to its members. Trinity operates more like a public institution: process oriented and committed to care for all regardless of their ability to pay. Business operations are not its top priority, and neither is the social status of its members.

The major barriers to the successful merger of the two organizations are the steadfast separation of all clinical services and disagreement over the allocation of capital resources for new programs and services. New clinical services to be based at one hospital or the other can never get past the planning stage. Administrative resources are spent, but no program materializes in return.

Frustrated and angry with the system, a high-profile group of surgeons has begun plans for a physician-owned surgicenter. At about this same time, amid falling patient volumes and problems with accounts receivable at both hospitals, a major donor has withdrawn his $72 million pledge to the cardiology program at Sutton Memorial on the grounds that his pledge was to Sutton and not to RRVHS.

Unable to consolidate clinical services and demoralized by the constant conflict and financial woes, the RRVHS board finally agrees on something: to dissolve the merger. Within the first year following the dissolution of RRVHS, Continental Healthcare moves quickly to purchase both hospitals, which it then operates as separate healthcare facilities.

Case originally published in a slightly different format in Mistakes in Healthcare Management: Identification, Correction and Prevention, *edited by Paul B. Hofmann and Frankie Perry. Copyright © 2005 Cambridge University Press. Reprinted with permission.*

ETHICS ISSUES

Roles of governance and management: Were the roles of governance and management being played out during the merger of Trinity and Sutton Memorial into RRVHS appropriate and consistent with the mission of the two hospitals? Were the actions of the principals involved in the best interests of patients and others served?

Fear-based action: Was the decision to pursue a merger based on a well-thought-out plan for the betterment of healthcare in this community? Or was it fear based and motivated by a desire to retain power and prestige?

Culture issues: Did the two hospital boards give appropriate consideration to the culture, values, and ethical standards guiding their respective organizations and how they might mesh in the newly merged system?

Failure to include medical staff: Was a successful merger possible without involving the physicians in its planning and implementation? Was clinical integration possible without physician leadership?

Stewardship of community resources: Do the two organizations have an ethical responsibility to use community resources prudently for the good of the community?

Ethical responsibilities to employees: Do the administrators and governing boards of the two hospitals, and later those of the merged system, have an ethical responsibility to adequately inform employees about, and involve them in, decisions that are being made that affect their employment, their healthcare, and their community? Are employees key stakeholders in these proceedings?

DISCUSSION

Roles of Governance and Management

The RRVHS case is like a very bad play where the actors don't know their lines or the roles they should be playing. The governing boards of the two institutions began exploring the possibility of a merger on their own instead of initiating joint discussions that included management and medical staff. A more inclusive approach may have identified potential obstacles to overcome. Neglecting to include management and the medical staff in all discussions and planning doomed the merger to failure. Following the merger agreement, the RRVHS governing board blurred their lines of authority and responsibility even more as they began micromanaging the system and withholding needed financial information from the governing boards of the two hospitals.

The three standards of board responsibility as outlined by the Association of Governing Boards (2013) are detailed in Chapter 4. The American Hospital Association (AHA 2013) is clear about board responsibilities in its governance policy statement "On Distinguishing Policy from Operations," whose stated purpose is "to clarify the difference between the board's policy-making responsibilities and management's operational responsibilities." The policy statement reads in part as follows:

1. Policy may be generally defined as a recommended course of action, a guiding principle, or a procedure that is established to guide current and future decision making.

2. From time to time, the board will adopt and articulate policies that are designed to guide the work and decisions of management, employees, the medical staff, and the board itself.
3. The board will generally limit its policy making to broad, high level matters. The board will delegate to management and the medical staff the operational implementation of its policies, and it will hold them accountable for performance.

In simpler terms, the governing board's responsibility is to see the "why," whereas the "what" and "how" are management's job.

At RRVHS, administrative leadership should have played a major role in seeing that governing board members clearly understood their functions and responsibilities and had continuing education opportunities to keep abreast of changes in the field. Administrators also should have been active in the selection and engagement of the consultants to make certain that all obstacles, disadvantages, and barriers to the merger were explored along with the advantages and benefits. And finally, strong hospital leadership would have insisted on being an integral part, along with the medical staff, of all merger discussions and negotiations.

Had administrators from both hospitals been included in the merger discussions from the beginning, they could have ensured that the missions and values of their respective organizations were not compromised. Moreover, the participation of administrative and clinical representatives would have led to a broader and more balanced perspective on the situation. Board members sometimes have difficulty setting aside their self-interests and staying focused on what is good for the organization and for the community (Greene 2012). For example, because some board members may lose their places at the table when a merger occurs, decisions made solely by the board may be skewed by individuals' attempts to secure their positions.

Fear-Based Action

Although fear may be a great motivator, it rarely brings the success of a well-thought-out strategy and transitional plan based on community needs and mutually beneficial collaboration. The two organizations going into this merger had operated in isolation from each other for years. Neither knew anything about the other. The merger was like a marriage without a courtship. The consultants, if experienced in mergers, should have forewarned the organizations of the potential perils. Effective management, if involved, may have foreseen the difficulties. The governing boards, on the other hand, seemed too concerned about their own self-interests and power to recognize the problem.

Culture Issues

Healthcare managers know a lot about corporate culture. They know that the leadership of an organization is responsible for establishing the organization's culture. They know that a culture will accept or reject change, can create a negative or positive work environment, can promote teamwork or not, and can be ethical or not. A simple definition of culture is "the way we do things around here" (Scanlan 2010). Perhaps culture is much more than that. Certainly, culture consists of behaviors and how business is conducted, but it also encompasses values and beliefs and reflects how members of governance, workforce, and management in an organization think and feel. Culture is a guiding philosophy about what is right and what is important. Organizations considering a merger tend to function best when their guiding philosophies are aligned.

Scanlan (2010) maintains that "culture will eat strategy" and that "unresolved culture conflicts can cripple or terminate a merger." Accordingly, Scanlan cautions leaders to have a solid understanding of their own organizational culture and to know when cultural differences between organizations make a successful merger unlikely.

Sutton Memorial and Trinity had very different cultures and value systems. Their differences seem not to have been given the consideration they deserved, especially at the board level. Power is a difficult thing to share, especially when values clash. Symbolism can become a source of friction if one of the hospitals in the merger is perceived to have such symbolic advantages as being the source of the new CEO, having more representatives on the board, being where the system offices are located, or controlling how publicity about the new system is crafted.

Although Beckham (2012) agrees that culture is an important consideration when it comes to leadership and that "there may be occasions when culture is well-positioned to eat strategy," he cautions that "a view of culture as fixed, omnipotent and sacred engenders passivity on the part of leaders." He challenges leaders to execute strategies that may overpower or change culture.

Regardless of their views on the primacy of culture, effective leaders are mindful of their organization's culture and the need to nurture it in ways that promote teamwork, collaboration, and organization-wide commitment to mission. Lack of respect for the influence of culture may result in careless and wasteful use of resources and failure to fulfill ethical responsibilities to communities served.

Failure to Include Medical Staff

The exclusion of key physicians and medical staff leaders from discussions about the feasibility of a merger can only be described as ill informed and misguided.

Certainly, if the administrators of the two hospitals had been active participants in the discussions, they would have enlightened the boards about the need for physicians' insights, awareness of internal politics, and knowledge of the medical community, all of which are crucial to any clinical integration. Governing boards and administrators must never lose sight of the fact that healthcare is driven by physicians and that the success of a healthcare organization depends in large part on the quality and expertise of its clinical staff. A successful merger is impossible without "a strong and definitive plan for working with your medical staff" (Morrissey 2012).

Stewardship of Community Resources

The failed RRVHS merger is an example of what typically happens when personal ambitions and goals take priority over an organization's mission and the stewardship of community resources. Brown (2005, 206) argues that all hospitals "share a common bond—a covenant . . . to serve as stewards of valued community assets—local hospitals." The hospital board's fiduciary responsibility is to protect its organization's assets and to act in good faith on behalf of the organization, not for personal benefit. The governing board members at RRVHS were not attentive to their stewardship of community resources or protection of the organization's assets. Struggles for power and control over an extended period of time wasted resources and raised the additional ethical question of what happens to patient care programs when time, energy, and capital are diverted elsewhere. The failure to eliminate duplication of services squandered the assets of both the health system and the community.

Ethical Responsibilities to Employees

The *Code of Ethics* of the American College of Healthcare Executives (ACHE 2011) is clear about a healthcare executive's ethical and professional responsibilities to employees. Maintaining a safe work environment that is conducive to ethical conduct, proper utilization of employees' skills and abilities, and freedom from harassment and discrimination are critical to providing quality, safe patient care. Poor communication with employees creates an environment of uncertainty, dissension, and mistrust. When management does not communicate appropriately, pseudo-leaders do—often with rumor, innuendo, and false information. The anxiety and pessimism that result are inevitably reflected in exchanges with patients and coworkers.

Failure to recognize that employees are key stakeholders in the future of the merged organization ignores that the people who carry out the mission of patient care, whether directly or indirectly, are important contributors to the success of the organization. It also does not take into account that employees rely on the security of their employment and may be unable to relocate if they lose their jobs. Whereas administrators and board members may move on to other positions in other communities, employees are frequently locked into the community where they are employed for a variety of reasons.

Further contributing to the uncertain work environment is what appears to be the arbitrary firing of senior managers with the accompanying loss of corporate history, experience, and knowledge. Such upheaval fosters feelings that the organization lacks direction and that leadership cannot be trusted. Were the fired managers treated fairly and ethically?

Many of these problems could have been avoided by implementing a well-thought-out employee communication strategy and plan aimed at acquiring employee input into the process and buy-in to the merger.

Lessons Learned

Although RRVHS is an example of a failed hospital merger, the lessons learned from this case are valuable to healthcare executives and governing boards who may, in the future, need to consider merging their healthcare organization with another. A clear rationale, a comprehensive feasibility study, and a well-thought-out implementation plan are essential to success.

Even after a merger is finalized, important work still needs to be done if the merger is to achieve the anticipated benefits. Peregrine and Nygren (2013) suggest eight follow-up steps that will ensure that the goals of the merger are realized:

1. Appoint a new leader who is qualified to achieve the vision.
2. Restructure departments and services to gain efficiency and avoid redundancy.
3. Name the new organization; roll out the image and branding initiative to create a shared identity.
4. Articulate the values and behaviors that will characterize the culture.
5. Make it clear to all that change must occur.
6. Focus on the strategic plan.
7. Honor post-closing agreements.
8. Communicate often.

A leadership team representative of governance, administration, and the medical staff will be needed to successfully complete the merger implementation.

A new study commissioned by the AHA to analyze the impact of hospital mergers found that the number of mergers has been relatively small—only 316 mergers in six years (Stempniak 2013). However, as the Patient Protection and Affordable Care Act is implemented and the healthcare industry moves to more efficient systems that coordinate care and emphasize cost savings and population health, we can safely speculate that more mergers will be considered.

REFERENCES

American College of Healthcare Executives (ACHE). 2011. *Code of Ethics.* Updated November 14. www.ache.org/abt_ache/code.cfm#patients.

American Hospital Association (AHA). 2013. "On Distinguishing Policy from Operations." Governance policy statement. Accessed June 8. www.greatboards.org/pubs/Policy_on_Policy_vs_Operations.pdf.

Association of Governing Boards. 2013. "Three Standards of Board Responsibility." Accessed June 8. http://agb.org/knowledge-center/briefs/fiduciary-duties.

Beckham, D. 2012. "Overestimating the Importance of Culture." *Hospitals & Health Networks Daily* August 16. www.hhnmag.com/hhnmag/HHNDaily/HHNDaily Display.dhtml?id=9120001624.

Brown, F. 2005. "Failed Hospital Merger: Richland River Valley Healthcare System Commentary." In *Management Mistakes in Healthcare: Identification, Correction and Prevention,* edited by P. B. Hofmann and F. Perry, 201–14. New York: Cambridge University Press.

Greene, J. 2012. "A New Voice at the Table." *Trustee* 65 (3): 8–12.

Morrissey, J. 2012. "Life After a Merger." *Trustee* 65 (10): 8–12.

Peregrine, M. W., and D. Nygren. 2013. "Merger's Closed. What's Next?" *Trustee* April.

Scanlan, L. 2010. "Hospital Mergers: Pay Attention to Those Culture Issues." *Hospitals & Health Networks Daily* August 16. www.hhnmag.com/hhnmag/jsp/articledisplay .jsp?dcrpath=HHNMAG/Article/data/08AUG2010/081610HHN_Weekly_Scanlan &domain=HHNMAG.

Stempniak, M. 2013. "New Study Analyzes Impact of Hospital Mergers." *Hospitals & Health Networks Daily* June 3.

CHAPTER 11

When Patient Demands and Hospital Policies Collide: Hurley Medical Center

AN INNER-CITY HOSPITAL in a depressed area of the Midwest made the front *Case* page of the local newspaper with the headline "Nurse's Lawsuit Draws Protestors." *Study* According to the article, a nurse claimed that the hospital granted a father's request that no African-American nurses treat his baby, who was a patient in the hospital's neonatal intensive care unit (NICU). The nurse, who was African American, claimed that while she was working in the NICU, the child's father asked to speak to her supervisor and allegedly rolled up his sleeve to reveal a tattoo believed to be a swastika. A different nurse was assigned to the baby, and a note was posted on the assignment clipboard: "No African-American nurse to take care of baby."

The lawsuit alleges that on the following day, the hospital made a decision to grant the father's request. The hospital's CEO publicly denied that the request was granted. Protestors rallied outside the hospital, claiming discrimination, and the president of the National Action Network said the hospital's actions were "an atrocity and a reversal of times" as well as "a manifestation of institutional racism." He went on to say that "the National Action Network will be calling for . . . all federal, state, and local dollars allocated to Hurley . . . [to] have a major-league string attached that the staff and administrators go through sensitivity training so that those policies will not ever occur again." He went on to call the hospital's actions a "powder keg that could set off the city" and to say that it was "unreasonable to believe that the supervisor . . . still would be employed" by the hospital.

Two weeks after the lawsuit was filed, the newspaper reported that the case had been settled. While the details of the settlement were not made public, the hospital's CEO said, "We regret that our policies were not well enough understood and followed, causing the perception that Hurley condoned this conduct." She indicated that the incident would be used in future training sessions to prevent it from happening again.

The political director of the National Action Network was quoted as saying, "We won't go away like a plaintiff in a lawsuit. We're here until the institutional practices of Hurley stop and they behave in a manner that's in the best interest of the community." The president of the state chapter of the National Action Network said about the hospital's leadership, "We would like to see that they make sure their staff is culturally competent. . . . It needs to be very clear in their procedures and policies that this type of behavior warrants a reprimand."

Sources: Adapted from Adams (2013a, 2013b); Aldridge (2013); and Ridley (2013).

ETHICS ISSUES

Patients' rights: Does a patient's bill of rights give patients—or, in the case of minors, parents and guardians—the right to select their caregivers in a healthcare facility?

Patient safety: What actions can Hurley Medical Center take to ensure the safety and security of patients and parents in the NICU?

Ethical responsibilities to employees: What actions can be taken to ensure employee safety? What considerations must be given to avoid the development of a hostile work environment? Is discrimination a legitimate concern?

Adherence to hospital policies: Are hospital policies being followed? Are those policies well known to the employees?

Organizational implications: What are the organizational implications of the hospital's actions? How will they affect staff morale and perceptions of management? Public relations and community image? Medical staff referrals? Staff productivity?

Cultural competency: What is management's responsibility to promote cultural competency through education with respect to both the patient population and the workforce?

Community values: Does hospital administration have a responsibility to be aware of community values and how they may affect the organization and influence the outcome of management actions?

Legal implications: Is the hospital legally liable for discriminatory behavior by its employees? What about for a hostile work environment?

DISCUSSION

An Open Secret

Chapter 1 notes that mistakes are often the result of the barrage of decisions that must be made by well-meaning managers who are pressed for time and strained by the demands of the job. Decisions are often made without the benefit of thoughtful reflection and the consultation of others that may be needed. Sufficient time may not be given to the unintended consequences that may occur. The situation at Hurley may have been such a case.

Fault finding is easy for people who are not confronted with the stressful clinical demands of an intensive care unit and the human emotions inherent in life-threatening situations. To malign an entire institution and its policies and procedures without knowing all of the facts can be a mistake. The only information available to the public in this case is in news reports about the initial incident and the comments and reactions that it elicited. Consequently, the discussion in this chapter is based on some assumptions and explores the issues that arise under those assumptions.

Chapter 2 discusses the interrelation of ethics and management and how the two cannot be separated when decisions are being made. The Hurley case involves an intersection of ethics, patient rights, and the law. A discussion of the resulting management challenges must take all three areas into consideration. Above all, this case presents a learning opportunity for all healthcare leaders because no organization is exempt from charges of discrimination based on race, age, sexual orientation, or other factors.

The incidence of requests for racially preferred caregivers in healthcare is much higher than commonly known. Paul-Emile (2012) calls it an "open secret," saying, "Patients routinely refuse or demand medical treatment based on the assigned physician's racial identity, and hospitals typically yield to patients' racial preferences. This widely practiced, if rarely acknowledged, phenomenon . . . poses a fundamental dilemma for law, medicine, and ethics." Paul-Emile concludes that although accommodating a patient's racial preferences appears to violate antidiscrimination laws, a conflict remains between "patient autonomy and accepted notions of racial equality." Others have called the accommodation of requests based on racial preferences a form of institutional racism (Aldridge 2013).

The *Code of Medical Ethics* of the American Medical Association (AMA 2008) prohibits physicians from refusing to treat patients on the basis of race, but no policy exists for handling race-based requests from patients. A recent University of Michigan study found that "a third of providers felt patients perceive better care from providers of shared demographics, with racial matching perceived as more important than gender or religion" (Padela et al. 2010). Some believe that requests for racial preferences are quietly honored and do not come to the attention of the public (Karoub 2013a).

In the barrage of published opinions that followed the Hurley incident, almost all of the legal and medical experts who weighed in agreed that honoring racial preferences violates antidiscrimination laws and is morally wrong. One opinion stood out as more pragmatic than theoretical. Susan Goold, MD, a University of Michigan professor of internal medicine and public health, said, "In general, I don't think honoring prejudicial preferences . . . is morally justifiable . . . [but] there may be times when grudgingly acceding to a patient's strongly held preferences is morally OK" (Karoub 2013a). She indicated that in some cases, such as those involving rape or violence, honoring patients' racial preferences might be preferable to forcing caregivers on them who might exacerbate their health condition.

Clearly, this multidimensional problem has no simple answers. Managers must struggle with the legal and moral challenges of situations like that at Hurley while exercising caution not to compromise patient and employee safety and the integrity of the healthcare organization.

Patients' Rights

In 1973, the American Hospital Association (AHA) published "A Patient's Bill of Rights," which delineated a patient's rights and responsibilities when cared for by a healthcare organization, and it amended this document in 1992 (Patient Talk 2013). The Joint Commission subsequently defined an accreditation standard requiring healthcare organizations to present patients with a copy of their rights. Hospitals throughout the nation soon adopted and distributed the AHA's bill of rights, and many developed their own and posted them on their websites. Several states enacted legislation requiring a patient's bill of rights as well. The attorney general's office in Michigan, where Hurley Medical Center is located, has posted the "Michigan Patient Rights and Responsibilities in State Licensed Facilities" on its website (State of Michigan Attorney General 2013), and Hurley has one posted on its website as well (Hurley Medical Center 2013).

The AHA, state of Michigan, and Hurley documents do not grant patients, guardians, or family members the right to choose or reject an organization's assigned caregiver. The patient responsibilities listed on Hurley's website, however, do specify that patients must follow hospital rules and regulations and respect the rights of other patients and staff members. None of the many documents defining patient rights entitles patients or family members to dictate which healthcare staff are assigned to their care. In the opinion of Larry Dubin, a Michigan law professor, "The patient's father has the right to select the hospital to treat the child. The father does not have the right to exercise control over the hospital in discrimination of its employees" (Erb 2013).

Patient Safety

The primary concern of hospital staff must be the safety and well-being of the patients in their charge. Nurses are especially aware of their responsibility in this regard. In the Hurley case, the safety of the newborn in question and the safety of the other patients and parents in the NICU must be the top priority. Indeed, the hospital's CEO reported that the father's swastika tattoo "created anger and outrage in our staff" and that supervisors raised safety concerns (Karoub 2013b). Given those concerns, Hurley staff might have moved the conversation with the father to a quiet place outside the NICU, with a second staff member in attendance. Having a witness to the conversation could be helpful in the future, and a smaller audience might have tempered the father's demands.

The second person serving as witness could have been the administrator on call, the nursing supervisor, or the patient advocate, depending on the shift and time of day. That person could have informed the father that it is against both hospital policy and the law for the hospital to discriminate against its employees. The person conducting the meeting also could have emphasized the specialized expertise and training of the NICU staff and explained that the safety of his newborn would be ensured by having all NICU staff available to handle any problem that may have arisen.

If the father persisted in his request, the next step might be to refer him to his child's doctor or suggest that he consider transferring his infant to another hospital—under Hurley's patient's bill of rights, a patient, parent, or guardian has the right to choose a healthcare facility. The feasibility of a transfer would depend, however, on the condition of the newborn and the availability of an NICU at another location. If the charge nurse believed that the father's tone and demeanor suggested that the conversation could become heated, security could be alerted. However, caution must be exercised to avoid any action that may escalate hostility.

Ethical Responsibilities to Employees

Hospital management has ethical and legal responsibilities to ensure a safe working environment for all employees. In this case, the moral and legal demands may conflict. Lance Gable, a law professor at Wayne State University, observed, "Maybe [the hospital's] explanation is an accurate description of what happened— the supervisor was scared of the father of this patient and made a decision that was ill advised. It might have been the right thing to do for the safety of the staff, and it still might be a violation of antidiscrimination laws" (Karoub 2013a). Indeed, the laws regarding workplace discrimination are clear. The safety of the nurse in this incident must be protected. Multiple phone and e-mail messages left for her were not returned, so their content remains undetermined. She also had her listed phone number disconnected as a matter of caution (Karoub 2013a).

Management cannot ensure that caregivers will not encounter potentially volatile situations from time to time. Unfortunately, bigotry and prejudice cannot be eliminated. Management can and should, therefore, prepare employees with conflict management skills. Such training may be especially important for frontline caregivers and their supervisors, who regularly face emotionally charged situations. Management has a responsibility to equip staff to assess circumstances and know when to get help in defusing potentially volatile encounters.

Healthcare leaders must both abide by the law and ensure the safety of employees. They must take steps to create a nonhostile work environment that is secure and free from discrimination. As the Hurley case illustrates, this task can be difficult indeed. The ability to anticipate situations in which patient and family demands may conflict with hospital policies and the foresight to prepare staff to deal with them effectively are the marks of a superior manager.

Adherence to Hospital Policies

Hospitals must not only abide by government antidiscrimination laws but also establish internal antidiscrimination policies that apply to patients, clients, and employees. At Hurley, the decision to accede to the father's demands would appear to violate internal hospital policies, and, in fact, hospital officials admitted that it did (Karoub 2013a).

Educating employees about hospital policies is a daunting task. The orientation of new managers undoubtedly includes discussion of the organization's policy manuals, standard practices, mission, vision, and values. Disseminating that information throughout the employee ranks is difficult, however, and requires effective communication strategies, attention, and repetition. Case-based staff education and training can be especially useful in driving home the rationale and importance of hospital policies and chain-of-command reporting mechanisms. Employees need to know when and how to seek advice and help in the clarification and enforcement of policies. Just knowing a policy and being able to state it to a patient or a family member is not enough. Unless patients and families understand why a policy exists and how it benefits them, they will view it as just a bureaucratic barrier to something they want. The importance of having well-informed, skillful staff to explain policy cannot be overlooked.

Organizational Implications

Some unintended consequences of staff actions in this incident were immediate; others may be more long-term. The gathering of protestors outside the hospital, international media response, lawsuits, staff confusion, mistrust of management, and fear of unsafe working conditions all occurred immediately and required enormous amounts of legal, public relations, administrative, and staff time, energy, and dollars. The long-term effect of diverting those resources from patient care and other more beneficial activities cannot yet be determined. The effect of the incident and its aftermath on the hospital's image and the community's trust cannot be measured as yet. For example, will it affect physician referrals or patient admissions? Perhaps the most critical and immediate responsibility facing Hurley's administration is to repair and strengthen employee–management relationships, trust, and commitment to the regeneration of the hospital's image.

Cultural Competency

As the US population continues to become more culturally diverse, much attention has been devoted to the need for organizations to train their employees in cultural competency. Accrediting and licensing agencies, marketing experts, business consultants, and lawyers tout the organizational benefits of having a culturally competent workforce. In healthcare, the evidence suggests that patients' health status improves when they are cared for by culturally competent caregivers. Healthcare costs and liability may decrease as well (Schulte 2010).

Leaders must be culturally competent in the management of their employees and provide employee education programs that foster respect for individual differences and awareness of actions that may be deemed discriminatory or illegal on the basis of race, gender, age, disability, national origin, or religion. For their part, employees need to be aware of actions that may be offensive to coworkers. For example, posting the note on the assignment board saying that no African-American nurses were to care for the newborn at Hurley most likely humiliated the assigned nurse and other staff in the NICU. Cultivating staff sensitivity to the effect of such actions on coworkers' feelings can eliminate those behaviors and foster a more positive and productive work environment.

Better understanding and appreciation of individual differences can strengthen employee loyalty and commitment to organizational goals and success. Employees will feel more vested in the organization and more confident in their ability to handle potentially difficult situations.

Community Values

Experienced managers have learned that prevailing community values have a significant effect on an organization's public image and how its actions are judged. Those values may be heavily influenced by religion, socioeconomic status, politics, and the like. In a working-class community—especially one that is heavily unionized like Flint, Michigan, where Hurley is located—people will sympathize with workers and support their legal rights. Hospital administrators must therefore consider carefully the consequences of their actions and how they will play out in the community. When governing boards are representative of the local demographics, members will be quick to criticize actions that do not reflect community values.

Legal Implications

Several court decisions have addressed issues of discrimination similar to those at Hurley. A 2010 decision by the US Court of Appeals for the Seventh Circuit, for example, held that the federal Civil Rights Act prohibits nursing homes from making staffing decisions based on residents' racial preferences (Karoub 2013a). In that case, nursing assistants claimed that complying with residents' racial preferences created a hostile work environment for them. The court agreed, saying that the nursing home could have warned residents on admission that "discriminatory requests and/or harassment of employees would not be tolerated, informing employees of their right to complain about such conduct, and . . . discharging a racially hostile patient" (Starr and Murphy 2011). In this ruling, the court also found that hiring based on gender preference was permissible under Title VII.

In 2005, a federal lawsuit was filed in Pennsylvania by three African-American employees of Abington Memorial Hospital who claimed that they were prevented from treating a pregnant white woman by her male partner, a member of a white supremacist group, who used a racial slur while refusing to let African-American caregivers treat his pregnant partner. The hospital honored the man's request, citing fear for the safety of its employees. The case was settled out of court, and the hospital admitted no liability.

In yet another recent case, rather than go to court, a healthcare organization agreed to pay damages to the Equal Employment Opportunity Commission and to implement policies and provide training to ensure that a patient's racial preferences are not honored over and above an employee's civil rights (Starr and Murphy 2011).

Whether lawsuits are won or lost, they are costly in terms of dollars, stress, time, and, most important, employee relations and public image.

REFERENCES

Adams, D. 2013a. "Flint Hurley Medical Center Lawsuit Settled; Nurse Glad It's a Learning Tool." *The Flint Journal* February 22.

————. 2013b. "Flint's Hurley Medical Center, Nurse, Settle 'No-Black-Nurses' Lawsuit." *The Flint Journal* February 22.

Aldridge, C. 2013. "Nurse's Lawsuit Draws Protesters." *The Flint Journal* February 19.

American Medical Association (AMA). 2008. "Potential Patients." Opinion 10.05 of the AMA *Code of Medical Ethics*. Updated June. www.ama-assn.org//ama/pub/physician-resources/medical-ethics/code-medical-ethics/opinion1005.page.

Erb, R. 2013. "Nurse Sues After Hospital Grants Dad's Racial Request." *Detroit Free Press* February 18.

Hurley Medical Center. 2013. "Patient Rights and Responsibilities." Accessed July 8. hhs.hurleymc.com/?id=529&sid=1.

Karoub, J. 2013a. "Lawsuits Highlight Challenge of Patients Who Refuse to See Doctors or Nurses of Different Race." *The Associated Press* February 22.

————. 2013b. "Race-Based Nursing Under Fire." *San Francisco Chronicle* February 28.

Padela, A. I., S. M. Schneide, H. He, Z. Ali, and T. M. Richardson. 2010. "Patient Choice of Provider Type in the Emergency Department: Perceptions and Factors Relating to Accommodation of Requests for Care Providers." *Emergency Medicine Journal* 27 (6): 465–69.

Patient Talk. 2013. "American Hospital Association Management Advisory: A Patient's Bill of Rights." Accessed June 6. www.patienttalk.info/AHA-Patient_Bill_of_Rights.htm.

Paul-Emile, K. 2012. "Patients' Racial Preferences and the Medical Culture of Accommodation." *UCLA Law Review* 60 (4): 462–504.

Ridley, G. 2013. "Nurse Sues Flint's Hurley Medical Center over Claim She Was Barred from Treating Infant Because of Her Race." *The Flint Journal* February 18.

Schulte, M. F. 2010. "Diversity in Healthcare: Leading Toward Culturally Competent Care." *Frontiers of Health Services Management* 26 (3): 1–2.

Starr, G. S., and P. J. Murphy. 2011. "Patient Choice Versus Employee Rights: Conflicting Obligations?" *Connecticut Law Tribune* January 24.

State of Michigan Attorney General. 2013. "Michigan Patient Rights and Responsibilities in State Licensed Facilities." Accessed June 6. www.michigan.gov/ag/0,4534,7-164-18156_18152-47223--,00.html.

CHAPTER 12

Legal Perspectives

Walter P. Griffin

Illegal actions may be unethical.
Unethical actions may be legal.
—Anonymous

ALTHOUGH THE GENERAL public may view *ethical lawyers* as an oxymoron, when contending with healthcare issues lawyers must be aware of the ethical implications in addition to the legal ones. Although unethical behavior may not be illegal per se, the fine line between unethical and illegal is easily crossed. Lawyers are responsible for ensuring that their clients understand the differences between illegal actions and unethical ones.

As illustrated throughout this book, those differences are not always obvious. Lawyers learn through professional training and experience that court rulings establish the distinctions between illegal, unethical, and appropriate actions and that those distinctions are fluid and continually subject to change. A legal opinion provided by an attorney one day may be revised, reversed, or confirmed by a court of competent jurisdiction the next day. In the complex, multijurisdictional US legal system, lawyers must stay abreast of the latest court rulings and how those rulings might affect their clients. Timing is crucial. A court decision promulgated one year may be superseded by a new decision the next year. That definitions of right and wrong can continually change seems improbable, and yet such changes can be seen throughout history.

PARADISE HILLS MEDICAL CENTER

The events at Paradise Hills Medical Center illustrate a basic legal principle: Hospitals may be held responsible for the actions of their employees—in this case, a medical physicist whose miscalculations caused excessive levels of radiation to be administered to 22 oncology patients.

The legal and ethical questions are whether the institution has an obligation to notify the patients of the mistake, even though the results may not adversely affect the patients; whether the ordering physician should be informed of the mistake and allowed to decide if the patients should be notified; or whether hospital management could simply do nothing. From a legal point of view, the doctrine of fraudulent concealment is important. An institution or physician who withholds possibly detrimental medical information from a patient may establish the basis for a claim of fraudulent concealment. For example, a surgeon who knows that a sponge was left in a patient during surgery and does not tell the patient about the mistake has fraudulently concealed a fact on which a lawsuit could be formulated.

In the case of Paradise Hills Medical Center, each patient who received an excessive dose of radiation has a cause of action based on medical negligence. To fraudulently conceal the mistake would not only establish a separate cause of action but also indefinitely extend the statute of limitations that might otherwise bar legal action after a specific amount of time. Therefore, to conform with the law, the hospital should notify the patients. That notification would also satisfy ethical obligations.

However, one question remains: Who is responsible for notifying the patients—the institution or the ordering physician? The institution may discharge its legal obligations by notifying the ordering physician of the error on the theory that the physician is acting as the outer ego of the patient, but doing that may not fulfill the hospital's ethical responsibility. If an institution exists to benefit the public, it has a responsibility to be open and forthright. A lawyer discharges his legal obligation by informing the hospital's management that patients must be notified of the error through either direct communication with the patients or communication with the patients' physicians. The hospital's ethical responsibility may not be met, however, unless the hospital has direct contact with the patients. Whether a patient was actually harmed or whether the likelihood of future harm is very low is irrelevant.

QUAL PLUS HMO

The governing board committee's position at Qual Plus HMO leads to legal and ethical questions concerning the authority and action of the institution itself. A clear conflict of interest exists when a member of the governing board committee participates in decision making about bids for construction when that member has a financial interest in the outcome. The COO had knowledge of the conflict and had a legal duty, based on his employment by a public corporation, to request that the member refrain from participating in construction-related committee matters and to inform the CEO of the conflict. In this case, he did object to the committee's motion that final bids be invited, and he did inform the CEO, who refused to discuss the committee's action.

Legally, the COO had discharged his duties. His lawyer would advise him to document the events and proceedings. However, from an ethical point of view, the CEO and the COO should have submitted the issue to Qual Plus's ethics committee or informed the governing board directly. As noted, the COO did attempt to present the issue informally to the ethics committee and was rebuffed. The COO should have formally requested the ethics committee to consider the issue, forcing a decision for or against his opinion. His ethical responsibility would have been discharged once that decision was made. If the ethics committee rejected the formal request and made no decision, an ethical argument could be made that the COO was required to communicate directly with the governing board. Although the CEO looked unfavorably on that approach, the COO may not be protected from litigation if the board member's conflict of interest later becomes public knowledge. The COO must give top priority to performing the duties and responsibilities spelled out in his job description. By allowing a fraudulent bidding process to proceed, the CEO exposed himself to legal liability, and because the CEO acted as the outer ego of the health maintenance organization, the organization itself then became liable.

The appropriate method of addressing the conflict of interest would have been for the COO to formally request the ethics committee to look into the matter and resolve it. This case is a perfect example of the need for an ethics committee to facilitate the fair and impartial adjudication of internal ethical violations. The COO should not have retreated when his informal request was rejected. The COO was responsible for ensuring the integrity of the governing board committee's actions and had an ethical responsibility to expose any known conflicts of interest. Even if revealing the conflict might have put the COO's job in jeopardy, the governing board should have responded impartially. Once informed of the possible conflict of interest, the board had a legal responsibility to investigate the situation and decide how to deal with it. That decision, no matter what it was, would have shielded the COO if, at a later time, a third party had exposed the conflict of interest. To avoid his legal and ethical dilemma, the COO should have fully disclosed the conflict of interest to all levels of authority.

ROLLING MEADOWS COMMUNITY HOSPITAL

The situation at Rolling Meadows Community Hospital is filled with ambiguities. The lawyer listening to the CEO's description of his relationship with the postgraduate fellow could only wonder why the governing board would consider the CEO's actions detrimental to the institution. Although the CEO was imprudent in disclosing his personal feelings for the fellow and his assumptions about the future, he addressed the situation in a timely manner.

Because an employee–employer relationship had arguably not yet been established, the primary question remaining would be whether the CEO's decision was discriminatory because the fellow, as a female, was a member of a protected class. From a legal perspective, if the CEO does not hire another person to fill the position that the fellow sought or declares that the organization no longer needs such a position, proving that he violated any statute or common law would be extremely difficult. Similarly, the fellow could not claim sexual harassment because she has no evidence of sexual contact or a hostile work environment. Moreover, it appears that the fellow did not voice her disapproval of the CEO's covert or overt actions. In fact, from a legal perspective, a jury might be persuaded that the CEO's actions were actually intended to avoid the possibility of a future claim.

A more disturbing aspect of the case is the action of the governing board. Any decision the board made that might adversely affect the CEO's career could be legally actionable. Although the CEO is undoubtedly an at-will employee, various legal theories could be used to maintain a legal action against the institution for discharging the CEO under these circumstances. (For reference, an at-will employee is one who is employed at the discretion of the employer and may be discharged under any circumstances for any reason.)

UNIVERSITY HOSPITAL

In the University Hospital case, the basic principles are clear-cut, but the actions required by those principles are open to interpretation. A second-shift operating room (OR) supervisor, who had great respect for the attending trauma surgeon, faced a situation that forced her to choose between clear legal principles and strong personal loyalties. The applicable legal principles were that as the second-shift OR supervisor, she had a legal duty both to stop an intoxicated trauma surgeon from performing surgery and to contact the second-call trauma surgeon if the original trauma surgeon did not arrive promptly to assist the resident in lifesaving surgery. In addition, in her managerial capacity the OR supervisor may have had an ethical duty—to the community at large—to report the intoxication of a trauma surgeon to her superior.

The OR supervisor also arguably had a legal obligation to report the incident because the hospital was responsible, on the theory of respondent superior, for the actions of a trauma surgeon whom it supplied in an emergency situation. Whether the surgeon was an employee of the hospital or was acting as an independent agent does not make a difference.

Another issue is whether the supervisor had a responsibility to stop the resident from performing surgery. If the resident had a license to practice medicine in the state where University Hospital is located, the OR supervisor did not have a legal responsibility to stop the resident from performing surgery. However, she may have had legal responsibilities to notify the patient's relatives that life-threatening surgery was being performed by a resident, to obtain permission to proceed because the patient was unconscious and thus unable to consent, and to contact the second-call trauma surgeon because of both the delayed arrival and the inebriation of the original trauma surgeon. By obtaining consent from the patient's relatives and by notifying the second-call trauma surgeon, the supervisor would have discharged both her ethical and her legal obligations. By taking any other actions she could have exposed the hospital to liability for allowing a resident to perform surgery, even though it may have been justified in an emergency, and she would certainly have exposed the hospital to liability for her failure as a supervisor to notify the second-call trauma surgeon when no supervising trauma surgeon was present. The hospital, in all likelihood, would not have been held responsible for the behavior of the intoxicated trauma surgeon because he did not perform the surgery—at least if the hospital was unaware of any previous episodes of intoxication.

This discussion assumes that the resident was licensed to practice medicine in the state where University Hospital is located and, therefore, did not violate licensing laws. It also presumes that a licensed resident can practice medicine and surgery under the statutes of the state. However, whether the resident was competent to perform the surgery creates legal exposure for University Hospital. From a legal standpoint, the question would be whether the resident, under the hospital's procedures and regulations, had privileges to perform surgery. From an ethical standpoint, an issue would be whether the patient's life-threatening condition demanded action even if the required privileges had not been extended to the resident. Clearly, the resident expected that an attending physician would be present to oversee the resident's performance of the surgery. The attending physician's presence would have been mandatory if the resident lacked the necessary privileges, but the ethical considerations would have remained the same. Ethically, the resident had to intervene. The resident may have no personal liability because a life-threatening emergency demanded intervention with or without the extension of privileges or proof of competency. Nonetheless, the resident should have instructed the OR supervisor to contact the second-call trauma surgeon. And to ensure future patient safety, the resident should have informed the director of the residency program about the trauma surgeon's intoxication.

HILLSIDE COUNTY MEDICAL CENTER

Knowledge of the legal definition of *standard of care* as it applies to healthcare is essential to the analysis of the Hillside County Medical Center case. The term refers to the standard that a reasonable physician would adhere to when providing medical care in his specialty under similar circumstances that other specialists in that same field would adhere to nationally.

A similar standard applies to medical institutions because their liability is created through their employee physicians, agent physicians, and other providers of medical care. Depending on the individual caregiver's expertise, either a professional standard or an ordinary negligence standard may be used, but the institution is still responsible for its employees.

A hospital's need to reduce its workforce because of economic difficulties or labor unrest is no defense for a breach of the standard of care. Legally, a reduction in workforce requires an equal reduction in the number of patients. The legal and ethical responsibilities of medical care providers are the same under these conditions. Legally, providers of medical care are required to follow the standard of care, and ethically they must give patients adequate care for their medical conditions. Simply stated, when too many patients have too few medical providers, the result is a breach in both ethics and the standard of care.

"Do no harm" remains the legal and ethical basis for evaluating the actions of medical care providers.

METROPOLITAN COMMUNITY HOSPITAL

Metropolitan Community Hospital (MCH) faces a problem confronting many hospitals throughout the United States: a shortage of nurses. How the hospital reacts to the shortage could result in both ethical and legal complications detrimental to the hospital's mission.

MCH is located in an urban area that is perceived to have a high crime rate. As a result, potential nursing recruits tend to believe that employment at MCH could be risky. Other deterrents include tensions between physicians and nurses, the poor management style of the board, and the schism between foreign-born and US-born nurses.

Although those issues are not legal in nature per se, each has the potential to escalate into a legal problem. For example, a patient could file a lawsuit claiming that because of the shortage of nurses he received inadequate care and suffered an unnecessary medical complication. If the nurse-to-patient ratio in MCH's medical/surgical unit is 1 to 12 and the standard in the United States is considerably lower, the patient could have a basis for his claim. The plaintiff then would be required to prove a causal relationship (proximate cause) between the nursing shortage and the complication he experienced.

The board and the chief nursing officer in particular need to focus on meeting the national standard for the nurse-to-patient ratio. Anything less than that creates a legal quagmire.

Another area of legal concern is the relationship between the physicians and nurses. The law is clear that an institution is responsible for its administrative staff when charges of harassment are levied. Most states have statutes directly related to the establishment of such a claim. The administration has a duty to educate its staff about the nature and ramifications of harassment and to implement measures to alleviate the risk of harassment claims.

HEARTLAND HEALTHCARE SYSTEM

In today's market, information technology (IT) is at the heart of providing efficient and cost-saving healthcare. The creation of an interconnected medical information system that includes direct connections to the offices of private physicians and computerized physician order entry is a complex undertaking for any healthcare system. Unfortunately, at Heartland Healthcare System, the project became even more complex because personal ambitions created legal and ethical problems.

The new chief information officer (CIO) disregarded a reputable IT consulting firm's advice about upgrading the existing system and, with the CEO's approval, pursued his personal ambition to build an enterprise system that would be the envy of the Midwest. From a legal perspective, the CIO disregarded the reports of the consultant and ventured into an area in healthcare for which he did not have the proper credentials. Personal ambition continued to drive the implementation as the CIO relied increasingly on the same independent contractor and refused to consider further evaluation by other IT vendors. Legally, failure to use a formal bid process to evaluate the system or to purchase additional equipment is highly unusual and open to criticism. A formal bid process should always be the avenue for the purchase of equipment and obtaining additional reviews.

It is unlikely that the CEO and CIO in this case would be legally liable under these circumstances, but this possibility cannot be excluded. The CIO ignored resources at his fingertips, including input from nursing staff and physicians, which undoubtedly undermined the possibility of success in enhancing the information technology. However, there is a difference between poor decisions and negligence. Actions would have to be far out of the norm for someone in their positions to be considered negligent.

RICHLAND RIVER VALLEY HEALTHCARE SYSTEM

The merger between Trinity Medical Center and J. Blair Sutton Memorial Hospital brought together two organizations with very different philosophies, boards, and cultures. These types of mergers are difficult to carry out, and the formation of the Richland River Valley Healthcare System (RRVHS) was no exception. The attempt to blend such different organizations raised significant legal and ethical issues.

Each board of directors was bound to its corporate culture and determined to maintain the philosophy and goals of its own institution. The two boards' duty to govern was not abrogated by the formation of a third board. Although power could legally be transferred to the merged board, the responsibilities for managing the hospital system still rested with the boards of the two institutions. Consequently, either the two hospitals' corporate cultures needed to be amalgamated or each board had to be allowed to continue to pursue its own interests.

Unfortunately, both boards abandoned their legitimate roles as governing bodies even though the establishment of the RRVHS board did not relieve them of board responsibility. That abandonment was obvious when the hospital boards allowed the RRVHS board to order the new CEO to terminate the senior administrators of both hospitals, erasing vital corporate memory at a critical time. They also accepted the RRVHS board's decisions to assume financial oversight of both hospitals and to stop providing them with operating budgets and routine financial reports. As a result, the hospitals were deprived of the resources they needed for operations and growth. The RRVHS board's financial control also led to disagreements over the allocation of capital resources for new programs and services and rivalry between the two hospitals over where new clinical services would be based.

Governing boards have legal and ethical responsibilities to maintain focus on their respective institutions' goals and culture and to take the actions necessary to ensure the ongoing soundness of their institutions. The RRVHS merger failed in part because of all three boards' lack of attention to the important role that corporate culture plays in every organization and the RRVHS board's unwillingness to provide the hospitals with the resources required for the efficient and profitable delivery of healthcare.

HURLEY MEDICAL CENTER

As events in the Hurley incident unfolded, several attorneys were interviewed and their opinions reported in the media. These legal perspectives are documented in the discussion of the case in Chapter 11.

PART III

Addressing Structural Issues That Affect Ethical Decision Making

CHAPTER 13

Deciding Values

Joan McIver Gibson

Isolation is the worst possible counselor.
—Miguel de Unamuno, Spanish philosopher

DECISIONS WHETHER TO tell patients the "whole" story (including uncertainty, ambiguity, and bad news) to honor professional responsibility, to minimize legal liability, to provide safe and high-quality care, and to enhance programmatic and institutional financial health (not to mention survival) are values based. That is, they reflect what matters to the decision maker(s) in a given situation.

Indeed, we would be hard pressed to come up with any decision or issue (public, private, or professional) that is not at bottom defined by values—our beliefs about what is useful, important, worthwhile, or desirable. Certainly, the issues at Paradise Hills Medical Center (Chapter 3) are defined by values. So how should healthcare executives, board members, and other managers, whose main "products" are decisions, apply this observation?

In a culture that still feels the effects of the nineteenth-century positivist separation of "fact" from "value," we find ourselves without a robust language or strategy for seeing, naming, and working with values. We are confident that as long as we are dealing with facts, we can make progress. And so we search for "hard" data to lead the way. In the Paradise Hills case, would a right decision become clear if we had more conclusive data on the adverse effects of the accidental radiation, or if hospital policy were clear-cut as to who the ultimate decision makers are, or if the hospital had an in-depth analysis of projected market share

This chapter describes a values-based decision-making process and tool developed by Joan McIver Gibson, PhD, and her colleague Mark Bennett, JD, of Decisions Resources, Inc. The authors' book A Field Guide to Good Decisions: Values in Action *(Westport, CT: Greenwood Publishing Group, 2006) explains the entire process and includes cases and work tools.*

over the next five years? Probably not. The decision makers still must navigate a sea of conflicting interests and values.

As soon as someone raises the specter of a values discussion, however, many people fear a slide into the black hole of private, subjective, and interminable discussion. Such discussions are not helpful when things need to get done. This chapter introduces a process of values-based decision making for executives and managers in healthcare institutions. The process also is transferable to virtually every decision-making facet of life: professional, public, and private.

THEORY AND HISTORY

Are values really separable from facts? Do values enter decision making only when we specifically invite them in? Scientists and philosophers over the past half century have dropped the fact–value dichotomy as outmoded and unhelpful at best, and as wrong at worst. They observe that all reasoning—from the beginnings of language development through complex theory building—is the attempt to create, reflect on, and communicate meaning. Reasoning is the process of making meaning, or valuing. To label something as "factual" is to make a very strong claim about its importance, status, utility, and reliability—that is, about its value (Polanyi and Prosch 1975).

How do we discern the values dimension of an issue or a decision? What vocabulary do we need for capturing values and crafting decisions that appropriately reflect those values? Expanding our understanding of sources and types of values and their historical evolution in Western philosophy may help.

VALUES: SOURCES AND TYPES

Professions, organizational culture, law, religion, social customs, family, and personal experience communicate important values (see Exhibit 13.1). What matters to us comes from the areas of strong influence in our lives. Consider the relative weight we place on these sources of interests and values. Sometimes, when faced with otherwise intractable conflicts among values, we make choices based on what we consider an influential source for values. For example, how should the Paradise Hills CEO weigh the relative influences of professional, personal, and community values? Should values issuing from one of these sources trump the values from the others?

Another related strategy is to recognize that decision makers project various roles and approach decisions on the basis of these roles. Cases present themselves differently depending on the disciplinary "lens" through which we view them. Our roles grow out of our professional, social, and personal identities and entail specific perspectives or lenses that refract according to the types of values important to a given discipline or role (Exhibit 13.2). Consider the following perspectives:

- **Legal.** What does the law require?
- **Scientific.** Is the explanation comprehensive, coherent, and simple?
- **Economic.** Is this distribution of resources the best one available?
- **Social.** Does this policy respect the values and traditions of our diverse community?
- **Aesthetic.** Do things fit together and run efficiently and smoothly?
- **Moral.** Is it the right thing to do?

Exhibit 13.1: Sources of Values

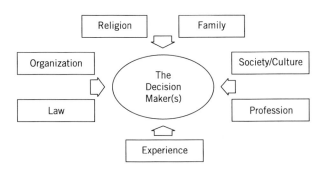

Exhibit 13.2: Examples of Values by Type

Economic	Context	Scientific
• Profitability • Efficiency • Frugality • Financial Security	We hold values that we use in making decisions. These values come from different sources. We have listed common values by type to assist you in identifying the values that you use in your work to make decisions. These types of values are not exclusive. For example, honesty is a religious value, a moral value, and a scientific value. We incorporate differing types of values to form our own unique set of personal values.	• Accuracy • Objectivity • Honesty • Knowledge

Aesthetic		Legal
• Beauty • Creativity • Simplicity • Elegance		• Justice • Equality • Freedom • Order

Personal	Your Personal Values Related to Work	Social
• Inner Harmony • Competence • Reliability • Happiness		• National Security • Cooperation • Responsibility • Loyalty

Religious	Institutional	Moral
• Charity • Sanctity of Life • Fidelity • Compassion	• Quality • Leadership • Teamwork	• Autonomy • Respect • Trustworthiness • Responsibility • Beneficence • Truth Telling • Integrity • Nonmaleficence • Justice/Fairness

This list is suggestive, not exhaustive, of the ways we unpack, label, and reorganize the variety of interests and values embedded in a single issue or decision.

Finally, history helps. In the United States, our contemporary set of values is a microcosm of more than 2,000 years of history. For example, reviewing the cumulative Western (primarily Anglo-Saxon and European) heritage, we see certain markers that signal different approaches to values. This tradition is but one of many cultural and historical strands that contribute to the American tapestry of values (see Exhibit 13.3).

In ancient Greece, virtue mattered most, at least to Plato and Aristotle (compare the Josephson Institute Center for Youth Ethics "Character Counts!" initiative). The question was, "How do I personally cultivate virtuous character traits?"—that

Exhibit 13.3: Major Historical Developments in Ethics

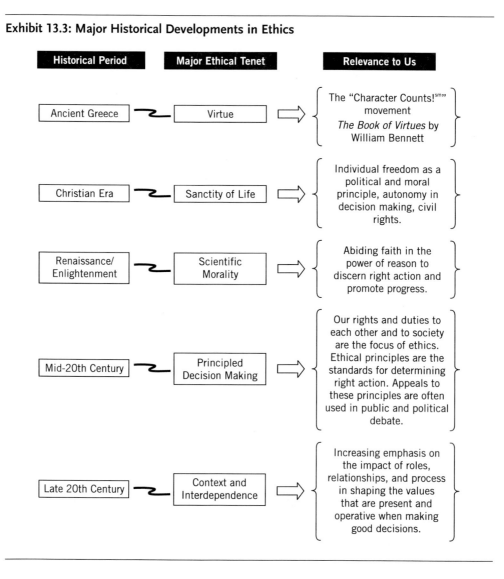

Historical Period	Major Ethical Tenet	Relevance to Us
Ancient Greece	Virtue	The "Character Counts!ˢᵐ" movement *The Book of Virtues* by William Bennett
Christian Era	Sanctity of Life	Individual freedom as a political and moral principle, autonomy in decision making, civil rights.
Renaissance/ Enlightenment	Scientific Morality	Abiding faith in the power of reason to discern right action and promote progress.
Mid-20th Century	Principled Decision Making	Our rights and duties to each other and to society are the focus of ethics. Ethical principles are the standards for determining right action. Appeals to these principles are often used in public and political debate.
Late 20th Century	Context and Interdependence	Increasing emphasis on the impact of roles, relationships, and process in shaping the values that are present and operative when making good decisions.

is, "Who should I be?" rather than, "What should I do?" Plato and Aristotle believed that a morally good person with right desires, motivations, or intentions is more likely to understand what should be done, more motivated to perform required acts, and more likely to form and act on moral ideals than someone without such virtuous traits.

At the beginning of the Christian era, two fundamental values were added: the sanctity of life and the importance of the individual person. Regardless of faith, the obligation to protect life and the intrinsic worth of persons as autonomous agents are values and imperatives that continue to drive American law and social policy.

During the Renaissance and Enlightenment, science, reason, and moral philosophy joined forces. The scientific values of simplicity, coherence, and comprehensiveness in explanation were extended to other disciplines (e.g., social theory, religion, art). These eras were characterized by a deep faith in the power of reason and the promise of progress, and morality was an important—perhaps the primary—object of rational inquiry. Faith in reason as the guide to right action continues, even (perhaps especially) as we lament its absence.

In the twentieth century, the application of reason to moral values became more systematized, even as it was separated from scientific and "factual" inquiry. Just as science, in one of its dimensions, is systematized explaining, so is moral philosophy (ethics) systematized valuing. One way moral philosophy is systematized is by extracting and abstracting from individual cases—those evermore general and encompassing reasons, standards, and justifications for what constitutes right actions. We call these most general and broadly applicable standards *principles*. This system of analysis and decision making took hold in medical ethics especially.

A principlist approach to valuing and ethics

- identifies the fundamental standards of right conduct, such as autonomy, respect for persons, beneficence, justice, truth telling, and professional responsibility and integrity;
- argues the moral importance of such standards; and
- applies each standard (where necessary) to a given situation.

How we justify these principles and the actions they support is important. Do we look to these standards themselves for self-evident value or to their consequences? Is there something about respect for persons and telling the truth that is intrinsically valuable, regardless of the circumstances or outcomes? Or should we calculate the consequences and seek the greatest good for the greatest number of people? The former approach is a formalist approach, the latter utilitarian. They are not mutually exclusive, and both are helpful.

The task, however, is not simply and mechanistically to follow or apply certain principles (for example, a code of ethics) to a given case, as one might follow a recipe, but rather to see how these standards help us understand and develop the moral dimension of a decision.

Toward the end of the twentieth century, as principlist ethics focused on formulating and impartially applying universally binding moral principles, contemporary philosophers began to observe that universal principles are inadequate for practical guidance—that abstract formulations and hypothetical cases that separate moral agents from the particularities and uniqueness of their individual lives and circumstances (and moral problems from social, historical, and contextual realities) are often less than helpful.

For example, telling the truth is important. Yet, sometimes it is not clear what the truth is, or what meanings different "messengers" might communicate, or to what extent quality patient care and safety might be compromised if a program is shut down. Unique circumstances, players, and environment are moving targets to be reckoned with. Context matters.

VALUES-BASED DECISION MAKING: A CONTEXTUAL APPROACH

A contextual (not to be confused with relativistic) approach to values-based decision making accommodates general principles, uniqueness, and particular details by focusing on roles, relationships, and process. The elliptical diagram in Exhibit 13.4 illustrates the approach. Features of the decision-making ellipse include the importance of context; the frames we and others bring to a situation; working with values by naming, clarifying, and weighing them; deciding on the basis of these values; and communicating the decision accurately and thoroughly along with the reasons behind it.

Context

Cases arise and decisions are made in specific contexts. Decision makers must see the full context, history, tradition, current conditions, and institutional values as well as the specific people, roles, and relationships that are at work. They must promote values and argue for their relative weight. Any decision involving Paradise Hills Medical Center must consider its history and role in the community, the current business climate, the institution's role as a teaching hospital, and the various roles and relationships of the respective players (physicians, CEO, board members, community at large). Effective decision makers understand the influence of context and use it to their advantage.

Exhibit 13.4: Decision-Making Ellipse

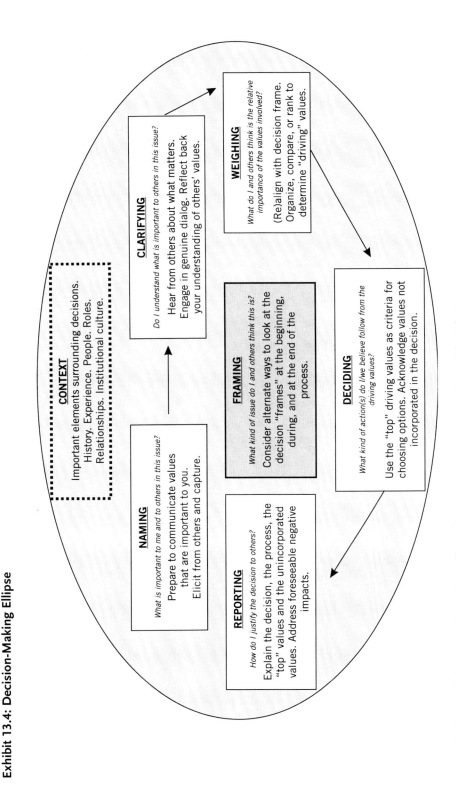

CONTEXT
Important elements surrounding decisions. History. Experience. People. Roles. Relationships. Institutional culture.

NAMING
What is important to me and to others in this issue?
Prepare to communicate values that are important to you. Elicit from others and capture.

CLARIFYING
Do I understand what is important to others in this issue?
Hear from others about what matters. Engage in genuine dialog. Reflect back your understanding of others' values.

WEIGHING
What do I and others think is the relative importance of the values involved?
(Re)align with decision frame. Organize, compare, or rank to determine "driving" values.

FRAMING
What kind of issue do I and others think this is?
Consider alternate ways to look at the decision "frames" at the beginning, during, and at the end of the process.

DECIDING
What kind of action(s) do I/we believe follow from the driving values?
Use the "top" driving values as criteria for choosing options. Acknowledge values not incorporated in the decision.

REPORTING
How do I justify the decision to others?
Explain the decision, the process, the "top" values and the unincorporated values. Address foreseeable negative impacts.

Framing: What Kind of Issue Do I Think This Is?

Each of us comes to any decision with a first take on what kind of issue is involved. We might initially consider the Paradise Hills case to be an issue of public relations; or perhaps one of liability exposure, institutional survival, or professional fiduciary responsibility; or maybe simply a matter of telling the truth. Different parties bring different initial frames to the decision (see Exhibit 13.4). Frames are neither right nor wrong; they simply are. The Talmud reminds us that "we see the world not the way it is, but the way we are."

We need ways to simplify and structure all the information "noise" that surrounds us. Our brains are hardwired to use categorical frames to bound what is "in" (relevant, important) and "out" (irrelevant, less important). Frames usually exist below our awareness and often remain untested and unexamined. Frames are not accessible for problem solving and decision making. Worse yet, they may impede our ability to see root causes of conflict. When frames are understood, appropriate, and flexible, they serve us well in dealing with difficult decisions and challenging situations. When they are hidden, unduly rigid, or based on flawed assumptions, they limit our ability to make wise decisions and may cause us to react to complex situations in an overly simplistic manner.

In decision making, frames determine who should participate; how the decision or question is formulated; what principles, values, and standards are applicable; what information is relevant; what is at stake; what the range of acceptable outcomes is; and how we should treat each other.

The main task of the framing step is to consider alternative ways to define the problem or structure the question, both at the beginning and throughout the decision-making process. Key framing questions include

- What kind of decision is this?
- What assumptions are we making?
- What boundaries do I (we, they) put on this question?
- Who are the people involved?

Specific framing activities might include

- periodically stepping back during the decision process and asking if we have the question, issue, or problem framed well;
- consulting with possible stakeholders about ways to frame the issue;
- listing three to five different ways to ask the question; and
- soliciting feedback from key people about the best way to approach the problem.

Naming and Clarifying: Do I Understand What Is Important to Me and to Others in This Issue?

The real brainstorming part of the process involves identifying the interests and values held by stakeholders. The goal of this step is to generate a comprehensive list of values described in everyday language, avoiding jargon. Questions that prompt useful values answers include

- What really matters in this issue?
- What is important here that we need to look at?
- What do you think our duties and obligations are in this situation?
- What worries you about this issue?
- When we look back on this decision one year from now, how will we know we did the right thing?
- If your teenager were watching us make this decision and asked why we did it, what would you say to her?

In the Paradise Hills Medical Center case, answers to the question "What is important?" might include (1) that Paradise Hills protect its good reputation; (2) that quality care and patient safety remain paramount; (3) that past, current, and future patients and families be able to trust the healthcare professionals at Paradise Hills; (4) that the hospital enjoy a strong economic position in the local healthcare community; and (5) that physicians honor their fiduciary duties to patients.

As values are named, others need to understand what they mean to the holder. Frequently, our stated values are merely the visible tip of their larger meaning. Listening well—not merely waiting to speak—is essential. Skills for avoiding "serial monologues" and creating dialogue include

- "reflecting back" one's understanding of someone's stated values;
- avoiding jargon by finding fresh ways to express values; and
- using the services of a facilitator to ensure a full, fair, and productive discussion.

When an individual's position is honored and allowed to take root in open dialogue, the health of the decision-making process is enhanced. Meanings are clarified, and participants feel they have been heard and may even be willing to let go of certain strong positions that might otherwise impede agreement. Even when full consensus is not possible or is not the goal, comprehensive naming and thorough clarification are necessary for decisions to last.

Weighing: What Do I Think Is the Relative Importance of the Values Involved?

A comprehensive list of interests and values is usually too long to be fully and equally honored. For example, profit, fiduciary responsibility, quality and safety, public reputation, professional autonomy, organizational mission, and increased market share are not entirely compatible. The question thus becomes: If we cannot equally honor all of these important interests, which are the most important? Put another way: If we do nothing else, we must make certain that _____ (fill in the value).

Values can be weighed and prioritized in several ways. Sometimes an "advocacy round" helps. Each participant speaks, briefly but strongly, to the value he thinks is most important. Other techniques include multiple voting, weighted multiple voting, and rank ordering. The rule of thumb is always to use a method that fits the situation. Patterns and agreement begin to emerge, at which point—and only at this point—decision options should be considered.

Deciding: What Actions Do I Believe the Most Important Values Warrant?

This process is not meant to replace full-blown decision-making processes already in use. Rather, it highlights a dimension of decision making that is routinely overlooked in much decision-making theory and practice: the values base. At the point in any decision-making process where alternative options are generated and considered, each option should immediately be tested against the prioritized list of values. The goal is to develop a decision that is genuinely driven—not just "spun" or superficially rationalized—by the identified top values. The coherence between a decision and its stated reasons must be genuine.

Communicating: How Do I Justify the Decision to Others?

Decision makers may feel that they work through many of the steps described so far as a matter of course and that their decisions are strong and sound for that reason. Chances are, however, that the communication of their decisions and the reasons behind them leave something to be desired. People who deserve to know should be informed about the grounds for a decision. First, who actually made the decision? This information should not be communicated by leading with, "It was decided that. . . ." How was the decision approached, and who was involved? What did the decision makers struggle with? What was most important in making the final decision? Finally, what is the decision?

Some decision makers prefer the "bottom line" approach, starting with the decision and working backward through the justifying reasons. Others prefer a more contextual or narrative approach that concludes with the decision. The components of a complete report are the same, however, and the common goal is to explain and justify the decision to stakeholders. Consider the two following Decision Summary Forms.

Form 1:
State the decision in direct, simple language. Be clear about who owns the decision. *(I/the executive committee have decided to _____.)*

Describe the most important values that drove the decision. *(Ultimately, we believe that _____ and _____ had to drive our final choice.)*

Directly address the downside of the decision—that is, what you do not like about it. *(There are some parts of this decision I do not like, such as _____.)*

Describe applicable values that could not be honored, and indicate the reasoning behind your judgment that other values were more important in this situation.

Address any negative effects of the decision on stakeholders. Pay particular attention to those who were not fully consulted in the decision process.

Form 2:
Describe how you approached the decision. Provide some brief highlights of the decision process—what steps you took, who was at the table, whom you consulted, and what level of time and effort was involved. *(Let me give you a sense of the road we took to get to this decision: _____.)*

Be candid about the downside of the decision.

Describe applicable values that could not be honored. Address the negative effects of the decision on the stakeholder.

Describe (using everyday language) the values that drove the decision.

State the decision in direct, simple language. Be clear about who owns the decision.

CONCLUSION

Decisions made with integrity are comprehensive, coherent, and transparent (see Exhibit 13.5). First, the decision maker has made a good-faith effort to consider the full range of interests and values (comprehensive). Second, the decision is logically grounded in the values considered to be the driving values; that is, the stated basis for the decision genuinely supports the decision (coherent). Third, the decision maker communicates the decision to those who deserve to hear it in a sincere,

Exhibit 13.5: Triangle Representing Decisions Made with Integrity

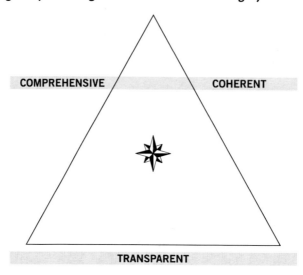

forthright manner. The decision maker is willing to stand up and be open and accountable to stakeholders by exposing the reasoning for the decision. Doing so requires a willingness to be tested, questioned, and judged by others (transparent).

This values-based decision-making process rests on certain important assumptions, observations, and hypotheses. All choices and decisions are driven by values—by what matters. Contemporary business approaches to ethics and integrity often focus on avoiding wrongdoing or breaking the law. Many decisions, however, are not about right versus wrong but rather right versus right (competing "goods"). Decisions are effective and enduring when they are based on clearly identified values, are made efficiently, have the resources and support to be fully implemented, and produce positive results that significantly outweigh the negatives. Durable decisions usually follow thorough dialogue, consultation, and collaboration.

POSTSCRIPT

The following tool is useful for a "values analysis on the fly"—when time is short but values still must be considered.

1. **Come prepared to speak directly to the values dimension of the decision.**
   • If you know the issue ahead of time, ascertain what frame you bring and what values you think are most important, and be prepared to communicate them.

- Encourage others to think ahead of time about their frames and values.
- Create the expectation that this kind of "homework" will be done.

2. **Commit to an advocacy round.**
   - Ask everyone in the room to explain his or her frame and values.
   - Avoid jargon and encourage ordinary language that captures the values in context.
   - Listen well and check in with people as they explain their values.
   - Record the frames and values where everyone can see and refer to them.
   - Weigh these values for relative importance.

3. **Return to the values list as appropriate.**
   - As issues and options are explored, consider which values each choice honors.
   - Craft decisions that are genuinely driven by the values that are most important in the situation.

4. **Report your values-based decision.**
   - State the decision and name the values that drove it.
   - Acknowledge the values that could not be honored.
   - Explain values priorities.

REFERENCE

Polanyi, M., and H. Prosch. 1975. *Meaning*. Chicago: University of Chicago Press.

CHAPTER 14

The Ethics of Managing People

Frankie Perry

THE CASES AND ethical dilemmas presented in this book have one thing in common—they all deal with the interrelationships of people and the different values, special interests, and goals that each person brings to the workplace. That the cases involve conflicts and ethical dilemmas should come as no surprise.

The cases presented are illustrative of the myriad interpersonal and professional relationships, diversity issues, external challenges, and management behaviors that predispose an organization to conflicts and ethical dilemmas. Paradise Hills Medical Center is an example of the complex relationships between physicians who deliver patient care and administrators who manage the delivery of that care. Qual Plus HMO examines the governing board's relationship with top management and probes whether top management does, literally, "serve at the pleasure of the board." Rolling Meadows Community Hospital looks at the superior–subordinate relationship and the dynamic of professional power. University Hospital explores professional relationships and the complexities of interaction with colleagues. Hillside County Medical Center demonstrates the importance of the relationships between management and unions and management and the medical staff, especially in times of financial crisis. Metropolitan Community Hospital explores the dynamics of physician–nurse relationships and a culturally diverse workforce. Heartland Healthcare System looks at the causes and effects of a lack of interdisciplinary integration. Richland River Valley Healthcare System shows what happens when the roles and responsibilities of governance and management are not clearly defined. Hurley Medical Center is a reminder to managers that they have ethical responsibilities to employees as well as to patients, some of them guaranteed by law. All of these cases point out why managers at every level need to follow ethical practices in managing people and how critical interpersonal relationships are in healthcare.

Healthcare managers often find the management of people to be the most difficult part of their jobs. Mastering skills in finance, planning, marketing, information systems, and the like is less difficult for most managers than dealing with the problems and conflicts that people introduce into the work environment. Complicating things even further is the diversity of today's workforce and the different values, ethics, and cultural perspective that each employee brings to the job.

Healthcare, with its preponderance of professionals and clinicians, introduces yet more ambiguities into this environment. Clinicians and professionals typically bring their own codes of conduct to the workplace and most often manifest their primary loyalty to their professions and the patients and clients they serve. Although commendable, this does not always translate to strong ethical practices in relationships with staff or colleagues. Dual lines of authority in the healthcare setting further complicate the role of the healthcare manager and her management of people. No wonder healthcare managers often want to just get the job done without the time-consuming messiness of having to negotiate, motivate, coordinate, evaluate, delegate, educate, and communicate with people.

What does all of this have to do with ethics? Healthcare managers usually are acutely aware of their ethical responsibilities to patients, clients, the organization, and the community. For the most part, they know what business practices are considered ethical. Too often, however, they overlook their ethical responsibilities to the people they manage. They may give lip service to the concepts of justice, honesty, loyalty, and fairness but do not necessarily apply these concepts in their day-to-day management of the people who report to them. Successful executives routinely practice ethical principles and management strategies that reflect these concepts. These executives have found that practical strategies that reinforce and routinize ethical principles can be incorporated into the daily management of people. Ethical principles should be integrated into management practices relating (but not limited) to management style, role modeling, culture, recruitment and hiring practices, performance evaluations, conflicts in the workplace, team building, mentoring and staff development, communications, workforce diversity, unions, firing practices, and references.

Some readers may think, "This all has merit, but isn't this stuff the responsibility of human resources? Isn't my time better spent focusing on the financial viability and competitive advantage of the organization?" Smart managers know that by ethically managing their people, they will be doing just that.

MANAGEMENT STYLE, ROLE MODELING, AND CULTURE

Healthcare managers at whatever level in the organization have control over their sphere of influence and would undoubtedly be surprised at how their personal management style and the ethical standards practiced in their area of responsibility (no matter how large or small) affect the organization as a whole. How employees within a department relate to other departments often determines whether projects are completed on time and within budget. How employees relate to one another within a department and with others throughout the organization sets the tone for how employees relate to patients, clients, and customers. A departmental culture that encourages ethical behavior and civility among coworkers contributes greatly to a corporate culture that expects the same standards. Each manager must nurture such a culture in his sphere of influence. While top management in an organization largely dictates the tenor and standards of the corporate culture, a department manager who abdicates responsibility in this matter is naïve and irresponsible.

"Pillars of excellence" exist in every organization. Close examination reveals that these departments or programs have a strong ethical culture. Their managers have clearly defined expectations for the ethical conduct of their staff and serve visibly as role models of these prescribed standards of conduct. The effect of culture on ethical behavior must not be underestimated. A recent National Business Ethics Survey spanning more than ten years reported that "organizational culture was more influential in strengthening ethical behavior" than were ethics training, compliance programs, and the like (Gilbert 2013, 60).

The work environment helps create the organizational culture. Healthcare managers have an ethical obligation to create a safe work environment that fosters ethical behavior and is free from harassment and coercion, especially coercion to perform illegal or unethical acts. The work environment must also be free of discrimination of any kind so that all employees are treated fairly and equitably. This includes fair compensation for work done, equitable opportunity for advancement, and honest and fair performance appraisals and rewards using the same standards for all employees.

Ethical healthcare managers are committed to promoting the implementation of programs that assist employees in times of need and provide confidential access for grievances. Providing confidential mechanisms for reporting such situations as employee impairment or sexual harassment and dealing with these issues with, for example, treatment or referral for impairment or disciplinary action for harassment are marks of an ethical organization managed by leaders who are willing to confront such issues head-on.

A significant and especially troublesome problem is workplace negativity, which can be insidious, contagious, and extremely detrimental to the organization if not recognized and addressed early on. A negative working environment can lead to poor morale, staff turnover, accidents, and—worst of all—medical errors and patient and family complaints. Topchik (2004) lists five causes of negativity in the workplace:

1. Poorly implemented change
2. Punishment of excellent performers (by giving them more work) and reward of poor performers (by giving them less)

3. Lack of learning environment
4. Challenges to security or stability
5. Inappropriate motivational strategies

Most of these causes of workplace negativity can be addressed with strong, effective employee communications and fair human resources practices.

When scarce resources threaten the fiscal viability of a healthcare organization, some executives look to workforce reduction as the only quick fix to the bottom line. Because hospitals are particularly labor-intensive organizations, downsizing may make financial sense, but the ethical implications warrant caution. The healthcare organization that achieves financial stability on the backs of its employees will most certainly not enjoy long-term success. Employee burnout and unsafe patient care are significant risks.

Furthermore, in times of financial crisis, an ethical healthcare executive will think twice before accepting a substantial bonus or salary increase in the face of massive employee layoffs. During the recent recession, Wall Street executives were criticized for taking bonuses as their companies went bankrupt. In an interview, economist Paul Volcker was asked if the ethics in the banking industry were worse today than in the past. His response left no doubt: "[In the past] you didn't have these huge compensation practices, bonuses were not considered appropriate, people didn't raid each other for talent. . . . There has been a loss of discipline about what is right and natural and ethical" (quoted in Gelb 2012). Renowned management consultant and author Peter Drucker has cautioned against excessive executive compensation and advocated that CEO salaries be no more than 20 times that of the average worker in the enterprise (Wartzman 2008). More than that, he said, will undermine morale and make teamwork difficult to foster. Some reported CEO salaries are more than 300 times that of the average worker in the company. In the context of healthcare, CEO salaries should be evaluated in comparison to the average nurse in the organization. Drucker clearly stated that he thought that excessive CEO compensation and bonuses during layoffs were "morally unforgivable" (Wartzman 2008).

Outsourcing is yet another practice that requires careful analysis if it means that cost savings are achieved as result of "cheap labor"—low wages, no benefits, and poor working conditions. A number of US corporations have been criticized for outsourcing jobs to overseas sweatshops, and their public image has suffered as a result.

Whether a healthcare executive practices participative management, continuous quality improvement, management by objective, management by walking around, or whatever the latest trend is, the importance of honesty, justice, loyalty, and fair play does not change. As seasoned executives know, a manager is most often a hybrid of styles. Some situations call for participation, others for a benevolent dictator. Seasoned executives also know that managers must be adaptable, because not all employees respond alike to the same management style. Research has suggested that effective managers—those who get the results they want—have learned to use different styles strategically at different times. These managers have a high level of *emotional intelligence,* which is "the ability to manage ourselves and our relationships effectively and consists of four fundamental capabilities—self-awareness, self-management, social awareness, and social skills" (Goleman 2000).

Given the mass of ethical violations in corporate and political society (including healthcare) that reflect hedonism, adding self-discipline to that list may be wise. While management style may vary with each employee, an ethical manager will make certain that such issues as performance expectations and appraisals, compensation, discipline, promotion, and educational opportunities are consistent across the board. Experienced managers know that favoritism predictably produces staff dissension and a loss of respect and effectiveness for the manager. Above all, employees want to be treated fairly and honestly.

Equitable treatment can be especially challenging when situations requiring disciplinary action arise with outstanding employees who are well liked by the manager. Disciplining high performers is hard, especially if you like them. But failing to do so adversely affects staff morale, productivity, and teamwork and lowers the bar for standards of conduct for all employees. Applying different standards to different employees may also set the stage for future litigation, if inconsistent discipline is applied in similar situations.

Micromanagement should be avoided. If performance expectations are adequately explained and necessary skills taught, managers can expect employees to function satisfactorily with appropriate supervision. If the employee is unable to perform, counseling or additional training may be warranted, perhaps even a probationary period or reassignment to a position for which the employee is better suited. Micromanagement over an extended period of time can be detrimental to the employee and counterproductive for the manager. The employee may lose interest in improving his output and abdicate responsibility for his work product, knowing that the manager will be closely reviewing all aspects of his work. Over time, the micromanaged employee may become a victim of learned helplessness and suffer an erosion of confidence, motivation, and productivity. The manager's productivity may suffer as well, as she spends time and effort micromanaging that could be better spent on other managerial duties.

Personnel policies—whether corporate or departmental—should be constructive, not punitive. They should be developed with the goal of motivating employees and improving work performance, not just oriented toward poor performers, rule breaking, and disciplinary actions.

Effective leaders insist on programs that reward accomplishments that achieve organizational goals and that recognize individuals, teams, and the employee population as a whole. Enlightened leaders invest in the surveys and conversations needed to learn what recognition programs and celebrations have value among their employees (Perry 2012). Haden (2012) lists four rewards more powerful than money:

1. Asking employees for ideas on how to do their job better
2. Asking for help in solving a problem
3. Creating short-term, informal leadership roles to solve a problem
4. Teaming up—taking on a task or education session together

Although employees, clinicians, and management staff may be motivated by different things, three general truths about human nature remain constant (Perry 2012):

1. The workplace is a social setting. People want to enjoy work and to look forward to coming to the workplace each day.
2. Most people want to do a good job (those who don't should be fired or reassigned) and want recognition, public or private, for a job well done.
3. People want their opinions about work to be solicited and valued.

Motivating people to rise to their full potential and to the level of performance needed to achieve organizational success is what produces results. "Management is getting people to do what needs to be done. Leadership is getting people to want to do what needs to be done" (Bennis 1999).

Above all, a wise manager never underestimates the power of example. The ethical manager consistently practices the standards of conduct that she wishes all employees to emulate. Employees and staff look to management to determine what is acceptable behavior and what is valued. Actions that a manager takes or does not take on a day-to-day basis are considered the behavioral norm.

RECRUITMENT AND HIRING PRACTICES

Some of the most important decisions a manager will make involve employee hiring. Individuals drive an organization, create the culture, and determine whether the organization succeeds or fails. The task of hiring staff should therefore be taken very seriously. Wrong choices can be costly to an organization in more than just financial terms.

Getting the right people on board will make a manager's job and the achievement of organizational goals much easier. Collins (2001, 41) says that "executives who ignited the transformations from good to great [companies] did not first figure out where to drive the bus and then get people to take it there. . . . they first got the right people on the bus (and the wrong people off the bus) and then figured out where to drive it."

Inexperienced managers sometimes look to hire staff who are easy to control. They may be afraid to hire someone smarter than they are, lest they lose full authority. Experienced managers know that to achieve organizational goals, they need to hire bright people for key positions who will bring needed skills and talents to the tasks at hand.

Smart managers seek out prospective recruits who possess integrity and strong character in addition to knowledge, skills, talents, and experience. Knowledge and skills are much easier to teach than integrity and character. Managers often look for new employees who they believe will fit well in the organization and get along with others. Equally important is that the employees be interesting and pleasant and have a positive attitude about work and life in general. Positive employees of strong character contribute greatly to productivity, morale, and an ethical work environment.

Granted, a manager may not always be able to intuit or even observe these attributes on interview. For this reason, interview teams should be used whenever appropriate, and they should ask the candidates similar questions and allow them to answer expansively. Scenarios can be presented to candidates during the interview that include subtle ethical dilemmas and the candidates asked how they might handle the situations.

When interviewing candidates, the hiring authority must pay attention to resumes and applications. Although the human resources staff may be responsible for checking education, licensure, certifications, and the like, managers responsible for hiring decisions must make sure that these qualifications have been verified. Attendance at a university does not mean that a degree was granted. A certification or license that has not been renewed may no longer be valid.

Russell and Greenspan (2005, 85–86) tell us that "hiring the right person to do the job is a challenge. . . . It is an even more difficult decision for any manager to replace an existing staff member who is unable to do the job well that he or she was hired to do. . . . The biggest mistake that managers consistently make is to recognize that they have the wrong person in a key position and fail to do something about it." Replacing an ineffective employee is especially difficult if the manager has strongly advocated for him or has boosted salary and benefits to recruit him. The recruitment process is brief, so paying careful attention to the interview process and involving key staff members are important.

When interviewing potential employees, the manager has an ethical responsibility to be honest and candid about the organization, its financial status (if appropriate), salary, benefits, job security, corporate culture, expectations of the position, and so forth. Employment is an implied contract, if not a written one, and neither party should experience any surprises. In the case of a top management position, the candidate may be relocating and making a substantial financial commitment for herself and her family. Withholding the fact that the position may be short term is unfair and dishonest, to say the least.

Another area of ethical ambiguity in recruitment is the issue of salary inequities. A manager may offer a candidate a higher salary to join the organization than what the organization is paying an existing employee working in the same capacity. Often justified as a recruitment strategy, this questionable practice raises issues of fairness, loyalty, and justice.

If qualified, existing employees should be allowed to apply for any promotion or other opening that occurs in the organization. Internal candidates should be given fair and equal consideration for these opportunities. If an internal candidate is not offered the available position, an explanation should be provided to that person so that performance areas may be strengthened or developed.

PERFORMANCE EVALUATIONS

Ethical organizations give employees clear, accurate, and current job descriptions and a thorough explanation of what is expected from them in the position. In addition, ethical organizations provide employees with the resources they need to satisfactorily perform the job, including knowledge and skills development. Ethical healthcare managers further ensure a working environment that properly uses the skills and abilities of each employee.

Regularly scheduled performance evaluations are an important part of the manager's role and responsibility to each employee. Some managers may procrastinate when it comes to this task because they feel uncomfortable discussing areas where the employee needs to improve. However, late performance evaluations, especially those that delay salary increases, will only make employees think that management is indifferent to their needs and places little value on their contributions. Delayed evaluations are also unfair to the employee, who may want guidance on how to further develop skills and improve job performance.

In addition to regularly scheduled performance appraisals, the manager should provide ongoing candid feedback on job performance that helps employees grow and master skills. Holding back what could be constructive comments and "blindsiding" employees with criticism at an annual performance review are unfair. Most people want to do a good job and need clear direction on what is required and expected of them. Managers who assume that employees always know what and how to do what is expected of them may be doing themselves and the employees a disservice. Managers who wish to nurture an ethical culture should also reward ethical conduct and remedy questionable behaviors as part of the performance evaluation.

Probationary periods for newly hired employees can benefit both the organization and the employee. They allow the organization ample time to ensure the new employee is working out and meeting the expectations of the job, and they give employees the opportunity to clarify what is expected of them and to ask for resources if needed.

Finally, a skilled manager is aware that employees garner pay for work (salary) and pay from work (self-esteem, respect, a sense of contribution). The skilled manager seeks to identify what activities provide this kind of gratification to each employee reporting to her and attempts to distribute assignments accordingly. Although each employee must have his fair share of less pleasant tasks, he will tackle these tasks with more enthusiasm knowing that gratifying assignments will come later.

MANAGING CONFLICT IN THE WORKPLACE

Conflict in the workplace is inevitable. Experienced managers know that some conflicts are valuable to the organization because they help identify issues and lead to innovative solutions. Similarly, workforce diversity may sometimes cause conflict, yet having a variety of knowledge, experiences, values, attitudes, and viewpoints produces solid solutions to problems. Diverse perspectives can help managers anticipate others' perceptions as well as the possible unintended consequences of actions under consideration.

Other conflicts, however, can be costly to the organization in terms of employee absenteeism, turnover, loss of productivity, and morale or to the organization's reputation as a nice place to work. Some conflicts can affect patient and client services, and others may even result in litigation. Although the manager may experience conflicts with coworkers, the boss, and patients or clients, more often the manager has to deal with (and has the most control over) conflicts among subordinates. Therefore, what follows are practical strategies for preventing conflict and productive actions that a manager can take when conflict does occur.

Management practices that preempt conflict among subordinates and simultaneously help achieve desired goals include

- clear policies and procedures;
- systems and structures for addressing employee concerns;
- diversity education to help employees understand and appreciate differences in communication or work styles;
- clear delegation of authority and accountability;

- conflict management training;
- informal employee events where employees can get to know one another;
- celebration of team accomplishments;
- performance evaluations that assess an employee's ability to function in a team;
- giving credit where it is due;
- fair and equitable compensation;
- role-modeling acceptable behavior;
- codes of conduct for staff interactions;
- strong, two-way employee communications; and
- candidate interviews that present conflict scenarios or such questions as the following:
  —Why did you leave your last job?
  —How did you get along with coworkers?
  —What kind of conflicts have you dealt with?
  —How did you deal with them?

In contrast, the following management behaviors provoke conflicts among subordinates and should be avoided:

- Constant rule changing
- Playing the blame game
- Micromanaging
- Playing favorites
- Putting off addressing unsatisfactory job performance

Managers must also be keenly alert to employee behaviors that may be toxic to a well-functioning work environment and effectively deal with them without delay. Problem staff include

- the condescending, self-righteous employee who must be right at all costs and resists any change unless it is her idea;
- the capable employee who frequently undermines coworkers or the organization;
- the naysayer who always has a reason why something won't work;
- the drama queen (or king) who insists on making much ado about nothing; and
- the gossipmonger who thrives on others' or the organization's misfortunes.

Employees guilty of such behaviors must be made to understand how the behaviors affect coworkers and the productivity of the team. They may not be aware how others perceive them. These employees, especially those who are otherwise competent, must be shown that these behaviors are not only unprofessional but also detract from the good work they do and can be career limiting. Failure to address toxic behaviors can hurt the corporate culture. They can be contagious or, if left unchecked, can become the accepted norm.

When conflict occurs, the manager should take a step back and determine if the conflict is one that needs to be dealt with. Not all conflicts need fixing—some will fix themselves. The manager should ask himself, "Does this conflict really matter? Is it temporary? Will it resolve itself? Do I really have any control over it?" On the other hand, conflicts that disrupt the workplace or involve bullying, disrespect, sexual harassment, a hostile work environment, or the like require immediate attention. The manager also needs to make sure that conflict resolution takes place at the appropriate level. Sometimes conflicts that should be resolved at a supervisory level find their way to a higher manager. When that occurs, the manager may offer advice to the supervisor but must resist personally dealing with the issue and return it to the appropriate level for resolution.

A common characteristic of inexperienced managers is the tendency to avoid conflict altogether. The danger here is that avoidance may give the impression that the manager condones the actions, and if left unattended, minor conflicts can turn into major ones. Equally dangerous is jumping in too quickly to fix whatever problem may arise. Understandably, managers want things to run smoothly and problems solved quickly. Although sometimes a quick fix is indicated, at other times the manager may need to allow employees the flexibility and freedom to solve the problem themselves.

When a manager determines that conflict management is his responsibility, certain rules of engagement may be helpful. He should take time to think through how best to deal with the conflict, decide what he wants to accomplish or gain by resolving it, and get all of the facts. Often, the truth lies somewhere in between what one person believes to be true, what the other person believes to be true, and what actually is true. Once he has all the facts, the manager may wish to seek advice from a trusted colleague. If the conflict is process related, he should request a root-cause analysis to identify and remedy process breakdowns. When resolving a conflict between subordinates, the manager must

- remain objective and never take sides;
- address the issues, not the people;
- clarify the roles and responsibilities of those in conflict;
- be flexible and open to ideas;
- look for potential compromise; and
- show those in conflict how they will benefit by resolving the dispute.

After the conflict has been resolved, the manager must encourage those involved to move on and focus on goals.

TEAM BUILDING

Most managers spend considerable time talking about the importance of teamwork. Many even arrange team-building exercises or seminars for their employees, often led by high-priced consultants. However, some managers, while ostensibly advocating teamwork and recognizing its benefits, act in ways that sabotage the very teamwork they wish to achieve in their sphere of influence.

To promote teamwork, managers must model behaviors that nurture it. They must teach employees who lack the needed skills how to participate in healthy debate, how to practice civil disagreement, and how to discuss controversial and not-so-controversial issues as a team, seeking acceptable resolutions to problems. Employees should be encouraged to think independently and express ideas freely. Employees who always agree with the boss contribute little to the discussion. Managers must reward team play so that employees place value on it. Managers must articulate the organization's goals and must structure action plans and reward systems that focus on teamwork in the achievement of goals and organizational success.

Managers who wish to encourage teamwork must never show favoritism or allow employees to gossip, belittle coworkers, or make disparaging comments about others' work. Some employees mistakenly believe that making coworkers look bad makes them look better. By remaining indifferent to negative comments, managers silently acquiesce to such criticism. Instead, managers must articulate clearly that such behaviors are unacceptable and counterproductive.

Providing equal "face time" and attention to all team members is another way a manager can foster teamwork. Sometimes a well-intentioned manager will adopt an open-door policy only to find that one or two employees take advantage of this unlimited access to the boss, to the detriment of the other team members. Reasonable and equitable access to the boss fosters teamwork and encourages more interaction among coworkers for problem resolution.

MENTORING AND STAFF DEVELOPMENT

Mentoring and staff development are not just nice things to do if you have the time. They are built into the culture of ethical organizations.

Employees cannot be expected to meet the requirements of the job without the resources needed to accomplish the tasks assigned. Knowledge, skill, and guidance are just as critical as budgeted dollars. As more clinicians enter management ranks, administrators must ensure that they are provided with the preparation that will ensure they succeed in their new roles. This preparation may take the form of management education or specific seminars on topics, such as staff performance evaluations or finance and budgeting, where the clinician may have little previous experience. Time spent mentoring these new managers on the way things get done, the politics of the organization, and the chain of command is time well invested.

Outstanding performers who are promoted to management may need special attention. They may micromanage their subordinates because the subordinates' job is what they previously did well and were rewarded for.

On occasion, an employee who is a superstar in one aspect of his job (e.g., computer technology) may be deficient in another (e.g., customer service). If the employee does not respond to counseling, a manager has options. She can fire the employee, which might be the easiest but not necessarily the best course of action, or she can look for ways to build on the employee's expertise and use it to the organization's advantage. Reassignment may be a more ethical way to deal with an employee who has something of value to contribute.

ETHICAL IMPORTANCE OF EMPLOYEE COMMUNICATIONS

The critical role that communications play in management, employee relations, organizational culture, and meeting organizational goals cannot be overstated. The role of communications is especially evident in the event of a new administration, work reductions, layoffs, mergers, and acquisitions of organizations. Anything that threatens the status quo or existing stability of the organization will have a personal effect on the job security of individual employees, wherever they may be in the corporate hierarchy.

Nothing causes more anxiety than uncertainty, and once people have information—good or bad—they can mobilize their personal resources to plan or take action. In times of change, ethical managers make sure that their employees and staff have as much information as they need. Failure to provide information will result in informal communication networks filling in the vacuum with rumor, speculation, and false conclusions, creating a work environment that is sure to have a negative effect on productivity. Although managers often are justifiably frustrated by having to repeat the same information several times to their employees, management is closer to, and has a better understanding of, situations. Employees need more time to process information and determine the effect it may have on them. Reinforcing the information will build trust between the workforce and management.

"The medium is the message" is the oft-quoted admonition of Marshall McLuhan (2003), a widely recognized expert on communication theory. He advanced the notion that the medium used for communication influences how the message is perceived. In today's cyberspace world, that idea bears remembering. E-mail communications have become the norm. They are quick and convenient, and they have a role. They save enormous time by eliminating telephone tag. But they also foster information overload, especially when an inordinate number of messages are mass-copied.

For important issues, alternative methods of communication need to be considered. Electronic communications are not as effective as face-to-face communication. They do not convey the tone or tenor of a message and do not allow for dialogue or immediate response from the recipient. Without immediate response, points cannot be clarified, questions asked, or information delivery adjusted to better achieve the intent of the addressing message. The anonymity of electronic communications may entice some people to say things they would not ordinarily say face-to-face or to say them with an unintended lack of civility that may put the recipient on the defensive. The actual identity of the sender may not be known, only the computer of origin. Unless the sender requests confirmation, he has no assurance that the intended recipient even received the message. Particularly troublesome can be occasions when a sensitive message unintentionally becomes part of a long chain of e-mails with many readers or just gets lost in a barrage of messages. Finally, the confidentiality of electronic communications is not guaranteed. Steve Jobs, master of the digital universe, required his staff to have face-to-face meetings rather than electronic ones because he believed they fostered more creativity (Isaacson 2011).

Ethical managers practice two-way communication with their employees. They seek employees' opinions and ideas. They encourage civil disagreement and debate. They listen carefully to and learn from employee comments rather than disregard them out of hand. Nancy M. Schlichting, CEO of Henry Ford Health System in Detroit, says, "I attend new-employee orientation, give out my e-mail address, and tell employees to let me know if they have concerns about whether we are meeting our standards" (quoted in Rice and Perry 2013, 35). Ethical managers care what their employees think and work to develop employee communication strategies that build a community of shared values.

WORKFORCE DIVERSITY

Building a community of shared values is challenging in a diverse workforce. Diversity has many faces. In today's multicultural society, healthcare managers must be aware of ethnic, cultural, generational, and religious differences among employees as well as different life experiences, economic status, sexual orientation, and disabilities.

In addition, multidisciplinary, multicultural healthcare professionals bring their personal codes of conduct, values, and biases to the workplace (Rice and Perry 2013).

Ethics begin with the way one interacts with people. Understanding the perspective of others and the lens through which they see the world greatly enhances the success of these interactions. Cultural competency training is not just important in the care of patients; it also must be addressed in relationships, supervision, and management of employees. An ethical healthcare executive fosters inclusion and collaboration, avoids tokenism, expands networking and mentoring opportunities for minority managers, and eliminates structural barriers that prevent women and minorities from moving up the ranks of the organization.

Above all, healthcare managers must practice ethical leadership in their day-to-day actions and in their employee relationships if they expect a diverse workforce to know the standards for acceptable conduct in the organization. Ethical managers must not let personal prejudices or moral judgments influence their evaluation of an employee's job performance. They must see to it that human resources policies are fair and nondiscriminatory and that respect is shown for cultural differences. Effective communications take into account cultural and generational differences. Managers must ensure clarity and meaning of language to avoid misunderstandings. Methods of communication with younger employees may have to be adjusted to meet their affinity for technology.

Living with and managing demographic diversity has become a central theme of the twenty-first century (Dunn 2010, 490). Effective healthcare leaders develop strategies to recruit, motivate, retain, and mobilize a multicultural workforce to support the mission of the organization. They promote and support diversity initiatives oriented to both their employees and their patient populations. They work to secure a workforce that is representative of the community's demographics. As Piper (2012) writes, "For an organization to fulfill its social contract to provide high-quality, cost-effective, and safe healthcare, it must satisfy the needs and manage the expectations of those who directly deliver these services."

WORKING WITH UNIONS

This discussion is not intended to be a primer on labor relations, but a few observations about working with unions merit mention. Although labor unions are declining nationally, unions are still prevalent in some geographic areas. Areas with substantial union membership in industry or government also tend to have a union presence in healthcare. The US Bureau of Labor Statistics reports that while union membership has decreased across all industries, union membership in healthcare has been steadily increasing (Elliott 2010). Close to one million healthcare workers were union members in 2009, and registered nurses were a large number of this group. This trend has been linked to the loss of control that nurses feel as a result of staff reductions, other cost-saving measures, and the uncertainty of health reform.

Money is not the primary reason that nurses unionize. Their efforts focus on improving patient safety, increasing nurse staffing ratios, advocating for patients' rights, and having a stronger voice in public policy. Administrators must recognize these motives and not assume nurses are motivated by self-interest. If management's desire is to deter unionization, paying attention to the nurses' goals could accomplish this aim. Working with unions has its challenges, but lessons can be learned from the experience. Some managers fear losing all control when unions enter the picture, but the key words in labor relations parlance are negotiation and bargaining.

Successful negotiation requires that both parties understand what the other wants to achieve, why the organization exists, and how organizational success benefits both parties. Successful negotiations that arrive at reasonable, fair contracts and that benefit the organization begin with trust and the ability to find common ground. When either party enters into negotiations in an adversarial posture, the discussion soon breaks down and resembles more of a power struggle than a desire to reach agreement. Unions often see management as interlopers into an organization that their members have helped build. Unions think that managers simply move up the career ladder and on to other communities, whereas unions and their members are vested in their community long-term. Effective leaders work hard to dispel this perception of management and are attentive to the image and interpersonal skills of staff who represent management in negotiations.

Management must be tough in negotiations, always with the best interests of the organization guiding their decisions—especially on issues that may threaten the organization's long-term success. Concessions granted out of fear of a strike are not always in the best interests of the organization, the community, or the union members themselves. Some automotive industry observers have remarked that this was a problem with General Motors—that management sacrificed the long-term viability of the corporation to avoid strikes and enjoy short-term profits. Successful negotiations involve bargaining that produces safe working conditions and fair compensation for work done and that ensures both the short- and long-term ability of the organization to fulfill its mission and obligation to the community.

Working with unions has aspects that many managers find burdensome and time consuming—requirements such as documentation of unsatisfactory performance and counseling, progressive discipline, timely performance evaluations, justification for firing, job descriptions that are current and consistent with assignments, and so forth. For inexperienced managers, these requirements may actually provide direction for dealing fairly and objectively with unsatisfactorily performing employees. Using these guidelines for terminating employment for unsatisfactory performance can bring clarity and objectivity to the process and prevent litigation.

In fact, the consistent practice of fair, equitable human resources policies is likely the best way to avoid unionization—and potential litigation. Segal (2011) says that "employment at will" does not mean that employees can be terminated at whim and warns that a claim of unfair treatment can lead to litigation. Managers in at-will employment organizations commonly make the ten following mistakes when dealing with problem employees:

1. Failing to notify employees that their jobs are on the line
2. Failing to confirm the corrective action in writing
3. Failing to state that the final warning is, in fact, final
4. Focusing on the cause of performance problems, such as illness, depression, and so forth
5. Focusing on intent rather than outcome
6. Using labels rather than describing behaviors
7. Overstating the risks of retention
8. Ignoring the comparators
9. Delaying the inevitable
10. Failing to provide dignity and respect

Segal (2011) says that when managers focus on what they assume to be the cause of the problem, such as illness or depression, they may set the stage for a disability claim. Focusing on intent is irrelevant because it can't be proven; using labels like "bad attitude" does not define what must change; and other employees who display similar behavior must be treated the same. This advice is good whether managers are working with unions or in organizations that enjoy employment at will.

When working with unions, managers should remember that unions have a vested interest in the organization's fiscal viability and that the challenge may be to enter into negotiations to find and exploit that common ground.

FIRING PRACTICES

Rarely does a manager relish the idea of firing an employee. When appropriate remedial measures do not produce satisfactory job performance, retaining an underperforming employee is unwise and unfair. A manager does no one any favor by not firing an employee who is not doing his job. It is unfair to coworkers who have to pick up the slack; to clients or others who are directly or indirectly affected by the poor performance; to the organization that is paying a wage for unsatisfactory work; to the manager who has to spend time and energy cleaning up after a poor performer; and to the underperforming employee himself, because it keeps him from moving on to a more satisfactory employment arrangement. The organization may suffer in other ways as well; tolerating poor performance lowers the bar and the standards for what is acceptable.

The firing of an employee should be done with honesty, clear explanation, fairness, and respect and in a way that enables the employee to retain as much dignity and self-respect as possible. Much has been written on firing practices, severance packages, liability protection, and the like. While the "what is done" is important, the "how it is done" has ethical implications. Honesty, fairness, and respect must characterize the process. Although they may not remember the words that were said, people will always remember how the conversation made them feel.

PROVIDING REFERENCES

Within the boundaries of the law and any post-employment agreements, reference information should be accurate, honest, and fair. Fear of litigation has prompted some employers to provide no more information than dates of employment and position held. To those checking references, this reticence may unjustly imply that the employee was fired or asked to resign or was an unsatisfactory performer. Given that not all employees are a perfect match with the position they held in the organization, honest responses to inquiries need not provide elaborate detail. Some questions are more appropriately answered by the former employee himself—for example, "Why did this employee decide to seek other employment?" Answering such questions based on personal assumptions is unwise, and questions such as these should be referred to the employee.

If references are being sought regarding a current employee, managers must be equally fair and honest. If the employee is valuable to your organization, you may be reluctant to give a glowing recommendation, but honesty must prevail.

When providing references, the manager generally focuses on the employee. However, the manager must be fair to the reference checker and his needs as well, even though he is usually a stranger. Ethics applies to all situations and to all relationships.

REFERENCES

Bennis, W. 1999. *Managing People Is Like Herding Cats.* Provo, UT: Executive Excellence Publishing.

Collins, J. 2001. *Good to Great.* New York: HarperCollins.

Dunn, R. T. 2010. *Dunn and Haimann's Healthcare Management*, ninth edition. Chicago: Health Administration Press.

Elliott, V. S. 2010. "Unions for Health Care Workers Are Growing." *American Medical News* February 22.

Gelb, L. H. 2012. "Oh, Those Greedy Bankers." *Newsweek* September 24.

Gilbert, J. 2013. "A Reflection on Everyday Ethics." *Healthcare Executive* 28 (1): 60–63.

Goleman, D. 2000. "Leadership That Gets Results." *Harvard Business Review* 78 (2): 78–90.

Haden, J. 2012. "4 Rewards That Are More Powerful Than Money." Inc. Posted February 7. www.inc.com/jeff-haden/4-employee-rewards-that-are-more-powerful-than-money.html.

Isaacson, W. 2011. *Steve Jobs*. New York: Simon and Schuster.

McLuhan, M. 2003. *Understanding Media: The Extensions of Man. Critical Edition.* Berkeley, CA: Gingko Press.

Perry, F. 2012. *Healthcare Leadership That Makes a Difference: Creating Your Legacy.* Self-study course. Chicago: Health Administration Press.

Piper, L. E. 2012. "Generation Y in Healthcare: Leading Millennials in an Era of Reform." *Frontiers of Health Services Management* 29 (1): 16–28.

Rice, J., and F. Perry. 2013. *Healthcare Leadership Excellence: Creating a Career of Impact.* Chicago: Health Administration Press.

Russell, J., and B. Greenspan. 2005. "Correcting and Preventing Management Mistakes." In *Management Mistakes in Healthcare: Identification, Correction and Prevention*, edited by P. B. Hofmann and F. Perry, 84–102. New York: Cambridge University Press.

Segal, J. A. 2011. "At Will but Still Armed." *Hospitals & Health Networks Daily* March 24.

Topchik, G. 2004. "Purging Workplace Negativity." *Executive Update* February.

Wartzman, R. 2008. "Put a Cap on CEO Pay." *Bloomberg Businessweek* September 12.

CHAPTER 15

Ethics Issues in Managed Care

Richard H. Rubin

OVER THE PAST few decades, the field of medical ethics has become increasingly important in both medical education and clinical practice. The expanding role and presence of medical ethics has manifested itself not just in the escalating number of books and journal articles on this topic, but also in the percentage of medical schools that now include training in medical ethics as part of the standard curriculum and the growing number of hospitals nationwide where ethics committees meet regularly to resolve perceived ethical dilemmas.

The past few decades have also seen the evolution of managed care to become a major factor in the delivery of healthcare in the United States. Although the term *managed care* refers to a rather heterogeneous group of institutions, a feature common to all managed care organizations (MCOs) is a systematic approach to controlling what has been a progressive escalation in the country's healthcare costs over the past half century.

The increasing prominence of both medical ethics and managed care has resulted in a number of well-publicized collisions, if not a head-on crash, between the two. The reason the two have collided has largely been their different perspectives of the moral universe and the social good. Medical ethics, undoubtedly influenced by the civil rights and consumer rights movements, has placed great emphasis on patient autonomy—the notion that each patient has a right to be treated with respect and dignity as well as to make all decisions related to her healthcare (the goal being an "optimal outcome" as defined by the fully informed individual patient). Thus, the focus has been on the primacy of the individual patient and physicians' responsibility to be advocates for their individual patients.

Managed care, on the other hand, has clearly concerned itself with not only the health of individual patients but also the collective health of a defined population—namely, the MCO's membership or so-called medical commons. The question of what should take precedence in the physician's mind—the individual patient or the collective medical commons—is at the crux of many disagreements between physicians and MCO managers. These often-wrenching ethical dilemmas have been complicated by the addition of still another element into the equation—the fact that the majority of MCOs are now of the for-profit variety, with a fiduciary responsibility to their shareholders.

Some have proposed that the potential for conflict among these various constituencies (individual patients, the medical commons, and shareholders) make the for-profit MCO model so ethically suspect as to have no rightful place in the US healthcare system. Others, meanwhile, contend that the currently dominant for-profit model is the most realistic and efficient means of achieving one of managed care's most overarching goals—that is, some semblance of ongoing control over the nation's healthcare costs.

While this debate rages on, physicians and managers in the managed care setting continue to face ethical challenges in their day-to-day work lives. This chapter sorts out some of these commonly faced ethical dilemmas and offers useful and practical guidelines for both physicians and managers. It also aims to provide both physicians and managers with some appreciation of the issues faced by their counterparts and to help each group gain a better understanding of the other's thinking and perspective.

This chapter will address seven questions:

1. What are the relevant principles of medical ethics?
2. What are the relevant principles of business ethics?
3. What ethics issues are commonly faced by physicians practicing in a managed care setting?
4. What ethics issues are commonly faced by managers in the managed care setting?
5. What are the legal ramifications for both physicians and managers in the managed care setting?
6. What ethical guidelines can be offered to physicians practicing in a managed care setting?
7. What ethical guidelines can be offered to managers in the managed care setting?

RELEVANT PRINCIPLES OF MEDICAL ETHICS

The task of medical ethics is to analyze and optimally resolve ethical dilemmas that arise in medical practice and biomedical research. Medical ethics is not a static, rigid entity; on the contrary, disagreements among acknowledged experts are common. Much of medical ethics has concerned itself with end-of-life issues and medical decision making in the case of incapacitated patients. Focusing on the issue at hand, however, the following six principles of medical ethics have special relevance to managed care:

1. **Autonomy.** Autonomy refers to (1) a person's right to be fully informed of all pertinent information related to his healthcare and (2) a person's additional right, after being so informed, to choose among or to refuse the available treatment options. Autonomy also implies a respect for the dignity and intrinsic worth of each individual person.
2. **Beneficence.** Beneficence is the commitment to "do good." It usually refers to the physician's obligation to work for optimal health outcomes for individual patients (although what constitutes an "optimal outcome" in a given situation is a decision that the competent, informed patient will help the physician determine).
3. **Nonmaleficence.** The flip side of beneficence is nonmaleficence—the commitment to "do no harm."
4. **Fidelity.** Fidelity is the notion that the physician should be faithful and loyal to the individual patient. It also implies that the physician will, if necessary, subordinate her own interests to serve the patient's interests.
5. **Veracity.** Veracity, or truth telling, refers to the physician's responsibility to be truthful to the individual patient, avoiding deception and disclosing to the patient all information relevant to the patient's health.
6. **Justice.** In the realm of healthcare, justice implies that all patients should be treated fairly, without regard to their race, ethnic background, socioeconomic status, or educational level. *Distributive justice* refers to the related notion that the allocation of limited healthcare resources should be determined on a fair and equitable basis.

All of these principles represent values that most thoughtful members of society would regard as worthwhile. However, even a brief consideration of the principles reveals how two or more of them could easily come into conflict and how two ethically astute physicians might differ in their viewpoints. For example, although practicing physicians typically think in terms of their responsibility to individual patients (including honoring the autonomy of individual patients), a public health physician entrusted to ensure the well-being of a wider community would be more likely to view distributive justice as an overriding ethical principle. The difference in perspective between the practicing physician and the public health physician reflects, in large measure, the parties that each regards as the major stakeholders affected by his decisions. In the case of the practicing physician, the major stakeholders are the individual patients the physician sees on a day-to-day basis. For the public health physician, the major stakeholders are the members of the community as a whole. In the real world of medical practice, ethical principles thus commonly come into conflict, with one's perspective typically determining which ethical principle one views as paramount in a given situation. The same situation is true whether the different perspectives are held by two physicians or a physician and a managed care executive.

RELEVANT PRINCIPLES OF BUSINESS ETHICS

Like medical ethics, business ethics is an example of what has been termed *applied ethics*—that is, ethics applied to a specific profession or occupation. Also like medical ethics, business ethics is a dynamic field where disagreement among acknowledged experts is commonplace. This disagreement may even extend to fundamental issues, such as what the goal of a business should be.

Many would contend that the obvious goal of any business enterprise is to be as financially successful as possible. Assuming the business enterprise is a publicly traded company, a related goal would be to maximize profits for shareholders. Under this model, the guiding ethical principle for corporate leadership would be, first and foremost, to reward its investors—those who have risked their own capital in the company's interest. To take this line of reasoning one step further, any deviation from the investor-first principle might well be viewed as unethical, especially if it ran contrary to what shareholders were led to believe.

Others would contend, however, that investors represent only one group of stakeholders that the corporate leadership needs to consider when making decisions. In this view (the second model), the needs of other stakeholders are also a rightful part of the equation. Such non-investor stakeholders include consumers, business partners, and employees. This so-called stakeholder model of business ethics is obviously more complex than the investor-first model and is one that many US businesses are now espousing.

In a third model, the corporate leadership might decide that the business enterprise should take on the additional role of enhancing the social good and allocate a percentage of its resources for that purpose. A number of US companies have followed this route, although they are hardly in the majority.

The three models described above illustrate the wide spectrum of thinking in business ethics. A major question in managed care, especially the for-profit model of managed care, has been whether healthcare should be considered just another business. The Woodstock Theological Center, a nonprofit research institute, convened a diverse group of executives, healthcare professionals, and ethicists to develop a consensus statement of ethical principles pertinent to the business aspects of healthcare. The Woodstock participants formulated the following six core principles (Woodstock Theological Center 1995):

1. **Compassion and respect for human dignity.** The Woodstock group affirmed that patient care is the primary goal and responsibility of healthcare enterprises. Furthermore, the group declared it would be unethical for healthcare providers to exploit the vulnerability of patients to enhance the organization's or a professional's income or profits.
2. **Commitment to professional competence.** All healthcare professionals, including physicians, nurses, and healthcare executives, have an ethical duty to continue their educational efforts and enhance their competence.
3. **Commitment to a spirit of service.** Healthcare professionals have a responsibility both to the community they serve and to individual patients. This responsibility extends to providing uncompensated or undercompensated care to the poor and needy.
4. **Honesty.** Healthcare professionals and executives have a responsibility to be truthful in their interactions, including their interactions with each other and with patients and families. Medical records should also reflect this commitment to truthfulness and accuracy.
5. **Confidentiality.** Information pertaining to the patient should be shared only with the express permission of the patient or legal guardian, except as required by law.
6. **Good stewardship and careful administration.** Healthcare professionals have an obligation to use health resources wisely, carefully weighing the relative costs and benefits of the available treatment options.

The similarities between the principles of medical ethics listed earlier and the Woodstock compendium of ethical principles for those in the business of healthcare are noteworthy but not surprising. "Compassion and respect for human dignity," for example, clearly resonates with the principles of patient autonomy, beneficence, and nonmaleficence. In addition, the principles of "commitment to a spirit of service" and "good stewardship and careful administration" both relate to the notion of distributive justice. Finally, the potential for conflict between several of the principles of medical ethics cited previously mirrors a similar potential for conflict in the Woodstock group's core principles. In the setting of limited healthcare resources and market competition, for example, can the "provision of uncompensated or undercompensated healthcare to the poor and needy" realistically coexist with "good stewardship and careful administration"?

ETHICS ISSUES FACED BY PHYSICIANS PRACTICING IN THE MANAGED CARE SETTING

Before examining ethical dilemmas faced by physicians in the setting of managed care, a brief discussion of ethics issues faced by physicians in the pre–managed care (fee-for-service) era might be beneficial. Otherwise, the reader might get the erroneous impression that ethical dilemmas for physicians only arose when managed care came on the scene.

As its name implies, in the fee-for-service model of healthcare delivery, physicians were paid a specific fee for performing a specific service, whether that service was an annual physical examination or bypass surgery. Although some older physicians might hearken back to the fee-for-service era as "the good old days," it was not free of ethical quandaries. For example, distributive justice was a major (if perhaps inadequately considered) problem, as the indigent and uninsured frequently could not afford the physician's fee and, except for charity care, were essentially shut out of the system. In addition, the physician's fidelity to the patient may sometimes have been compromised in a system where physicians were financially rewarded for providing services that might have been of questionable or only marginal benefit to the patient. Physicians' veracity (truth telling) may also have been less than optimal in the fee-for-service system if, for example, the physician just happened to be a part owner of the laboratory to which patients were referred for tests. Finally, in retrospect, nonmaleficence (the obligation to do no harm) may not have been observed as much as one would hope; one wonders how many patients in the fee-for-service system were ultimately harmed by procedures that were recommended for questionable or marginal reasons by physicians and surgeons who benefited financially from performing as many of those procedures as possible.

Unfortunately, ethical dilemmas for physicians appear to be no less common (and some would argue are even more common) in the setting of managed care. Many of these ethical quandaries are related to one fundamental question: In the managed care system, where should the physician's loyalty ultimately lie—with the individual patient, the medical commons, or the MCO itself? This fundamental question branches out into a number of others:

- Should the physician engage in the rationing of healthcare at the bedside of an individual patient?
- How should the physician respond when she believes that the patient requires the specific expertise of a consultant not on the MCO's panel of consultants?
- Under what circumstances should the physician prescribe medications not on the MCO's formulary, medications that might well be more expensive than those listed on the MCO's formulary?

- How much information related to diagnostic and therapeutic options should the physician disclose to the patient?
- How forcefully should the physician "fight" the MCO when the MCO makes a patient care–related decision with which the physician disagrees?

Rationing Care at the Bedside

A topic of ongoing—and often heated—discussion among medical ethicists is whether physicians should ration care at the bedside of an individual patient. Some would argue that a "new ethic" requires that the physician's level of concern about the medical commons be so pervasive as to influence the physician's recommendations to individual patients. Others, however, contend that to act in this manner undermines the very foundation of the patient–physician relationship—that is, the patient's expectation that the physician is the patient's advocate, recommending those diagnostic studies and therapeutic interventions that the physician believes are in the patient's best interest. After all, how can the patient trust the physician to give her proper care if he is primarily thinking about the welfare of the medical commons? One view is that physicians should not engage in rationing healthcare at the bedside of individual patients because it violates the physician's ethical responsibility of fidelity, an ethical responsibility that patients have rightfully come to regard as an underlying premise of the entire patient–physician relationship.

However, physicians should acknowledge the reality that healthcare resources are finite. Physicians can reasonably do this in at least three ways without violating the trust their individual patients have placed in them. First, physicians need to recognize that there is no ethical obligation to provide clearly useless or futile care, whether it is prescribing antibiotics for a viral illness or extending the life of a terminally ill patient with prolonged ventilator care. Second, all things being equal, physicians should prescribe the least costly among effective therapies. Why choose a more expensive quinolone antibiotic for an uncomplicated urinary tract infection, for example, when the inexpensive antibiotic trimethoprim-sulfamethoxazole will treat the infection just as well? Finally, the question of how best to enhance the well-being of the medical commons in an environment of limited healthcare resources is clearly a profound and entirely legitimate concern. This issue, and the related matter of priority setting, should be addressed in an ongoing, transparent, and careful manner at the MCO's highest policy-making level, with thoughtful input from physicians as well as from the MCO's membership.

Choice of Consultants

A common question that arises for primary care physicians in the managed care setting is whether a specialty consultant on the MCO's panel is the optimal consultant for a given patient's clinical condition. The following two cases illustrate such issues in everyday practice.

Case 1:
A 50-year-old MCO patient with an inguinal (groin) hernia asked his primary care physician to refer him to a surgeon in Canada who he heard had developed a new technique for hernia surgery.

Case 2:
A 74-year-old MCO patient with hearing loss and vertigo was diagnosed as having an acoustic neuroma, a relatively rare tumor of the acoustic (ear) nerve. Even though the MCO had contracted with a local neurosurgeon to handle all of the plan's neurosurgical procedures, the MCO's consulting neurologist advised the primary care physician to refer the patient to a nearby tertiary care medical center because the center had much more experience with the required neurosurgical procedure.

In Case 1, the primary care physician did not agree to the patient's request to be referred to the surgeon in Canada because the physician knew that the MCO's general surgeon was experienced in performing herniorrhaphy (hernia surgery) and that a high-quality outcome could be anticipated if the MCO's surgeon performed the operation.

In Case 2, however, the physician decided to refer the patient to the tertiary care center for the more specialized type of operation the patient needed. The MCO did not approve this referral at first, but after a series of appeals by the patient, the primary care physician, and the consulting neurologist consultant (and after the patient informed the MCO that he had hired an attorney to ensure his interests were safeguarded), the MCO reversed its initial decision. The patient subsequently underwent successful surgery at the tertiary care center.

If the physician has good reason to believe that the patient requires special expertise for appropriate care management, then the physician has an obligation to pursue the necessary out-of-plan referral with the MCO's administration.

Non-Formulary Prescriptions

In many respects, the issue of prescribing non-formulary medications is analogous to the situation just discussed—namely, referring the patient to a consultant not on the MCO panel. If the physician is convinced that a non-formulary drug is superior to its counterpart on the MCO's formulary, then the physician should serve as the patient's advocate and prescribe the non-formulary medication, explaining to the MCO's pharmacists and administration why he made that choice. In addition, physicians should work with the MCO's pharmacy committee to modify the MCO's formulary when they believe such action is in the best interest of patient care.

Disclosure of Information

Physicians should adhere to the ethical principle of veracity (truth telling), disclosing to the patient all information pertinent to the patient's care. This information includes all relevant diagnostic and therapeutic options, especially because an informed healthcare decision on the patient's part would be impossible if such information were withheld. Physicians should also disclose to the patient all relevant financial arrangements between themselves and the MCO (see below) because patients have a right to know about possible conflicts of interest, especially if such conflicts of interest could affect the care they receive.

In addition to their obligation to communicate in a truthful manner with patients and families, physicians also have an obligation to communicate truthfully with MCOs. Physicians should not try to "game the system" by providing MCOs with inaccurate or incomplete information, even when their rationale for doing so is to assist the patient in obtaining MCO approval for requested consultations, prescriptions, or other services.

Challenging the MCO's Decisions

Several of the scenarios mentioned can place the physician in the position of challenging decisions that the MCO makes. Without a doubt, this position can be uncomfortable for the physician—that is, being between the "rock" of fulfilling one's ethical responsibilities to the patient and the "hard place" of a potentially adversarial relationship with the MCO. The latter possibility is hardly a trivial issue. If the physician is a salaried employee of a staff model MCO, for example, the MCO could conceivably fire him for "not being a team player." In the more common situation, where the physician enters into contracts with a number of MCOs to ensure an adequate volume of patients, the MCO could decide to terminate its contract with him. Depending on the precise wording of the MCO–physician contract, such termination (known in the trade as "deselection") can often be accomplished with minimal notice and without explanation or due process. Physicians routinely walk a tightrope in the managed care setting, one that might cause them to be less than forceful in their patient advocacy role.

Financial Incentives and Disincentives

In addition to the threat of deselection, MCOs use another instrument to influence physician behavior. Most MCO–physician contracts feature clauses outlining financial incentives, financial disincentives, or both. Financial incentives and disincentives are meant to engage the physician (or physician group) more actively in the MCO's cost-containment efforts by using a "carrot or stick" approach. Successful cost-containment efforts over the contractual term will result in the physician (or physician group) receiving a monetary bonus, whereas incurring excessive patient costs will result in money being withheld (usually in escrow). If financial incentives and disincentives are modest or are based on the performance of a sizable group of physicians, physicians will likely not be influenced by these arrangements when caring for individual patients. When the financial incentive or disincentive is significant and based on the performance of an individual physician or a small group of physicians, however, the physician's financial interest may be pitted against the patient's interest in a direct and disturbing way, raising the suspicion, if not the reality, of physician misbehavior if the patient believes that her care is somehow being compromised.

Pay for Performance

Over the past decade, the term *pay for performance* (P4P) has been used increasingly by healthcare policy analysts and in the medical literature (Doran et al. 2006; Ryan and Blustein 2012). As the phrase suggests, P4P involves a financial incentive for assiduously following a set of recommended clinical guidelines or, even better, achieving optimal patient outcomes. P4P can be applied either at the macro level (to hospitals or groups of physicians) or at the micro level (to individual physicians). At the time of this writing, the published evidence is as yet inconclusive as to whether P4P actually leads to improvement in the quality of healthcare delivered. A number of ethics issues have also been raised about P4P, especially as it pertains to individual physicians and so-called targeted outcomes (e.g., average level of blood sugar control in a physician's panel of patients with diabetes). For example, will a physician's MCO profile be enhanced (and a financial incentive gained) if she "fires" sicker or more challenging patients—the very patients, arguably, who need help the most?

ETHICS ISSUES FACED BY MCO MANAGERS

MCO executives also face a variety of ongoing ethical challenges. Some of these ethical dilemmas are similar to those faced by physicians, whereas others are different.

Persuasive Advertising and Selective Marketing

In the world of advertising, veracity is usually not uppermost in the minds of those who produce radio, television, or print media commercials. The entire point of advertising, after all, is to present the product in the best possible light, and if some less-than-flattering details are left out in the process, that is to be expected. Unfortunately, in the case of MCOs, deceptive advertising can result in the prospective MCO member being misled—for example, when an ad implies that MCO members can see whichever specialist they please. The primary care physician is left with the responsibility of educating the new MCO member on how the plan actually works, including the fact that the "gatekeeping" primary care physician first has to make specialty referrals and the MCO member is usually restricted to seeing those consultants on the MCO's panel.

An issue closely related to advertising is marketing. From a bottom-line business perspective, a younger, healthier member is preferable to an older, sicker one. Some MCOs have been known to direct their marketing efforts to effectively exclude those members of the community who are most frail or infirm—for example, by holding sign-ups for seniors at dances or movie screenings, events unlikely to be attended by the bedridden, the housebound, or those requiring walkers or wheelchairs. Such selective marketing aimed at attracting the healthiest (and least costly) prospective members is like "cherry picking." Although advertising that is less than fully truthful and marketing that is selective might be accepted behavior in most businesses, ethical healthcare organizations should refrain from engaging in such practices.

Disclosure of Information

Honesty should be the rule for MCOs not only when dealing with prospective members but also when dealing with those already enrolled in the plan. Patients have a right to be informed of all pertinent diagnostic and therapeutic options related to their healthcare and the right to be informed of all financial arrangements between the MCO and its physicians (including incentives and disincentives) that could potentially affect patient care. "Gag rules," where physicians are instructed to withhold such information from patients, should be prohibited.

Financial Incentives and Disincentives

For MCOs (and physicians) to simply disclose information pertaining to financial incentives and disincentives is not enough. From an ethical standpoint, such incentives and disincentives must be based on the performance of a sizable group of physicians and not be of such magnitude as to place the physician's personal financial interests in direct conflict with the interests of the individual patient under his care.

Ensuring Quality

Although each individual healthcare professional has a duty to maintain a high level of expertise and competence, the MCO is responsible for making sure that its members are receiving high-caliber medical care. From an organizational stand-point, quality care can be accomplished in several ways:

- Contracting only with well-trained and suitably credentialed primary care physicians and specialty consultants who are highly regarded in the local or regional medical community
- Working with physicians to establish diagnostic and therapeutic guidelines that are evidence based, especially for commonly encountered conditions
- Soliciting thoughtful physician and pharmacist input when developing the MCO's drug formulary, with a periodic review process so that the formulary can be kept up to date
- Providing performance-based feedback to physicians using a carefully conducted and accurate profiling system and soliciting physician input in the profiling process
- Using patient satisfaction measures as an additional means to evaluate physician performance

Appeal Procedures

Either patients or physicians, acting in good faith, may on occasion disagree with the MCO's decisions, especially those related to patient care issues. MCOs need to have a clearly outlined appeal procedure in place. This appeal protocol should be logi-cal, reasonable, and fair and should not be biased against individual patients. These qualities are especially important when questions arise as to whether a particular innovative or experimental therapy is covered by the MCO, because medicine is an ever-changing field. In addition, the MCO must clearly state that it will never act in a punitive fashion or take retribution against either patients or physicians who challenge the MCO's decisions or who otherwise participate in the appeal process.

Confidentiality

Like any other healthcare organization, MCOs need to have systems in place to carefully protect patient confidentiality. This includes adherence to the provisions of the Health Insurance Portability and Accountability Act.

Allocation of Resources

Because healthcare resources are finite and MCOs must remain economically competitive in a market economy, priorities in allocating healthcare resources need to be established. MCOs should make these allocation decisions in an open man-ner, with input from physicians and the MCO's members.

Fostering the Social Good

Because of the predominance of the for-profit MCO model, the US healthcare system has had difficulty financing several domains that may be considered under the general heading of the social good. These include (1) medical education and the training of future healthcare professionals; (2) biomedical research; and (3) the care of the uninsured, who currently number more than 45 million. What role should MCOs (including for-profit MCOs) play in addressing such social concerns? The responsibility of healthcare organizations to promote the social good is not merely an issue raised by "ivory tower" ethicists. The *Code of Ethics* of the American College of Healthcare Executives (ACHE 2011), for example, says that

> the healthcare executive shall work to identify and meet the healthcare needs of the community . . . support access to healthcare services for all people . . . [and] apply short- and long-term assessments to management decisions affecting both community and society.

LEGAL RAMIFICATIONS FOR PHYSICIANS AND MANAGERS IN THE MANAGED CARE SETTING

Ideally, ethical guidelines should suffice in causing physicians and MCO managers alike to do the right thing. However, inappropriate behavior sometimes crosses a line and becomes not only ethically suspect but also legally negligent.

A landmark and still very illustrative case in the annals of managed care case law is *Wickline v. California*. Ms. Wickline was admitted to a hospital in California in the late 1970s for a peripheral vascular procedure. Following that procedure, her physicians recommended an additional eight days in the hospital for post-procedure care and observation. Ms. Wickline's insurer was MediCal (California's Medicaid program), which denied her physicians' request for eight days of additional hospitalization, approving a four-day stay instead. At the end of four days, Ms. Wickline was discharged. She subsequently developed complications that necessitated readmission and eventual amputation of her leg. Ms. Wickline did not sue her physicians, whom she regarded as her advocates, but rather MediCal, whom she blamed for the abbreviated initial hospital stay. In a lower court, Ms. Wickline won her suit and was awarded several hundred thousand dollars. MediCal appealed that decision, however, and in a 1986 ruling the Appellate Court reversed the lower court's decision. The ruling of the Appellate Court was noteworthy in two respects (*Wickline v. California*, 226 Cal. Rptr. 661 [Cal. App. 2 Dist., 1986]):

> Third-party payers . . . can be held legally accountable when medically inappropriate decisions result from defects in the design or implementation of cost containment

mechanisms as, for example, when appeals made on a patient's behalf for medical . . . care are arbitrarily ignored or unreasonably disregarded or overridden.

However, a physician who complies without protest with the limitations imposed by a third-party payer, when his medical judgment dictates otherwise, cannot avoid his ultimate responsibility for his patient's care. He cannot point to the healthcare payer as the liability scapegoat when the consequences of his own . . . medical decisions go sour.

The first paragraph indicates that a third-party payer—whether an MCO or a government program such as Medicaid—could be sued if its cost-containment policy resulted in medical harm, especially if the treating physician's legitimate objections were arbitrarily ignored or overridden. The second paragraph is clearly aimed at physicians working in managed care settings and emphasizes that the physician's ultimate obligation is to the individual patient and not passive acceptance of the third-party payer's cost-containment policies.

Since *Wickline v. California*, a number of other cases (e.g., *Boyd v. Epstein, Hand v. Tavera, Fox v. Health Net of California*) have involved the legal liability of physicians in the managed care setting or the legal liability of MCOs (Gosfield 1995; Moskowitz 1998). Although each of these cases is different from *Wickline v. California*, the common theme is that adverse patient outcomes resulting from cost-containment policies can place both the physician and the MCO at legal risk. MCO executives also need to be aware of yet another case, *McClellan v. Health Maintenance Organization of Pennsylvania*, in which the court ruled that the MCO in question had an obligation to select and retain only competent physicians.

Notably, despite the cases cited here, MCOs have been relatively protected from lawsuits in state courts for medical negligence because of the 1974 Employment Retirement Income Security Act (ERISA). The purpose of ERISA was to prohibit state regulation of employee pension plans and other employee benefit plans, including health benefit plans. Because most Americans in MCOs are enrolled through their employer, ERISA has effectively barred most MCO enrollees from suing their MCO for medical negligence in state courts (although it has not prevented patients from suing their MCO physicians in state courts). In their decisions in the 2000 case of *Pegram v. Herdrich* and the 2004 cases of *Aetna Health Inc. v. Davila* and *Cigna Healthcare of Texas Inc. v. Calad*, the US Supreme Court ruled to uphold ERISA, continuing MCOs' immunity from medical liability, at least in many of the situations commonly encountered. The issue of whether ERISA should be overturned or amended remains the subject of ongoing and intense political debate. ERISA's future will likely be decided in Congress, with the eventual outcome still uncertain.

ETHICAL GUIDELINES FOR PHYSICIANS PRACTICING IN THE MANAGED CARE SETTING

Physicians practicing in the managed care setting should consider the following recommendations:

- The physician–patient relationship is the cornerstone of the practice of medicine, and physicians should view their primary obligation as the provision of humane, high-quality care to their individual patients.
- Physicians are not obligated to provide care that is clearly useless. In addition, physicians have a responsibility to choose among the least costly of effective therapies.
- Any decisions regarding the allocation of healthcare resources should be made on a broad, policy-making level and not at the bedside of individual patients. Physicians have a responsibility to participate in these resource allocation decisions, bearing in mind the ethical principle of distributive justice.
- Physicians should be truthful in their dealings with patients and families. All information that might affect patient care should be disclosed, including (1) relevant diagnostic and therapeutic options and (2) all physician–MCO financial relationships that might affect patient care.
- Physicians should be truthful in their dealings with MCO management and refrain from attempts to game the system.
- Any financial incentives and disincentives should be limited in magnitude and should ideally be based on the performance of a sizable group of physicians rather than that of a single physician or a small group of physicians. The physician's personal interests should never result in the withholding of care that is medically necessary or medically advisable.
- Physicians have an obligation to maintain their professional competence and seek appropriate consultation for patient care issues outside their realm of expertise.
- Physicians should serve as advocates for a system of healthcare that (1) is based on humaneness, high-quality care, and optimal outcomes for patients and (2) does not place restrictions on access to medical care that is necessary or advisable.

ETHICAL GUIDELINES FOR MCO MANAGERS

In many respects, recommendations for MCO managers parallel those made for MCO physicians. For example, recommendations regarding truth telling, the fair and equitable allocation of healthcare resources, and the need for limited financial incentives and disincentives are germane to both physicians and MCO executives. Additional recommendations for MCO managers include the following:

- Refrain from engaging in misleading advertising or selective marketing, no matter how great the temptation.
- Establish and maintain systems within the MCO that aim to protect patient confidentiality.
- Ensure high-quality patient care by (1) selecting and retaining only high-caliber healthcare professionals, (2) working with physicians to establish diagnostic and therapeutics guidelines that are evidence based, and (3) providing performance-based feedback to physicians that is meaningful and accurate.
- Establish appeal procedures that are fair and free of punitive overtones.
- Consider carefully how the organization might contribute to the social good, including medical education, medical research, and care of the indigent or uninsured.

A BLUEPRINT FOR THE FUTURE: THE TAVISTOCK PRINCIPLES

Although this chapter's ethical recommendations to physicians and those to MCO managers overlap considerably, the current perception is that each constituency in the healthcare universe (physicians, MCO executives, or others) tends to view healthcare issues through its own particular lens, often hampering meaningful discussion and interdisciplinary cooperation.

In 1999, a group of interested parties, including physicians, nurses, healthcare executives, economists, and ethicists, convened to develop a set of mutually agreed-on ethical principles. Called the Tavistock Group because they initially met near Tavistock Square in London, these parties proposed the following seven principles (Davidoff 2000):

1. **Rights.** People have a right to health and healthcare.
2. **Balance.** Care of individual patients is central, but the health of populations should also be our concern.
3. **Comprehensiveness.** In addition to treating illness, we have an obligation to ease suffering, minimize disability, prevent disease, and promote health.
4. **Cooperation.** Healthcare succeeds only if we cooperate with those we serve, with each other, and with those in other sectors.
5. **Improvement.** Improving healthcare is a serious and continuing responsibility.

6. **Safety.** Do no harm.
7. **Openness.** Being open, honest, and trustworthy is vital in healthcare.

The Tavistock principles are similar in spirit to the principles outlined by the Woodstock group nearly a decade earlier. The tone of shared values and productive cooperation embodied in both sets of principles might one day replace the rancor and divisiveness that has all too often characterized discussion of the US healthcare system over the past few decades. Only time will tell if the for-profit MCO model will be able to adhere to these principles while simultaneously generating the level of profits that investors in other businesses typically expect. The passage of the Patient Protection and Affordable Care Act and the political controversy surrounding it have introduced an additional measure of uncertainty to the current US healthcare system. However, no matter what model of healthcare delivery prevails in the future, healthcare professionals of all stripes and at every level must make sure that the ethical underpinnings of patient care are honored.

REFERENCES

American College of Healthcare Executives (ACHE). 2011. *Code of Ethics.* Updated November 14. www.ache.org/abt_ache/code.cfm#patients.

Davidoff, F. 2000. "Changing the Subject: Ethical Principles for Everyone in Healthcare." *Annals of Internal Medicine* 133 (5): 386–89.

Doran, T., C. Fullwood, H. Gravelle, D. Reeves, E. Kontopantelis, U. Hiroeh, and M. Roland. 2006. "Pay-for-Performance Programs in Family Practices in the United Kingdom." *New England Journal of Medicine* 355 (4): 375–84.

Gosfield, A. G. 1995. "The Legal Subtext of the Managed Care Environment: A Practitioner's Perspective." *Journal of Law, Medicine & Ethics* 23 (3): 230–35.

Moskowitz, E. H. 1998. "Medical Responsibility and Legal Liability in Managed Care." *Journal of the American Geriatrics Society* 46 (3): 373–77.

Ryan, A., and J. Blustein. 2012. "Making the Best of Hospital Pay for Performance." *New England Journal of Medicine* 366 (17) 1557–59.

Woodstock Theological Center. 1995. *Ethical Considerations for the Business Aspects of Healthcare.* Washington, DC: Georgetown University Press.

CHAPTER 16

Evaluating Healthcare Ethics Committees

Rebecca A. Dobbs

THE HEALTHCARE SYSTEM in the United States continues to undergo radical changes in its structure, delivery and financing of services, and role in society. The current environment is characterized by an increased awareness of patient rights and responsibilities, increased treatment options, significant advances in biomedical technology, higher costs, and the powerful influence of insurers in healthcare delivery and decision making. The era is characterized by broad changes in not only the mechanics of healthcare delivery and financing but social values and public expectations as well. Newly raised ethical concerns stemming from resource allocation issues (e.g., rationing of care), scientific and technological advancements (e.g., human genetics), moral duplicity (e.g., assisted suicide), evolving financial arrangements (e.g., conflicts of interest, the Patient Protection and Affordable Care Act), and increased attention to quality and accountability (e.g., new quality measures and performance standards from the Centers for Medicare & Medicaid Services) pose new challenges for healthcare institutions and professionals.

In March 2010, the Patient Protection and Affordable Care Act and its amendment, the Health Care and Education Reconciliation Act, were signed into law, further affecting healthcare reform in federal and state programs (e.g., Medicare and Medicaid). Healthcare organizations will be challenged to transform into entities that provide high-quality care and services to a growing population amid increasing fiscal constraints. These challenges underscore the importance of a formalized, comprehensive ethics program to deal with an ever-changing healthcare delivery system, evolving societal expectations, and their effect on professional behavior.

Many healthcare organizations have already recognized the need for a comprehensive ethics program—one that goes beyond a mechanism for merely dealing with ethical concerns that arise in patient care. Historically, such programs have taken a variety of forms. Some healthcare organizations have chosen to use individual ethics consultants or bioethicists, some have written extensive ethics policies and procedures to be carried out by existing organizational committees or entities, and still others have formed ethics committees dedicated to the task of dealing with ethics issues as they arise. Some organizations have created positions for ethics officers or compliance officers to monitor the organizations' adherence to ethical standards.

Few organizations, however, have ventured into the realm of a fully integrated healthcare ethics program—one that monitors the ethical climate of the organization, proactively addresses potential ethics issues, aggressively manages ethical discourse in both the clinical and the organizational context, critically evaluates its overall effectiveness, and takes action to change the organization's ethical culture and processes. Efforts to create an integrated ethics program so far have primarily entailed the merging of existing organizational areas (e.g., compliance, accreditation, quality assurance, risk management, clinical ethics) under a single organizational title. Until a fully integrated healthcare ethics program matures enough to meet the growing ethical needs of healthcare organizations, the healthcare ethics committee (HEC) remains the primary vehicle for fielding ethics issues in healthcare organizations.

Historically, HECs have been acute care oriented but are increasingly being presented with primary care and outpatient issues that further blur the distinction between bedside (clinical) and boardroom (organizational) ethics. Hence, HECs may be called on to respond to an increasing number of organizational ethics concerns that cannot be disentangled from purely clinical ones.

HECs are powerful influences in healthcare decision making. Although formalized requirements for performance assessment and improvement have not been extended to HEC functions and processes, and no widely publicized or accepted performance standards exist to guide HEC activities, an increased level of scrutiny and accountability with respect to HEC composition, management, and functions can still be expected.

HEC FUNCTIONS

The work of HECs consists of three main functions: education, policy development, and case consultation.

Education

The ethics education function serves three principal audiences: the ethics committee itself, the organization's staff, and the community at large. Education of ethics committee members is widely accepted as a priority. Educational initiatives frequently focus on medicolegal issues, ethical theories and principles, the application of these theories and principles to ethics policy development and ethics review and consultation, committee functions and obligations, group processes, and communication skills. Educational goals may vary depending on the HEC's mission and objectives, committee member needs, organizational setting, and available resources. Ethics education provided in the organization frequently focuses on improving staff's understanding of general bioethical and medicolegal issues as they relate to medical treatment and patient care activities. Topics often include current issues in bioethics and the organization's institutional policies and procedures. Community education efforts focus on stakeholders that exist beyond the confines of institutional boundaries. Educational needs in the community can be addressed by providing local workshops on selected topics, conducting focus groups designed to share information and solicit input for policy development and revision, working with university faculty on curriculum development, working with legislators to develop new legislation, and testifying before legislative bodies. The success of community education depends largely on adequately identifying the needs and interests of the target audience and planning educational opportunities accordingly (Ross et al. 1993).

Policy Development

The second HEC function encompasses those committee activities related to the development, implementation, review, revision, and compliance assessment of ethics policies and guidelines. *Ethics policies* establish standards or define ethical boundaries within which specific activities must occur, whereas *ethics guidelines* are more flexible and less prescriptive by suggesting options in or alternatives to a given ethical situation. The level of HEC involvement in this function varies among healthcare organizations. Some HECs are directly involved in ethics policy/guideline activities, whereas others take on a more consultative role. Most HECs write policies and guidelines on well-documented topics for which broad societal consensus exists, but some HECs are venturing out into relatively uncharted waters by developing policies and guidelines on clinical issues such as organ transplant recipient criteria and organizational issues such as resource allocation during public health emergencies and disasters. The degree of HEC involvement in ethics policy development is determined largely by organizational culture, the composition and maturity of the committee, and its role in the organization and community.

Case Consultation

Ethics reviews and consultations are performed primarily to assist healthcare professionals, patients, and families or surrogates in sorting out treatment options, making informed decisions, or resolving conflicts. An *ethics review* is generally performed retrospectively to analyze a situation about which an ethical concern or issue has been raised. An ethics review can have a positive effect on future situations presenting a similar issue, but its timing prevents it from having any effect on the situation being studied. An ethics review can also be performed proactively in a hypothetical setting, an exercise that can help HECs and organizations work through ethical dilemmas before they occur. The ethics review can also provide useful inputs to the development, review, and revision of ethics policies and guidelines. An *ethics consultation,* on the other hand, generally refers to the analysis of a current ethical concern or issue by the parties involved to resolve the ethical dilemma. An ethics consultation can be performed by the whole committee, a consultation team, or an individual committee member or consultant (Ross et al. 1993).

An HEC can choose from among a variety of models (medical, legal, or educational) to guide an ethics review or consultation. The *medical model* emphasizes the medical expertise of physicians, nurses, and usually a chaplain in addressing clinical matters. The *legal model* treats the ethics review or consultation as a type of hearing, in which input is sought from the parties involved and attention is given to issues of due process. The *educational model* employs a multidisciplinary approach to explore the various ethical dimensions of a given situation. Selection of an appropriate model for an ethics review or consultation is based largely on the specific ethics issue and the special concerns of those involved (Ross et al. 1993).

Administration and Management

To the three widely accepted HEC functions, Dobbs (2000) added a fourth function—HEC administration and management. This function addresses activities related to infrastructure, strategic planning, the committee's composition and role in the organization, committee membership criteria, resource allocation, and performance evaluation. HECs across the country vary greatly in mission, structure, role in the organization, scope of activities performed, and formality of internal processes. Little has been written in the literature regarding HEC administration and management. Thus, HEC administration and management likely remains one of the most widely varied of the recognized HEC functions. Despite the scarcity of published data on evaluation strategies or performance standards and criteria, the need for HEC evaluation is necessary, in part, to enhance HEC credibility and to justify the commitment of increasingly scarce institutional resources. Information obtained from the HEC evaluation process can be used to

1. identify areas for improvement,
2. prioritize improvement activities,

3. assist in the strategic planning process,
4. plan resource requirements,
5. provide baseline data for future evaluation and benchmarking activities, and
6. document activities for internal management reviews and external accreditation surveys.

HEC EVALUATION STRATEGIES

Although many agree that critical evaluation of HEC processes demonstrates an organization's commitment to quality healthcare and attention to societal needs and concerns, no consensus has yet been reached about which approach is most suitable for conducting such an evaluation. Evaluation strategies commonly used to assess healthcare functions or programs include program evaluation, internal evaluation, and self-assessment. *Program evaluation* provides a highly structured analysis of program elements and activities by an external source. *Internal evaluation* provides an organizational perspective of a program's interrelated components and functions as measured by other members in the organization. *Self-assessment* provides an intimate evaluation of a program by those who are directly responsible for its planning, execution, and management.

Program Evaluation

Program evaluation is a process for determining the value or effectiveness of a program or program elements. It is typically classified as formative (process oriented) or summative (outcome oriented), depending on the type of information produced and how that information is used.

Formative evaluation assesses the process by which the program conducts its activities and is designed to improve the program and its management. A formative approach has certain advantages: (1) practitioners can develop performance standards and assessment criteria relatively easily, and (2) even when not fully validated, the standards and criteria can serve as interim measures of acceptable performance. The main disadvantage to a formative approach is that it may actually encourage dogmatism and perpetuate potential errors in what is determined to be acceptable performance (Donabedian 1980).

Summative evaluation focuses on the long-term effects of a program—its end product, how well it is functioning, and whether it has had any effect on given performance indicators. A summative approach also has certain advantages: it (1) discourages dogmatism, (2) reflects the contributions of all practitioners, and (3) provides a more direct assessment of the practitioner–customer relationship when customer satisfaction measures are included. Disadvantages of the summative approach include (1) the difficulty practitioners experience in specifying outcomes of optimal performance, (2) the ethics issue associated with waiting for adverse outcome trends to emerge before taking action, and (3) the challenge of drawing pertinent conclusions when outcomes are assessed without evaluating the related processes (Donabedian 1980).

Program evaluation is an integrated process of collecting and analyzing data using various scientific methods to determine the relevance, progress, efficiency, effectiveness, and impact of program activities. Five approaches to program evaluation are widely accepted: monitoring, case studies, survey research, trend analysis, and experimental design.

1. *Monitoring* is concerned with program progress and improvement and involves the comparison of program expectations with actual results. Even though monitoring may be viewed as mundane or nonscientific, it is particularly important for formative evaluation and critical to the evaluation of progress and continuous improvement.

2. *Case studies* rely more on the ingenuity, insight, and experience of the researcher than other evaluation strategies using more rigorous methods such as sampling and statistical techniques. Even though they are primarily qualitative in nature, case studies frequently employ a variety of quantitative data collection and analysis techniques.

3. *Survey research* has become a common evaluation strategy, particularly in the summative evaluation of programs, and is primarily either descriptive or analytic in nature. Descriptive surveys are used to produce an accurate depiction of the phenomenon being studied by describing a problem that requires some type of program activity, describing the program from the perspective of providers or participants, or describing the program's results from the perspective of the providers or participants. Analytic surveys are used to describe relationships between different aspects of the phenomenon by determining whether program participants who have different characteristics view a program more or less favorably or by determining whether the program has some differential effect on participants who have certain characteristics.

4. *Trend analysis* is an evaluation strategy for examining tendencies in performance indicators over time. It can be done in conjunction with monitoring to determine whether the introduction of a particular program has a causal connection to changes in the condition that the program was established to influence.

5. *Experimental design* is the most powerful program evaluation approach. It can be a complex undertaking even though the basic pattern is relatively simple: The state of a system is observed at a given point in time, an experimental

variable is introduced, and the state of the system is observed again to determine the effect of the variable on the system. Some experimental designs may be too complex for healthcare settings. However, designs that appear to be feasible and appropriate include pretest and posttest, pretest and posttest with a control or comparison group, multiple group pretest and posttest, and posttest only.

The selection of an evaluation approach does not dictate the use of the formative approach or the summative approach exclusively. Rather, a well-designed program evaluation may require a combination of approaches reflecting the nature of the information to be obtained and other requirements of the situation.

Internal Evaluation

Another evaluation strategy applicable to healthcare settings is internal evaluation. Performed by members of the group or organization under study, internal evaluation examines the organization as a set of interrelated components and functions. Data obtained from internal evaluation activities can assist the healthcare organization in

- preparing for compliance or accreditation reviews,
- meeting internal or external reporting requirements,
- identifying and documenting client or customer needs,
- describing programs and services,
- identifying program strengths and weaknesses,
- establishing program priorities,
- planning budgets,
- obtaining and maintaining financial support, and
- relating to external customer groups.

Self-Assessment

Social values in the current climate call for interdisciplinary team building, trust, responsibility, and accountability in healthcare organizations. Self-assessment is a process by which a healthcare organization or an entity within the organization evaluates itself to systematically monitor performance against established standards. Self-assessment may be used to evaluate compliance, effectiveness, or performance. Compliance self-assessments are generally performed on a routine, periodic basis in anticipation of an upcoming external evaluation such as an accreditation review or licensing board visit. Effectiveness self-assessments are often performed to identify system improvement opportunities. Performance self-assessments are differentiated from the other two by their direct observation and evaluation of a process or an activity. Even though a self-assessment may provide the organization with information about its strengths and weaknesses, it does not render a prioritization of improvement actions. The organization needs to review and prioritize improvement actions on the basis of its mission, goals and objectives, resources, and desired level of performance.

The primary steps of the self-assessment process are

- setting recognized standards,
- rating the standards,
- making changes necessary to satisfy the standards, and
- confirming achievement of the standards by external evaluators.

Self-assessment provides a snapshot of how well the organization meets stated requirements, establishes methods of program delivery that meet high professional standards, and monitors the quality of its services. Standards are written statements or conditions that specify performance expectations. Selection of standards for assessing HEC performance is an important, but often difficult, decision that an organization must make. Performance standards fall into three categories: outcome, process, and structure (Donabedian 1980).

1. **Outcome standards.** Outcome standards measure specific characteristics of services that an organization provides, define both desirable and undesirable results, and can be used to benchmark performance. Even though outcomes are the typical indicators of organizational effectiveness, they can present problems in interpretation. For example, outcomes reflect not only work performance but also the application of technology and other characteristics of the organization's internal and external environments. Thus, knowledge about causes and effects is relatively complete only when the organization can control its environment. In the case of healthcare ethics outcomes, many factors beyond the HEC's locus of control (e.g., legislation, organizational policies, social norms, cultural influences, individual preferences) can have a significant impact on the services being provided and outcomes produced. Outcome measures associated with HEC functions (particularly ethics review and consultation) tend to be controversial because of the broad range of ethical resolutions and the lack of consensus on any single best one.

2. **Process standards.** Process standards specify how an organization's performance capabilities are operationalized. Clearly defined processes reduce process variation, leading to more predictable outcomes. Even so, full compliance with process standards is not expected because a certain degree

of variation may be justifiable in some situations. Process measures assess the quantity or quality of organizational activities with respect to effort rather than effect or achievement. Process measures may be more valid measures of organizational performance because they directly assess performance values. However, process measures assess conformity to a given standard, not the adequacy or correctness of the standard. Surveys, interviews, direct observations, and documentation reviews can be used effectively to evaluate HEC functions from a process perspective.

3. **Structure standards.** Structure standards define the rules under which the organization is governed and services are rendered. They are the absolutes of the organization and cannot be situationally modified. Structure standards assess the organization's capacity to perform effectively and are based on relatively stable organizational features or individual characteristics presumed to have an impact on organizational effectiveness (accreditation rating; professional staff licensure; available tools and technology; human, physical, and financial resources). Structure standards are especially useful in the planning, design, and implementation of healthcare programs. However, structure is relevant only to the extent that it can increase or decrease the probability of good performance. Appropriate structural measures of HEC functions include identifying the presence of (a) mechanisms for conducting ethics consultation, formulating ethics policies, and communicating information to patients and surrogates; (b) written policies; (c) library holdings on ethics subjects; (d) budget allocations and personnel to support education; and (e) ongoing ethics assessment.

Donabedian (1980) suggests a certain ordering of these performance measures (structure → process → outcome) based on fundamental functional relationships between them. In essence, structure (prerequisites, organization, resources) affects process (content, configuration, rendering of services), which affects outcomes (end product, effects of services provided).

As an evaluation strategy, self-assessment is the most desirable platform because it is executed by those who are the most knowledgeable and have the highest degree of control over healthcare ethics programs—HEC chairpersons and members. Self-assessment incorporates the most beneficial elements of program evaluation (formalized structure) and internal evaluation (organizational focus) to provide a comprehensive analysis of HEC functions.

PRACTICAL APPLICATION

If HECs are to be recognized as credible components of the healthcare system, organizations must be willing to evaluate performance, document success, identify opportunities for improvement, and ensure customer satisfaction. When properly planned and executed, almost any evaluation approach can be used effectively to assess HECs. The common elements of successful evaluation endeavors are objectivity, management support, an ability and willingness to change, and a commitment to improvement. The following are practical tips for conducting an HEC evaluation:

1. **Discuss the proposed evaluation activity as a committee.** Get the group's support and commitment, and seek volunteers to champion major tasks.

2. **Secure management support.** Identify the necessary organizational resources, and seek additional funding if needed.

3. **Design the evaluation effort.** Delineate clearly its purpose and scope. Will it be a comprehensive evaluation or will it focus on a specific HEC function or process? What evaluation approach (or combination of approaches) will be used? What key questions does the committee want to answer? Develop an evaluation timeline.

4. **Conduct the evaluation.** Because most HEC members are volunteers, time constraints will likely preclude the entire committee from participating in the evaluation. Consider identifying a small number of committee members who are interested in participating. Schedule time for the evaluation. The assessment of a major function or process can take several hours, but the actual time frame will depend on the scope and depth of the evaluation, the selection of participants, and their knowledge of the committee's historical background and current functions. Consider scheduling separate sessions for each functional area or process being assessed.

5. **Analyze the data.** The evaluation is intended to give the committee an opportunity to reflect on its activities and to generate topics for further discussion and consideration. If performance standards were developed, the committee does not yet need to perform at the level at which the standards were written. Performance standards provide a benchmark against which the committee's current level of development can be measured to plan improvement activities. Do not hesitate to seek an external interpretation of the data.

6. **Share the evaluation findings with the committee.** Review and discuss the findings with committee members.

7. **Document the findings.** Record the evaluation participants and processes used. Maintain evaluation files for other uses (historical records, benchmarking progress, accreditation surveys, budget preparation).

8. **Report the findings.** Decide what will be reported—major findings, data and results, alternatives, or recommendations? Determine in what format

the findings will be reported—formal written report, executive summary, oral briefing with charts, newsletter or journal article, or group discussion? Decide how widely evaluation findings will be distributed—who are the intended users, and who else could benefit from the data being generated?

9. **Take action on the findings.** Develop an action plan and timeline to address the findings. Prioritize activities. Seek volunteers to champion major tasks. Track action items, and provide regular progress reports to the committee. Keep management informed on progress, as required. Seek additional resources, as needed.

10. **Start planning the next HEC evaluation.** Revising the process and instruments used for the most recent evaluation while critical comments are still fresh will make the next evaluation flow more smoothly.

REFERENCES

Dobbs, R. A. 2000. "Self-Assessment of Hospital Ethics Committees in New Mexico: A Study in Process Improvement." PhD diss., Walden University, Minneapolis.

Donabedian, A. 1980. *Explorations in Quality Assessment and Monitoring: The Definition of Quality and Approaches to Its Assessment, Volume 1.* Chicago: Health Administration Press.

Ross, J. W., J. W. Glaser, D. Rasinski-Gregory, J. M. Gibson, and C. Bayley. 1993. *Health Care Ethics Committees: The Next Generation.* Chicago: American Hospital Publishing.

CHAPTER 17

Prevention and Treatment of Substance Use Disorders Among Healthcare Professionals

J. Mitchell Simson

HEALTHCARE MANAGERS MUST be able to identify an impaired healthcare professional and understand what assessment, intervention, and treatment entail. Despite increased attention to physician impairment, the number of impaired physicians reported by colleagues appears to be much lower than the estimated number of physicians who become impaired (DesRoches et al. 2010).

Before examining this issue, however, relevant terminology should be defined. *Impairment* is "the inability to practice medicine with reasonable skill and safety to patients by reason of physical or mental illness, including deterioration through the aging process, the loss of motor skills or the excessive use or abuse of drugs, including alcohol" (AMA 1992). *Addiction* is "a primary, chronic disease of brain reward, motivation, memory and related circuitry. Dysfunction in these circuits leads to characteristic biological, psychological, social and spiritual manifestations . . . reflected in an individual pathologically pursuing reward and/or relief by substance use and other behaviors" (ASAM 2011).

The fifth edition of the *Diagnostic and Statistical Manual* (DSM-5), published in May 2013, combined the previous diagnoses of *substance abuse* and *substance dependence* into a single overarching diagnosis—*substance use disorder* (APA 2013). The severity of the disorder is now graded according to the number of criteria the individual meets. If the individual meets none or only one criterion, no diagnosis is made; if two or three, the diagnosis is mild; if four or five, moderate; if six or more, severe.

For example, the 11 criteria of an alcohol use disorder are as follows:

1. Missing work or school
2. Drinking in hazardous situations

3. Drinking despite social or personal problems
4. Craving alcohol
5. Development of tolerance
6. Withdrawals when cutting down or trying to quit
7. Drinking more than intended
8. Inability to successfully quit
9. Increase in alcohol-seeking behavior
10. Interference with important activities
11. Continued use despite health problems

THE IMPAIRED HEALTHCARE PROFESSIONAL

To help readers identify the healthcare professional impaired by a substance use disorder, the general characteristics of addicted physicians are described here. Although the exact prevalence of substance use disorders among physicians is unknown, an estimated 6 to 8 percent have drug use disorders and 14 percent have alcohol use disorders—figures that mirror those in the general population. Therefore, of the more than 800,000 physicians in the United States (75 percent male, 25 percent female), 64,000 will develop a drug use disorder and 112,000 will experience an alcohol use disorder (Baldisseri 2007).

The age at first presentation for treatment of addiction is bimodal—physicians in training and in early practice constitute the first wave, and physicians in mid- to late career constitute the second (Ries et al. 2009). However, from 1998 to 2007, the average age of physicians entering addiction treatment increased from 42.5 years to 48.0 years. More males enter treatment than females, in a ratio of between 6 and 10 to 1, which contrasts with a male-to-female physician ratio of only 3 to 1 (McGovern et al. 1998; Wunsch et al. 2007). Female physicians in treatment tend to be younger (average age 39.9 years versus 43.7 for males), have more medical and psychiatric comorbidity, and are more likely to use sedatives or hypnotics than males (Wunsch et al. 2007). Women are more likely than men to have suicidal ideation and more likely to have attempted suicide either under or not under the influence of drugs or alcohol. Addiction does not appear to account for any gender difference in employment problems or legal problems (Wunsch et al. 2007).

Many studies have examined the specialties of physicians receiving care in addiction treatment centers. Psychiatry, emergency medicine, anesthesiology, and family medicine predominate (Ries et al. 2009). An interesting correlation is that physicians in all of these specialties except psychiatry self-report higher levels of burnout (Shanafelt et al. 2012).

At the top of the list of drugs that are abused by physicians (and by the general population) is alcohol. In the general population, heavy drinking decreases with age; among physicians, however, it increases with age (McAuliffe, Rohman, and Breer 1991). Surgeons and emergency medicine physicians smoke more than other physicians do, but overall, physician tobacco use is decreasing (Buhl et al. 2011; Mangus, Hawkins, and Miller 1998). Cocaine use seems to be higher among physicians in surgical specialties who have medical access to it (ENT, plastics, head and neck, ophthalmology) and among emergency medicine physicians. The national plague of opioid abuse is reflected in physician use—opioids are the second most common drug that physicians abuse. Family medicine and obstetrics-gynecology physicians tend to abuse oral opioids, while anesthesiologists use the highly potent injectables (Seppala and Berge 2010). Anesthesiologists also abuse the injectables ketamine and propofol to which they have access (Bryson and Silverstein 2008). Marijuana abuse seems more prevalent in emergency medicine, family medicine, and anesthesiology. Psychiatrists report a higher frequency of unsupervised benzodiazepine misuse (Hughes, Baldwin, and Sheehan 1992).

Many other risk factors for physician addiction have been studied. Physicians have the same genetic predisposition as the general population—a family history of drug or alcohol dependence. Personality disorders have also been postulated as increasing the risk of drug use and abuse. A recent study that examined the role of personality disorders on physicians' rates of sobriety in the first two years following treatment did not find a significant relationship between personality and substance abuse (Angres, Bologeorges, and Chou 2013). Older studies examined such "personality types" as sensation seeking (McAuliffe, Rohman, and Wechsler 1984), perfectionist (Bissell and Jones 1976), compulsive (Udell 1984), and introverted and introspective (Yufit, Polock, and Wasserman 1969; Zeldow and Daugherty 1991). Physicians' work may, arguably, benefit from introspection and a certain amount of compulsivity. Physicians and other healthcare professionals are not immune to other medical, psychiatric, and emotional comorbidities that can include depression, bipolar disorder, chronic pain, and posttraumatic stress disorder.

Twenty years of research shows an increase in physician burnout. In surgeons who self-reported a major surgical error, the only factors that were independently associated with their perception of the cause of the error were burnout and depression (Shanafelt et al. 2010). To date, most efforts to reduce surgical errors look at systems errors that can be corrected by applying quality improvement matrixes, but individual factors such as burnout and depression need to be more fully identified and remedied. Despite evidence that self-disclosure of errors reduces medical liability, many physicians do not feel supported by their healthcare organization in disclosing errors.

IDENTIFYING AND REPORTING THE IMPAIRED HEALTHCARE PROFESSIONAL

How does a healthcare manager identify the impaired health professional? Sometimes they self-identify ("self-ID") after seeking treatment for their addiction on their own. Sometimes they "self-OD," as when an anesthesiologist is found unconscious from a sufentanyl overdose or an internist is hospitalized with acute pancreatitis resulting from alcoholism. Not uncommonly, the work site sees a behavioral change that is typically first reported by ancillary staff—rounding at irregular hours, irritability and explosive behavior toward support staff and colleagues, alcohol on the breath at work, disheveled appearance, intoxication without alcohol odor, significant weight gain or loss, depression, forgetfulness, drop in productivity, frequent job changes, and so forth. Sometimes, if the work site is the source of the abused drug via samples or diversion, the physician works additional shifts to increase access to that drug. Thus, the physician might mask the drug abuse by hiding his behavioral change in a cloak of increased productivity.

Dealing with an impaired colleague is a difficult, emotionally charged job for physician leaders and hospital administrators, who often have little training on how to handle such a situation (Seppala and Berge 2010). Regarding the hospital's ethical responsibilities in assisting the impaired physician, Darr (1991) states:

> Two themes must describe the context of the hospital's relationship with physicians: the primacy of the patient, and the trustees and managers as moral agents. The personal ethic of each trustee and manager, within the context of the hospital's organizational philosophy, provides a moral framework for the relationships among patients, physicians, employees, organization, and community. Managers especially are not, and cannot be morally neutral technocrats. Rather, trustees and managers morally affect and are morally affected by decisions made and actions taken. This means decision making is not value-free: there is a moral dimension to the decision's effect on its environment and all persons touched by it. Primarily, meeting the hospital's ethical responsibility to impaired physicians requires an inquiring mind and attention to detail. Those involved must ask whether the specific action contemplated violates the principles of respect for persons, beneficence, nonmaleficence, and justice.

Similarly, physicians have an ethical duty to report impairment in colleagues. According to the American Medical Association (2004):

> Physicians have an ethical obligation to report impaired, incompetent, and/or unethical colleagues in accordance with the legal requirements in each state and assisted by the following guidelines. . . . Physicians' responsibilities to colleagues who are impaired by a condition that interferes with their ability to engage safely in professional activities

include timely intervention to ensure that these colleagues cease practicing and receive appropriate assistance from a physician health program.

Nevertheless, not all physicians aware of an impaired colleague will report her to the appropriate authority. According to a recent study, only 64 percent of 1,891 surveyed physicians completely agreed that all instances of impairment or incompetence should be reported (DesRoches et al. 2010). Reporting was significantly correlated with type of practice organization: 76 percent of physicians practicing in hospitals and 77 percent of those in medical schools or universities reported an impaired or incompetent colleague to a relevant authority, whereas only 44 percent of physicians in solo or two-person practices did so. The reasons for failing to report an impaired or incompetent colleague included the following (DesRoches et al. 2010):

- "Thought someone else was taking care of it" (19 percent)
- "Believed nothing would happen as a result of the report" (15 percent)
- "Fear of retribution" (12 percent)
- "Believed it was not your responsibility" (10 percent)
- "Believed the person would be excessively punished" (9 percent)
- "Did not know how to report" (8 percent)
- "Believed it could easily happen to you" (8 percent)

Despite legal, ethical, and moral considerations to report impairment, a "culture of resistance to 'whistle blowing'" still exists (Scarpello 2012).

TREATMENT OF THE IMPAIRED HEALTHCARE PROFESSIONAL

Once a healthcare professional is identified as having some type of performance problem, a comprehensive assessment should be performed even if the physician resists. These multidisciplinary assessments can be conducted through physician health programs (PHPs) or as an outpatient evaluation undertaken over several days at a treatment program for health professionals. Such assessments typically include a full medical and psychological evaluation, neuropsychological testing, and drug testing (Ries et al. 2009). Most states have PHPs, which can be independent businesses, offices of state medical societies, or operated by state medical licensing boards (Gunderman and Grogan 2012). PHPs typically monitor physicians after they have completed their initial inpatient or outpatient treatment for addiction. Monitoring usually involves random drug testing, accessing or providing individual or group counseling, and interfacing with state medical boards and hospital physician health programs and credentialing committees.

A recent study of 16 different PHPs found that over the study period of five to seven years, 78 percent of addicted physicians were continuously abstinent and more than 90 percent were still practicing medicine (McLellan, Skipper, and Campbell 2008). Similarly high rates of success have been reported by hospital impaired-physician committees (Schwartz, White, and McDuff 2008) and PHPs (Buhl et al. 2011).

With the advent of the patient-centered medical home, even more stresses will be placed on primary care health providers. Increasing levels of stress coupled with a heavier workload may lead to a feeling of lack of control over one's practice life and a loss of meaning, both strongly associated with burnout. Krasner and colleagues (2009) report that an intensive educational program in mindfulness, communication, and self-awareness can improve physicians' feelings of well-being and attitudes associated with patient-centered care. They present a proactive approach to reduce psychological distress that aims to reduce burnout before it leads to personal or professional impairment.

CONCLUSION

The tasks set before the healthcare manager to identify and intervene with impaired physicians are complex. The organizational culture needs to be one that encourages confidential reporting of impairment and incompetence, and a clear procedure needs to be provided to staff and physicians for reporting impairment and incompetence confidentially without fear of retribution. Ongoing education about successful treatment of addictive disorders should be provided to staff and physicians so that they do not shirk their legal and ethical duties to report concerns about impairment. Hospitals also should support research and educational programs for their medical staff and for those in the community who may not understand how to confidentially report concerns about impaired colleagues. Finally, active programs should be in place to identify sources and reduce levels of stress, depression, and burnout among all staff.

REFERENCES

American Medical Association (AMA). 2004. "Reporting Impaired, Incompetent, or Unethical Colleagues." Opinion 9.031 of the AMA *Code of Medical Ethics*. Updated June. www.ama-assn.org//ama/pub/physician-resources/medical-ethics/code-medical-ethics/opinion9031.page.

———. 1992. "Reporting Impaired, Incompetent, or Unethical Colleagues." Report of the AMA Council on Ethical and Judicial Affairs. *Journal of the Mississippi State Medical Association* 33 (5): 176–77.

American Psychiatric Association (APA). 2013. *Diagnostic and Statistical Manual of Mental Disorders*, fifth edition (DSM-5). Arlington, VA: American Psychiatric Publishing.

American Society of Addiction Medicine (ASAM). 2011. "Definition of Addiction." Public policy statement. Issued August 15. www.asam.org/docs/publicy-policy-statements/1definition_of_addiction_long_4-11.pdf.

Angres, D., S. Bologeorges, and J. Chou. 2013. "A Two Year Longitudinal Outcome Study of Addicted Health Care Professionals: An Investigation of the Role of Personality Variables." *Substance Abuse* 7: 49–60.

Baldisseri, M. R. 2007. "Impaired Healthcare Professional." *Critical Care Medicine* 35 (2): S106–S116.

Bissell, L., and R. W. Jones. 1976. "The Alcoholic Physician: A Survey." *American Journal of Psychiatry* 133 (10): 1142–46.

Bryson, E. O., and J. H. Silverstein. 2008. "Addiction and Substance Abuse in Anesthesiology." *Anesthesiology* 109 (5): 905–17.

Buhl, A., M. R. Oreskovich, C. W. Meredith, M. D. Campbell, and R. I. Dupont. 2011. "Prognosis for the Recovery of Surgeons from Chemical Dependency: A 5-Year Outcome Study." *Archives of Surgery* 146 (11): 1286–91.

Darr, K. 1991. "Hospital's Ethical Responsibilities: Assisting the Impaired Physician." *Hospital Topics* 69 (1): 4–7.

DesRoches, C. M., S. R. Rao, J. A. Fromson, R. J. Birnbaum, L. Iezzoni, C. Vogeli, and E. G. Campbell. 2010. "Physicians' Perceptions, Preparedness for Reporting, and Experiences Related to Impaired and Incompetent Colleagues." *Journal of the American Medical Association* 304 (2): 187–93.

Gunderman, R. B., and K. Grogan. 2012. "Physician Impairment and Professionalism." *American Journal of Roentgenology* 199 (5): W543–W544.

Hughes, P. H., D. C. Baldwin, and D. V. Sheehan. 1992. "Resident Physician Substance Use by Specialty." *American Journal of Psychiatry* 149 (10): 1348–54.

Krasner, M., R. Epstein, J. Beckman, A. Suchman, B. Chapman, C. Mooney, and T. Quill. 2009. "Association of an Educational Program in Mindful Communication with Burnout, Empathy, and Attitudes Among Primary Care Physicians." *Journal of the American Medical Association* 302 (12): 1284–93.

Mangus, R. S., C. E. Hawkins, and M. J. Miller. 1998. "Tobacco and Alcohol Use Among 1996 Medical School Graduates." *Journal of the American Medical Association* 280 (13): 1192–93.

McAuliffe, W. E., M. Rohman, and P. Breer. 1991. "Alcohol Use and Abuse in Random Samples of Physicians and Medical Students." *American Journal of Public Health* 81 (2): 177–81.

McAuliffe, W. E., M. Rohman, and H. Wechsler. 1984. "Alcohol, Substance Use, and Other Risk-Factors of Impairment in a Sample of Physicians-in-Training." *Advances in Alcohol & Substance Abuse* 4 (2): 67–87.

McGovern, M. P., K. H. Angres, N. D. Uziel-Miller, and S. Leon. 1998. "Female Physicians and Substance Abuse: Comparisons with Male Physicians Presenting for Assessment." *Journal of Substance Abuse Treatment* 15 (6): 525–33.

McLellan, A. T., G. Skipper, and G. Campbell. 2008. "Five Year Outcomes in a Cohort Study of Physicians Treated for Substance Use Disorders in the United States." *British Medical Journal* 337: a2038.

Ries, R. K., D. A. Feillin, S. C. Miller, and R. Saitz. 2009. *Principles of Addiction Medicine,* fourth edition. Philadelphia: Lippincott Williams & Wilkins.

Scarpello, J. 2012. "Dysfunctional Doctors—Will Revalidation Help?" *Clinical Medicine* 12 (2): 111–13.

Schwartz, R., R. K. White, and D. R. McDuff. 2008. "Four Years Experience of a Hospital's Impaired Physician Committee." *Journal of Addictive Diseases* 14 (2): 13–21.

Seppala, M. D., and K. H. Berge. 2010. "The Addicted Physician: A Rational Response to an Irrational Disease." *Minnesota Medicine* 93 (2): 46–49.

Shanafelt, T. D., C. M. Balch, G. Bechamps, T. Russell, L. Dyrbey, D. Satele, P. Collicott, P. J. Novotny, J. Sloan, and J. Freischlag. 2010. "Burnout and Medical Errors Among American Surgeons." *Annals of Surgery* 251 (6): 995–1000.

Shanafelt, T. D., S. Boone, T. Litjen, L. N. Dyrbye, W. Sotile, D. Satele, C. West, J. Sloan, and M. R. Oreskovich. 2012. "Burnout and Satisfaction with Work–Life Balance Among US Physicians Relative to the General US Population." *Archives of Internal Medicine* 172 (18): 1377–85.

Udell, M. M. 1984. "Chemical Abuse/Dependence: Physicians' Occupational Hazard." *Journal of the Medical Association of Georgia* 73 (11): 775–78.

Wunsch, M. J., J. S. Knisely, K. L. Cropsey, E. D. Campbell, and S. H. Scholl. 2007. "Women Physicians and Addiction." *Journal of Addictive Diseases* 26 (2): 35–43.

Yufit, R. I., G. H. Polock, and E. Wasserman. 1969. "Medical Specialty Choice and Personality." *Archives of General Psychiatry* 20 (1): 89–99.

Zeldow, P. B., and S. R. Daugherty. 1991. "Personality Profiles and Specialty Choices of Students from Two Medical School Classes." *Academic Medicine: Journal of the Association of American Medical Colleges* 66 (5): 283–87.

CHAPTER 18

Ethics Issues in Graduate Medical Education

Clinton H. Dowd

THAT GRADUATE MEDICAL education presents ethical considerations is not surprising. The extent to which changes in the traditional paradigm for resident education have altered those considerations, however, may be more revealing.

Education of residents has traditionally been carried out in university settings, where a number of assumptions have been made:

1. After completing their residency, residents will leave to practice their craft elsewhere.
2. University-based teachers are rewarded for their scholarly activity first and their clinical practice second.
3. Post-residency fellows spend a significant amount of time supervising junior residents as a "price" for the advanced education that they are receiving.
4. The department chair and the medical school dean control most faculty funds, so that the faculty work for a contracted amount plus incentives. This compensation structure places tremendous control of the faculty's time in the hands of the university's leaders.
5. Protected faculty time is spent advancing scholarly activity, including supervising resident research. Nonclinical research faculty enhance this environment and are supported by both private and government research grants.
6. Residency program directors are the department chairs, although much daily supervision is delegated.

A number of changes in this traditional paradigm have occurred over the past few decades. Historically, subspecialty care was rendered in the university setting, and major entities in outlying regions referred cases to the university medical centers. To provide this care, fellowships were granted to an ever-increasing number of residents finishing their training. These fellowships provided the departmental clinical "grist mill" with junior faculty support at minimal cost to the university and allowed subspecialists to pursue their chosen clinical research and academic careers in a relatively unfettered manner.

Once a source of pride and power for medical schools, university medical centers became a financial drain as the federal government lowered reimbursement for medical education. University hospital faculty were forced out of their academic environment to compete for patient dollars from insurers. This competition was not limited to traditional university boundaries, and soon the battle began between university and community medical centers.

As subspecialists became more readily available in the communities, community medical centers ceased being the "poor stepchild" of medical education whose residents were considered inferior to university residents and whose faculty consisted only of "generalists" who could not function without the assistance of the university specialty faculty. The subspecialty faculty who moved to the community setting—often under the threat of dire consequences, such as not passing subspecialty board exams—found the clinical-oriented teaching environment to be a marked financial improvement compared with the university stipends of their mentors.

At many universities, research activity decreased because of the lack of formal fellowships. The university position was further eroded by a marked reduction in referrals from traditional nonuniversity medical centers. More and more faculty were forced to compete directly with their referral sources in outlying communities for patient dollars. In the resulting university–community teaching system, animosity could easily have been anticipated.

This chapter deals with the following ethics issues:

- Resident recruitment
- Resident evaluation
- Resident retention and discipline
- Faculty recruitment
- Faculty retention and discipline
- Hospital administration and resident education
- Research

Interpolated in the discussion are short cases that present ethics issues for the reader's consideration.

RESIDENT RECRUITMENT

Medical education programs recruit residents from allopathic and osteopathic schools throughout the United States as well as from a large pool of international graduates that includes both US citizens educated abroad and foreigners educated in other countries. Foreign residents often gain access to the United States but may not have visas or work permits to allow them to enter the medical education stream easily.

Each education program serves a certain patient population, whose diversity ideally will be reflected in the makeup of the residents in the program. This representation may be difficult to achieve and yet, if it is achieved, may have a long-term detrimental effect on the program as described in the following paragraphs.

For many years, the Residency Review Committees (RRCs) of the Accreditation Council for Graduate Medical Education collected statistics on the source of the residents in each program. Programs that contained many residents from sources that university programs did not traditionally employ were often viewed as weak and were subject to intense scrutiny by the RRC. The specialty boards routinely released information on "pass" rates by resident source (i.e., US medical graduate, osteopathic graduate, international graduate, US international graduate), which suggested that one group performed at a higher level of function than did another, regardless of the many considerations that played a part in that performance level.

The largest group of resident candidates are international graduates. Most programs, especially those that are attractive to US graduates, have responded to the almost overwhelming number of international candidates in the same manner: They give the applications at most a cursory evaluation, because subjecting them to the same in-depth review as applications from US graduates is impossible. The evaluators do not know the referees and may therefore question the validity of the reference. The examination system that judged the candidate is also unknown or poorly understood. During the interview process, international graduates' language skills may not be at the same level as those of US candidates. As a result, many popular programs do not evaluate all candidates on the basis of ability. Correspondingly, programs that are less popular—either because their location is perceived as undesirable (large, urban centers) or because they include less popular specialties (e.g., psychiatry, anesthesia)—have an overrepresentation of candidates perceived as being less desirable. The inference that the educational content of these programs is not up to standard because they recruit these residents may place the program in jeopardy with the reviewing bodies.

Most residency programs evaluate 10 to 15 candidates per position. A multitude of factors are considered:

- past experience with candidates from the same educational institution;
- references (now less common because of the RRC's computerized application process);
- direct experience with the candidate (i.e., elective externships);
- the residency program's gender composition; and

- professional pressures from administrators and colleagues seeking entrance to the program on behalf of friends, family, and acquaintances.

Few programs have a dedicated committee that reviews all candidates, so final selections are usually made on a "point count" of various parameters as assessed by a nonuniform set of evaluators. Given the inconsistencies and uncertainties of the system, it is surprising that issues of beneficence and honesty can be satisfactorily addressed as often as they are.

Case 1

A small program has the opportunity to recruit an international resident with impeccable credentials. However, if it does so, a majority of its residents will be of international origin. Will this disproportion have a negative effect on subsequent recruitment of US graduates? If a US candidate is available, should he be given preference even if his credentials are not as good? Should the fact that the parents of US graduates pay taxes have any bearing?

Case 2

A group of international physicians lobby to have residents of their ethnic origin and religion given preferential treatment during the recruiting process so that their families will have specialist physicians of similar backgrounds treating them.

Case 3

A candidate applies to a residency program. She has performed well on her examination but is dyslexic and must therefore, according to the Americans with Disabilities Act, be given extra time to accomplish assigned tasks. Should she be granted equal consideration for a place in the residency program?

RESIDENT EVALUATION

Residency programs need to be evaluated on an ongoing basis so that the progress of residents in training can be assessed and the quality of the teaching process appraised. The assessment needs to be standardized to some degree to create a benchmark by which all can be judged.

The faculty are responsible for assessing the clinical judgment and competence of residents. They usually accomplish this by means of written examinations administered during training. Written exams are extremely subjective, however, and reduce the assessment to a mere number that is much less valid than many would like to believe. As a result, assessments can degenerate into a popularity contest that pits one faculty member against another. Not many faculty members want to be the "bad guy" in the evaluation process.

Because programs must now credential graduates (particularly in technical areas) so that they may receive hospital privileges, the validity of the credentialing process is of paramount importance. Failure of the process can not only create significant medicolegal implications for the program but also result in harm to patients.

Case 4

After graduating from a program, a resident causes irreparable harm to a patient during a surgical procedure. An ensuing legal action determines that the residency program does not have documentation that the resident was capable of independently performing the procedure.

Case 5

On completion of the residency program, a resident applies for specialty certification. Despite several attempts, he fails to matriculate and consequently faces losing his hospital privileges and expulsion from HMO panels as a specialist. He files a lawsuit against the program for failure of its educational process to adequately prepare him for the examination and for his consequent financial loss.

RESIDENT RETENTION AND DISCIPLINE

Despite expectations to the contrary, not all residents accepted into a program identify successful completion of the residency as their highest priority. While most have little difficulty transitioning from medical student to resident physician, some struggle with the change.

Although resident compensation is perhaps less than it should be, the increase in disposable income, compared with what the resident was accustomed to as a student, is significant. Quickly, lifestyle changes occur: new cars, new spouses, new social status, and some free time without the immediate pressure of impending examinations.

These factors can distract the resident from what should be her primary goal— to get as much academic and technical education out of the program as possible. To achieve this goal, the resident must maintain and hone the habits of reading and intellectual inquiry learned in medical school. This learning must occur in an environment that is different from what the resident is used to and in places, such as the operating room, where senior mentors are more likely to talk about last night's football score or the most recent fine wine that they consumed. Harrison's *Textbook of Medicine* is pretty dull fare by comparison.

Not infrequently, new residents come from families that have not had the same opportunities for education and success that the resident is now experiencing. The resident does not know how to function in the newly assumed role of physician and may not receive the degree of family support that many of her peers enjoy. The new role may therefore create significant social pressure for her.

Despite an element of sleep deprivation, the junior resident can perform his daily duties without much intellectual effort: Rounds are made with senior residents and physicians, who make most of the major decisions and who plan subsequent evaluations and interventions. Although the junior resident may be asked some penetrating questions, more likely the questions will be directed at the medical student. By merely contributing to work output (e.g., histories, physicals, order input), being on time, and looking neat and tidy for rounds, the junior resident can potentially "slide" for a period of time until a rigorous evaluation exposes his lack of real progress as a physician. Lost ground is very difficult to make up when a deficit of information has been allowed to occur.

Although in many regards a lack of progress is the resident's problem, for several reasons it is also the residency program's problem:

- A resident who cannot carry her weight places a greater burden on colleagues.
- The time the faculty spend remedying the resident's deficiencies is taken away from other duties.
- The resident suffers a loss of respect among peers and faculty that may be difficult, if not impossible, to recapture.
- The resident loses confidence as a result of needing remediation.
- The emotional impact of failure can be devastating for the resident, resulting in severe depression and even suicide.
- Recruitment suffers as prospective residents, who hear about residents' failure and expulsion, fear that this fate might unjustly happen to them.

Once a resident has been identified as having deficiencies, these deficiencies must be corrected. Remediation must be accomplished within a reasonable time frame but over a sufficient period to allow the resident to assimilate the necessary material. If too long a time frame is granted, however, the resident loses valuable time in making further progress as a physician.

Subsequent evaluation must confirm that the resident has mastered the material. If the remediation process is unsuccessful, several important questions must be answered: How much time in the program should the resident be credited with? Does the resident have to be released from the program, or can she be allowed to resign? What is the program's continuing responsibility to the resident and to any program that might subsequently hire her?

These questions represent serious concerns for a program because, if the remediation process is not clear-cut and well documented, litigation will likely arise either on behalf of the former resident or on behalf of a patient alleging inappropriate treatment by an inadequately trained resident.

Of equal concern is the consequence—both personally as well as professionally—to the resident who has been dismissed. Will he be able to find a career in medicine that will be rewarding and allow the self-fulfillment that he sought on the first day of medical school?

In fairness to all, the deficient resident is not the only one affected during the remediation process: Other residents have to pick up the slack. If dismissal results, can a replacement be identified to fill the position so that call schedules are not permanently altered, potentially putting the program out of compliance with nationally mandated limits on resident work hours?

If the resident does not receive credit for the time spent in a program (especially a primary care program, where the number of years of training is clearly laid out), obtaining Medicare funding to allow him to complete any program may be difficult. This possibility could mean either that the resident is not compensated for a year or that a program has to pay the resident's stipend without remuneration from federal sources.

Case 6

A resident in the second year of his program takes the second-year national training examination and achieves only the fifth percentile. Earlier in the program, the resident had received counseling for marginal performance. The examination results become available to the program in late March, and the program allows the resident three months to remedy his deficiencies. However, subsequent examination shows no evidence of improvement. The decision to terminate the resident is deferred until September because of a number of exceptional circumstances. How should the action of dismissal be balanced with the impact on the resident, his fellow residents, and the program? What does a residency program owe a resident who is dismissed—another chance? Psychological counseling? Job placement? A favorable reference? Or a "no comment" response to inquiries from other programs?

FACULTY RECRUITMENT

For the most part, faculty recruitment has traditionally concerned subspecialists. These individuals are expected to perform research, provide their clinical expertise, and function as a traditional academic. Of lesser importance are expectations of financial self-sufficiency, regular clinical supervision of non-specialty clinical care, and private practice.

As described earlier in this chapter, the number of subspecialists has increased dramatically, and many who now practice in community medical centers compete for specialty cases with their former mentors at universities. In addition, because clinical demand for subspecialty expertise may be low in a small community, community-based specialists also compete with local generalists for private patient dollars while being subsidized by the local medical center.

The dramatic increase in the number of subspecialists pales in comparison with the amount of supervision of resident services that the federal government has mandated, however. Because they lack general experience, many subspecialty faculty refuse to provide day-to-day clinical supervision beyond their area of expertise. Their refusal is fueled in part by the legal environment, in part because these individuals are "specialists," and in part because such supervision interferes with the provision of private patient care for which they are very well compensated.

Faculty recruitment must therefore include generalists to provide supervision. To successfully recruit young, enthusiastic generalists who are at the peak of their productivity, their salary demands must be met—often by supplementing their salary with private practice dollars. The federal contribution to faculty compensation is inadequate to support the amount of supervision that the federal government requires.

Recruiting faculty to a residency program is even more challenging than recruiting residents because faculty need to be effective role models and teachers. Faculty have a profound impact on recruiting both residents and other faculty; even their gender and ethnic background will influence recruitment. Just as the resident group should reflect the patient population it serves, so should the faculty group reflect that diversity. When the faculty group mirrors the patient population, the faculty can model appropriate patterns of behavior and demonstrate cultural sensitivities that may otherwise be lacking.

FACULTY RETENTION AND DISCIPLINE

Both university and community medical centers offer extensive opportunities for faculty employment. In general, however, community-based faculty are more interested in providing patient care. Because few community medical centers have tenure-track positions, they provide less of a stimulus for research and academic writing than the university setting does.

Community-based faculty tend to be more difficult to control because the portion of their compensation that comes from the community medical center is only a relatively small component of their stipend. Furthermore, no dean resides over a community medical center, and the department chair has little authority except that to which the faculty voluntarily submit themselves. The hospital administration primarily exercises financial control, but they may be poorly equipped to effectively deal with disciplinary matters.

Traditionally, a large number of residents trained in a community setting will remain in that setting to establish or join a practice. Because community-based faculty are thus training their own future competition, they have little incentive to share cutting-edge knowledge or technology with residents who, once trained in the advanced techniques, will have no reason to refer their patients to their former teachers for specialized procedures. While teaching may be a stimulus for the faculty to acquire and maintain cutting-edge technology, given the vagaries of funding these technologies, that stimulus may be more apparent than real.

The retention of community-based faculty also presents challenges. Although many faculty are drawn to community-based programs because of the higher financial remuneration, which is balanced at the outset against the more relaxed lifestyle and reduced clinical load of the university setting, many faculty are also attracted by the opportunity to teach and carry out research in a clinical setting. Community medical centers need to recognize the diverse reasons faculty are attracted to community-based programs; otherwise, retaining them will be impossible.

Probably the most efficient way to retain faculty and avoid conflict is for the medical center administration to delegate the negotiation and control of faculty contracts to the program director or department chair. Although faculty physicians are ultimately accountable to the medical center, managing them efficiently cannot otherwise be achieved.

Case 7

In the course of building a new subspecialty faculty division, a community-based program recruits a senior member of a university department as the divisional director. As the division grows, a junior member is subsequently recruited. Although both have excellent academic credentials, the junior physician strives to augment the division's clinical activity without a corresponding increase in academic yield. Friction ensues, leading to a split between the two physicians. The hospital administration favors the junior physician because of the increase in clinical activity.

HOSPITAL ADMINISTRATION AND MEDICAL EDUCATION

As hospitals have grown in size and complexity, the use of professional managers has increased. Often endowed with credentials from prestigious business schools, these managers usually have little if any medical background. These professional managers bring a different perspective to the educational setting than the medical staff do. The ultimate responsibility of these hospital administrators is often fiscal viability and ensuring that the institution remains strong as compared with its competitors. This financial responsibility extends to residency programs.

At the same time, the residency program director and staff are responsible for medical education. Traditionally, medical education has been valued as a way to "give something back" to the medical staff, to enhance the prestige of the institution, and to ensure the medical staff remain current. Even the nonteaching medical staff may provide some clinical supervision and mentor residents under the direction of the program director.

The administrative intrusion into the medical education program is understandable but places the faculty in the position of working for two masters. Needed by the residency review committees for supervision and accreditation, the faculty are often required to adhere to administration demands because the administration pays their salary. In many cases, faculty salary contracts are created with little if any input from the program director. These contracts may also run contrary to the demands of quality resident education and frequently include time-consuming clinical duties, expanded programs outside the hospital, and nonteaching administrative responsibilities. Because the administration bears the ultimate financial responsibility for the institution, administrators hesitate to delegate contract responsibilities to the program directors, whom they may view as fiscally less competent. It is a wise hospital administrator who can travel the rocky road of allowing the program director to manage her faculty in a fashion that fulfills the institution's needs and keeps the responsibility for residency education in the hands of physicians.

RESEARCH

No discussion of ethics issues in graduate medical education would be complete without some mention of clinical research. Generally, three areas present ethical dilemmas:

1. Issues related to patient participants
2. Conflicts of interest
3. Intellectual integrity

Issues related to patient participants surround informed consent; patient confidentiality; and, most important, patient safety. Institutional review boards typically ensure that clinical trials and research studies are legitimate, appropriate, and safe.

Often less regulated are the areas of conflict of interest and intellectual integrity. Much has been written about concerns related to the industrial funding of clinical research and how much influence that funding may have on the products of research. Residency program directors and research staff must closely examine the methods that companies use to achieve their desired results. The study design, the study population, the comparable drugs and dosages used in the study, and the time durations used to effectively demonstrate adverse effects all affect the study results and must be appropriate. Sometimes clinical investigators may be more interested in their personal financial gain than in the methods employed (Bodenheimer 2000). Conflicts of interest on the part of clinical investigators are of special concern given the wide array of financial arrangements among hospitals, physicians, and suppliers to the healthcare field.

Equally important are the issues of intellectual integrity. Who controls the data, who authors the articles, and where the results are published are all significant questions that, if left unaddressed, may impinge on the integrity of the study results.

Teaching programs and the corporate world have good reason to work together in research. Such collaboration enhances income and resources for programs, opens up opportunities for resident physicians, and advances medical research and the development of new diagnostic and treatment modalities. However, program directors and administrators would be wise to ensure that appropriate policies and guidelines promote ethical standards of practice related to the conduct of all clinical research. For example, Cleveland Clinic requires all of its doctors to disclose their trade and industry relationships on its website so that patients can find out if their doctor is being paid for services by the company manufacturing the medications he is prescribing for them or the procedures he is ordering (Cosgrove 2013).

Globalization has introduced new ethics issues to medical research and clinical trials. Claiming that clinical trials in the United States and developed countries are too time consuming and costly, pharmaceutical companies are outsourcing some or all aspects of clinical trials to contract research organizations (CROs), which perform these studies in developing countries, such as India and China. These CROs can be commercial or academic (Mendivil 2012).

The Declaration of Helsinki is clear that potential subjects must be informed about all potential risks, expected benefits, and goals of the study and be notified that they have the right to deny or withdraw from the study at any time (WMA 2008). However, these guidelines are not always followed, for a number of reasons. Participants often lack education and the language skills needed to understand their rights and the risks of clinical trials. Payment for participation may be their only form of wages. In addition, the lack of any regulatory infrastructure in developing countries means little oversight of clinical trials (Mendivil 2012, 6). As for-profit organizations, CROs may take shortcuts to meet the pharmaceutical companies' need for lower costs and thereby secure future contracts with them.

Academic institutions and graduate medical education training programs that are affiliated with CROs need to pay particular attention to the ethical standards and guidelines that are being applied to research and clinical trials in developing countries.

REFERENCES

Bodenheimer, T. 2000. "Uneasy Alliance: Clinical Investigators and the Pharmaceutical Industry." *New England Journal of Medicine* 342 (20): 1539–44.

Cosgrove, T. 2013. "Transparency: A Patient's Right to Know." Institute of Medicine commentary. Published May 17. http://iom.edu/Global/Perspectives/2013/RightToKnow.aspx.

Mendivil, L. 2012. "Ethical Implications: Outsourcing of Clinical Trials by Pharmaceutical Companies." Student research paper for "Outsourcing of Professional Activities" course at the University of Arizona. http://next.eller.arizona.edu/courses/outsourcing/Fall2011/student_papers/finalluismendivil.pdf.

World Medical Association (WMA). 2008. "Ethical Principles for Medical Research Involving Human Subjects." Declaration of Helsinki. Amended October. www.wma.net/en/30publications/10policies/b3/.

CHAPTER 19

Ethics Issues in Disaster Planning

Rebecca A. Dobbs

SINCE THE 1990S, the Federal Emergency Management Agency (FEMA 2013) has issued numerous disaster declarations for terrorist events, hurricanes, tornadoes, wildfires, floods, winter storms, a bridge collapse, and pandemics that have further stressed the already-strained US healthcare system at the regional and national levels. Added to that, major emergency events affect healthcare delivery at the local level (e.g., utility disruptions, train derailments, chemical releases, epidemics, planned public gatherings). Such events serve as a stark reminder that the healthcare system is vulnerable to a variety of hazards and that comprehensive disaster planning needs to include deliberate preparedness for addressing ethical concerns.

In February 2003, the White House issued Homeland Security Presidential Directive 5, which directed the US Department of Homeland Security to develop and administer a single comprehensive system for preventing, preparing for, responding to, and recovering from a domestic event of any size or complexity. As a result, contingency-based planning was replaced with the National Incident Management System—an all-hazards approach intended to improve coordination and cooperation among entities at all levels, including federal, state, local, tribal, private sector, and nongovernment organizations. Current emergency management practice in the healthcare arena follows these nationally recognized principles and is structured around the four phases of emergency management: mitigation (prevention), preparedness (building capacity and resilience), response (mobilizing assets to stabilize the incident), and recovery (returning to a new normal).

For the purposes of this chapter, an *emergency* is defined as any hazard resulting in an event that causes a disruption in normal operations. Emergency events are classified as natural (e.g., tornado, epidemic), technological (e.g., utility failure, transportation accident), or human (e.g., terrorism, labor strike). An emergency event can significantly disrupt the hospital's ability to provide care or services; compromise the environment of care; or result in a sudden, radically changed, or increased demand for services. A *disaster* generally refers to an emergency event resulting in large-scale or widespread damage or destruction; numerous casualties or fatalities; drastic change to the environment; or marked degradation of the economic, social, and cultural aspects of life.

Ethical concerns can arise during an emergency event of any cause, size, or complexity. Healthcare practitioners must work closely with emergency management planners and coordinators to ensure that a mechanism is in place to proactively identify and adequately address potential ethics issues during all phases of emergency management. Understanding how ethical values can be integrated into the emergency management paradigm will help with this process.

ETHICAL DECISION MAKING DURING A CRISIS

Based on experiences gained during the SARS (severe acute respiratory syndrome) pandemic, the University of Toronto Joint Centre for Bioethics (2005) developed ten substantive values and five process values to guide ethical decision making during a crisis:

- Substantive values
    1. **Individual liberty.** Restrictions to individual liberty should be proportional, necessary, and relevant; employ the least restrictive means; and be applied equitably.
    2. **Protection of the public from harm.** Required actions that impinge on individual liberty should assess the imperative for compliance, provide incentives for compliance, and establish review mechanisms.
    3. **Proportionality.** Actions that restrict individual liberty should not exceed what is necessary to address the actual risk or critical needs of the community.
    4. **Privacy.** Individual privacy may be overridden during an emergency to protect the public from serious harm.
    5. **Duty to provide care.** Health professionals must weigh their duty to provide care against obligations to their own health and that of their families.
    6. **Reciprocity.** Society has a duty to support those taking extraordinary measures for the public good and take steps to minimize disproportionate burdens.
    7. **Equity.** During an emergency, care normally available to all patients on an equal basis may be curtailed or deferred.

8. **Trust.** Confidence in decisions being made requires transparency and thoughtful communication.
9. **Solidarity.** Collaboration and a shared vision are essential in and among healthcare institutions.
10. **Stewardship.** Resource decisions are intended to achieve the best patient and public health outcomes given the situation.

- Process values
  1. **Reasonable.** Credible, accountable people must be able to provide the rationale for actions taken.
  2. **Open and transparent.** The decision-making process must be open to scrutiny and publicly accessible.
  3. **Inclusive.** Stakeholders should be involved in the decision-making process.
  4. **Responsive.** New information should be incorporated into the decision-making process with a mechanism to address disputes and complaints.
  5. **Accountable.** Decision makers are held accountable for their actions and inactions.

Even though these values were defined specifically for a pandemic influenza outbreak, they could easily serve as an ethical framework in any emergency event.

Emergency planners, policymakers, and healthcare professionals have many questions regarding the ethics and standards that apply to care decisions and care delivery during unusual or extreme circumstances. Some of the more prominent ones pertain to the duty of healthcare workers to respond during an event, disaster triage and the allocation of scarce medical resources, and altered standards of care.

Duty of Healthcare Workers to Respond

The American Nurses Association (ANA) reports that registered nurses "have consistently shown to be reliable responders, and their compassionate nature typically compels them to respond to those in need, even when it puts their own safety or well-being at risk" (Brewer 2010). However, the firing of 11 nurses and 5 staffers at a Washington, DC, hospital for not reporting to work following back-to-back snowstorms in February 2010 (Vargas 2010) emphasizes the need to identify and discuss such issues so that emergency plans, policies, and staff training reflect organizational expectations and so that resources can be made available to support worker compliance. Questions related to the duty of healthcare workers to respond include the following:

- How can workers travel safely to work locations?
- Could a risk of exposure to disease or dangerous elements bring harm to the worker or family members?

- Is physical security adequate at the work location?
- What if the worker's family members or dependents need assistance?
- Is a practitioner's license protected when working outside the normal work area or specialty?
- Is the healthcare worker legally bound to respond?
- What are the legal ramifications of not being able to provide adequate care because of limited or lack of resources?

Brewer (2010) contends that these concerns and unanswered questions represent a gap in the nation's disaster preparedness and response systems. The ANA is currently partnering with government groups, nongovernment organizations, and employers to promote policies and laws that enable healthcare workers to respond confidently so that the needs of the US public can be met during a disaster. For example, the Uniform Emergency Volunteer Health Practitioners Act—model legislation developed by the National Conference of Commissioners on Uniform State Laws—is being promoted nationally to streamline the deployment of licensed healthcare workers to areas of declared emergency. It also (1) provides legal safeguards for practitioners acting within scope and in good faith, (2) clarifies interstate practice differences, and (3) deems the legal scope of practice authority to the state requesting the practitioners.

Ongoing, concerted efforts by federal and state governments, state agencies, and healthcare organizations are essential to resolving these issues. According to Brewer (2010), the role of federal government should be to establish the vision for seamless, coordinated, and safe response efforts; state legislatures, planners, policymakers, and response agencies should create nonpunitive environments that enhance healthcare worker efficiency and capacity to provide ethical care in response efforts; and employers should ensure that emergency plans meet the medical needs of the community in a system that protects healthcare workers and volunteers.

Disaster Triage and the Allocation of Scarce Medical Resources

Scarce medical resources include physical items (e.g., medical equipment and supplies, pharmaceuticals), services (e.g., diagnostics, treatments, nursing care, palliative care), and healthcare personnel (e.g., physicians, nurses, lab technicians, other essential workers in healthcare settings) (Phillips, Knebel, and Johnson 2009). Disaster triage may be used to ration or reallocate limited resources when healthcare providers cannot meet all care needs or provide care equitably. Therefore, disaster triage protocols that are medically acceptable and ethically defensible need to be developed in advance of emergencies to support provider decision making, create other forms of care for patients, and anticipate the ensuing behavioral health needs of healthcare professionals (ANA 2008).

The process of developing disaster triage protocols should be transparent and open. Stakeholders (including healthcare providers and the public) should assist in identifying, clarifying, and prioritizing ethical values to promote public confidence in the fairness of critical medical decisions that may need to be made quickly. Disaster triage protocols must then be used consistently to ensure ongoing public trust and cooperation (ANA 2008). Employing disaster triage protocols and allocating scarce medical resources in an emergency can be very distressing to healthcare professionals who are trained to provide unconstrained emergency care for all patients. Therefore, training for healthcare professionals is essential to ensure they are prepared to function in situations where they may be called on to provide care only to those who are likely to recover as a result of receiving that care (ANA 2008).

The allocation of scarce resources during a major emergency event must be conducted in a manner that is different from usual circumstances but appropriate to the situation. Making the right decisions about the allocation of scarce resources will be instrumental to healthcare system survivability and optimal functioning during a major emergency and may ultimately contribute to the saving of many lives (Phillips, Knebel, and Johnson 2009).

Little information is available to assist medical planners and policymakers in developing formal standards or guidelines for the allocation of scarce medical resources during major emergencies. A review of plans from 11 states and one US territory identified the following strategies for optimizing the allocation of scarce medical resources:

- Reduce or manage less urgent demand for healthcare services (e.g., limit hospital care to urgent cases).
- Optimize use of existing resources (e.g., redistribute patients on the basis of care needs).
- Augment existing resources (e.g., use alternate care sites).
- Implement crisis standards of care (e.g., provide essential interventions only).

Although the plans proposed these strategies to varying degrees, none included all four (Timbie et al. 2012). The only strategies available in the literature are efforts designed to develop guidance for specific events, such as the allocation of mechanical ventilators during a pandemic (New York State Department of Health 2007) or of scarce hemodialysis resources in the city of Seattle during the 1960s (Phillips and Knebel 2007).

Emergencies can quickly deplete the resources of healthcare entities and jurisdictions. Response activities often require the movement of people and resources from many locations to where they are needed. However, until an emergency is officially declared, legal and fiscal limitations may hinder the sharing of resources by the entities that possess them with those that need them. An emergency declaration may authorize interjurisdictional coordination efforts or suspend laws that interfere with such coordination during an emergency. Examples of existing interjurisdictional legal coordination between states, local governments, and foreign countries include the following:

- **States.** The Emergency Management Assistance Compact provides automatic license reciprocity to volunteer health providers deployed from other states, immunity from civil liability for harms to patients, and access to state workers' compensation benefits (US Congress 1996).
- **Local governments.** The Illinois Public Health Mutual Aid System agreement provides assistance in the form of personnel, equipment, supplies, and services between local health departments (Illinois Department of Public Health 2004).
- **Foreign countries.** The International Emergency Management Assistance Compact between several New England states and Canadian provinces has established protocols to share personnel and equipment in a major emergency (International Emergency Management Group 2013).

These formal agreements facilitate the real-time exchange of resources during emergencies under prespecified conditions. Other compacts, such as the Mid-America Alliance's (2009) mutual aid project involving ten midwestern states, authorize resource exchanges in the form of personnel, services, and equipment in urgent situations not meeting the governor-declared emergency threshold.

Altered Standards of Care

According to the Agency for Healthcare Research and Quality (AHRQ 2005) report on altered standards of care in mass casualty events, "the term *altered standards* has not been defined but generally is assumed to mean a shift to providing care and allocating scarce equipment, supplies, and personnel in a way that saves the largest number of lives in contrast to the traditional focus on saving individuals." Circumstances following a major emergency event may necessitate a change from accepted standards of care to altered standards of care as the result of (ANA 2008)

- a loss or severe disruption of essential services (e.g., power, water, supply chain);
- a loss of infrastructure (e.g., facilities, medical informatics);
- a personnel shortage resulting from transportation issues, worker or worker's family illness or injury, or unwillingness to report to work;

- the number of people affected by the emergency requiring community-level triage;
- a sudden increase in the number of patients in marked excess of capacity, with elevated Injury Severity Score, or other extreme conditions; or
- a relocation of care to an alternate facility not equipped for patient care.

In these types of situations, consequences can be severe if changes in care practices are not undertaken to mitigate loss of life or the exposure of patients and staff to unreasonable risks (ANA 2008). AHRQ (2005) suggested five principles for developing altered standards of care in response to a mass casualty event:

1. Keep the healthcare system functioning, and deliver acceptable quality of care to preserve as many lives as possible.
2. Implement planning that is comprehensive, community based, and coordinated at the regional level.
3. Ensure an adequate legal framework for providing health and medical care.
4. Protect the rights of individuals to the extent possible and reasonable under the circumstances.
5. Ensure clear communication with the public before, during, and after the event.

Before an altered-standards-of-care policy or protocol can be activated, a number of legal, policy, and ethics issues will need to be addressed (AHRQ 2005):

- What circumstances will trigger a change to altered standards of care?
- Who is authorized to make that decision?
- Under what legal statutory authority should the decision be made?
- Who assumes responsibility for directing emergency actions after the decision is made?
- What is the relationship between otherwise autonomous healthcare organizations and the incident management system?

Although health and medical professionals who are close to the event may make decisions that trigger the move to altered standards of care, the highest levels of authority necessary must implement policies that support the move to altered standards (e.g., professional scope of care, hospital licensure, liability protections) (AHRQ 2005).

A formal emergency declaration may activate certain statutory, professional, or regulatory provisions that provide legal protections. However, changes in care patterns may be necessary before such a declaration is made. In either case, the public must be informed about resource allocation, patient relocation, and other decisions that may lead to altered standards of care. Such communications should be coordinated with the appropriate public information structures at the local level (ANA 2008).

Extreme conditions may arise with or without warning as a result of a variety of hazards—natural, technological, or man-made—to which healthcare organizations are exposed. The entire healthcare workforce has a professional responsibility to be ready and willing to adapt and provide essential care under any condition. This responsibility can be better met if healthcare leaders and professionals consider relevant ethics issues in advance, address them in the planning process, prepare staff at all levels, and remain committed to delivering the best care possible no matter the circumstances (ANA 2008).

ALL-HAZARDS APPROACH

The all-hazards approach to emergency management does not literally mean preparing for all hazards. Rather, it provides a general framework to address any type of disaster that might occur. Hazards are generally categorized into three types: natural, technological, and human (man-made). *Natural* events are the result of forces occurring in nature or the environment (e.g., naturally occurring disease outbreak, flood, hurricane, tornado, blizzard, earthquake). *Technological* events are the result of accidents or failures involving processes or systems (e.g., transportation, utilities, telecommunications). *Human* events are man-made—intentionally caused by human intervention (e.g., terrorism, labor strike, bomb threat).

PHASES OF EMERGENCY MANAGEMENT

The four generally recognized phases of emergency management are mitigation, preparedness, response, and recovery. Activities in each phase contribute to the hospital's overall resilience—its ability to prepare for, respond to, and recover from an event of any size or complexity. Ethical dilemmas can occur at any point in the emergency management cycle. Therefore, a thoughtful application of ethics principles in each phase is important to ensure that ethical challenges are identified and appropriate courses of action are developed and implemented before an emergency event occurs.

Mitigation

Mitigation measures are activities that prevent an emergency event, reduce the likelihood of occurrence, or reduce an event's damaging effects. Administering immunizations and purchasing flood insurance are examples of mitigation activities.

The cornerstone of the mitigation phase is the hazard vulnerability analysis (HVA). The HVA is conducted to identify

- potential emergency events that could affect the demand for hospital services or the hospital's ability to provide those services,
- the likelihood of those events occurring,
- consequences of those events, and
- areas where the hospital may be vulnerable.

The HVA serves as the basis for developing emergency plans and procedures, conducting training and exercises, budgeting for and acquiring resources and assets, establishing external support agreements, and prioritizing mitigation and preparedness activities.

Much as an HVA identifies potential natural, technological, and human hazards and the hospital's vulnerability to them, an "ethics vulnerability analysis" enables the hospital to identify potential ethics issues as well as the consequences of not taking action to mitigate them. In a survey of 6,428 healthcare workers in New York City, Iserson and colleagues (2008) reported that willingness to work during a disaster varied by event type—ranging from a high of 84 percent during a mass casualty event to a low of 48 percent during a SARS outbreak. Therefore, a thorough assessment of a hospital's ethics vulnerabilities in the mitigation phase is instrumental to developing policies, plans, and procedures for eliminating or lessening their impact during an event. For example, the hospital should consider surveying all employees, not just healthcare practitioners, to determine their ability and willingness to respond to certain types of emergencies (e.g., hurricane, epidemic, radiological event). Some employees may be unable to respond during an emergency event because of family commitments (e.g., single parent with small children, caregiver for an elder dependent). Likewise, a survey of physicians and nurses could reveal misconceptions about policies related to disaster triage, allocation of scarce medical resources, or altered standards of care that could be resolved by additional training or by revising procedures during the preparedness phase.

The application of ethics principles in the mitigation phase can be accomplished by the following activities:

- Conduct ethics and legal audits of all emergency- and disaster-related plans, plan annexes, policies and guidelines, standards of care, treatment protocols, key processes (e.g., triage, admission, discharge, allocation of scarce resources), and external support agreements (e.g., contracts or memoranda of agreement with vendors, other healthcare entities, and public agencies) to identify areas requiring clarification or revision to address ethical and legal concerns. Some of these items, particularly processes or external support agreements, may be informal or unwritten. Consider formalizing and committing them to written form.

- Invite an ethics consultant or member of the hospital ethics committee (or its equivalent) to be a standing member of the emergency management committee (or its equivalent). Having this person available during discussions of proposed mitigation activities, HVA, and program review processes will ensure that ethics issues and concerns are identified before the planning process even begins.

- Mitigation activities (e.g., vaccination programs, quarantine, planned evacuation, inter-facility transfers) should have clearly defined and realistic goals, especially when they infringe on liberty, autonomy, or individual rights. Planners should work closely with stakeholder groups to explain the rationale for mitigation activities and strive to reach consensus on the least intrusive yet effective courses of action.

- Assess staff ability and willingness to respond to specific types of emergency events to determine what factors (e.g., safety concerns, fear of liability, family obligations) would limit their participation. Identify issues that require input and guidance from internal entities (e.g., legal department, risk management) as well as external entities (e.g., professional licensing boards, insurers, accreditation bodies). This information will be crucial in developing response plans and training initiatives.

Preparedness

Preparedness activities are designed to build and sustain capacity and capabilities by preparing the hospital and staff for response and recovery operations. Preparedness activities include planning, developing policies and procedures, stockpiling resources, conducting role-appropriate training for all staff, and testing capabilities through drills and exercises. Preparedness activities are defined and prioritized on the basis of hazards and vulnerabilities identified in the HVA.

In the United States, cultural individualism and ethical systems that stress autonomy, rights, and civil liberties directly affect the hospital's ability to develop ethically acceptable emergency plans and procedures. What may be perceived as inherently paternalistic directives must be fully explained and justified to stakeholders and the public. Consequently, the ethical acceptability of an emergency plan is a function of both its content and the process by which it was developed, debated, and ultimately approved. When properly executed, preparedness activities can actually become a form of social contract to which stakeholders have given their implied informed consent (Jennings 2008).

Hastings Center Fellows John Arras and Bruce Jennings have formulated seven ethical goals to guide the development, review, revision, and implementation of emergency preparedness plans (Jennings 2008):

1. **Harm reduction and benefit promotion that protect public safety, health, and well-being.** Public health emergency preparedness planning and response activities should protect public safety, health, and well-being. They should minimize the extent of death, injury, disease, disability, and suffering during and after an emergency.
2. **Equal liberty and human rights.** Preparedness and response activities should be designed so as to respect the equal liberty, autonomy, and dignity of all persons.
3. **Distributive justice.** Preparedness and response activities should be conducted so as to ensure that the benefits and burdens imposed on the population by the emergency and by the need to cope with its effects are shared uniformly and fairly.
4. **Public accountability.** Preparedness and response activities should be based on and incorporate decision-making processes that are inclusive and transparent and that sustain public trust.
5. **Development of strong as well as safe communities.** Preparedness and response activities should strive as a long-term goal to develop hazard-resistant and resilient communities. Such communities have robust internal support systems and networks of mutual assistance and solidarity. They also maintain sustainable and risk-mitigating relationships with their local ecosystems and their natural environment.
6. **Public health professionalism.** Preparedness and response activities should recognize the special obligations of some public health professionals and promote their competency, as well as coordination among them.
7. **Responsible civic response.** Preparedness and response activities should promote a sense of personal responsibility and citizenship.

These goals can be used to formulate answers to several ethical questions that will likely arise during the planning process:

- Who should be protected and to what level?
- How are budgets and planning priorities established?
- In what order should patients be evacuated? Which staff should remain behind with those who cannot be moved?
- When and under what circumstances should therapeutic efforts be stopped and shifted to palliative care to conserve scarce medical resources?

Solutions developed during the planning phase should be based on ethical analysis that can provide guidance during implementation even if the planned solutions must be altered in response to unforeseen circumstances (Timbie et al. 2012).

Emergency planning is an imperfect process. Unexpected events will occur, system failures will happen, and those with operational responsibility will be forced to make on-the-spot decisions requiring ethical judgments. Ethical considerations need to be explicit during the planning process so that, when those decisions must be made, they are consistent with the spirit of the ethical judgments that guided the planning process.

The application of ethics principles in the preparedness phase can be accomplished by the following activities:

- Actively engage the ethics representative during the planning process. Obtain an ethical perspective as plans, procedures, and external support agreements are being developed or revised. Seek guidance on resolving ethical conflicts.
- Identify the staff who will fill key response roles during an emergency event. Ensure that these personnel are trained to function in those capacities and that they understand the ethical components of those roles.
- Identify individuals and groups (e.g., elderly, disabled, medically underserved) who are particularly susceptible to harm or injustice during emergencies to ensure their needs will be addressed.
- Develop a support annex to the emergency operations plan (EOP) describing the decision-making process for the allocation of scarce medical resources and implementation of altered standards of care. (EOPs typically comprise a base plan followed by a series of incident annexes, support annexes, and resource annexes.)
  —Identify and describe the relevant ethical constructs. Be clear about how *disaster ethics,* which emphasize fair distribution of limited resources, differ from *clinical ethics,* which emphasize protecting the rights of individual patients.
  —Identify which triggers will activate the annex.
  —Describe how the annex will work in practice.
  —Describe the processes for withholding or withdrawing scarce resources (e.g., mechanical ventilators, IV fluids, medications) from a patient when clinicians determine that another patient is more likely to benefit from the resource.
  —Describe how existing resources will be fairly distributed during an emergency.
  —Justify why priority access to scarce resources may be provided to certain individuals or groups.

—Identify who was involved in developing the annex and the process used.

—Describe how the annex will be reviewed and revised. Make the annex available for public for review and comment.

- Provide role-specific ethics training (initial and refresher) for all employees. Managers, planners, and members of the incident management team will require a broad exposure to ethical principles and required actions, whereas healthcare practitioners will benefit from training that focuses primarily on clinical care issues. Even administrative and housekeeping personnel need a general understanding of planned response actions and the rationale behind them. Look for opportunities to incorporate ethics training into existing training offerings.

- Test the ethics components of emergency plans and procedures during periodic drills and exercises. Identify and document ethics questions and issues that arise so that plans and procedures can be clarified before they are needed for an actual emergency event. Provide follow-up training on any changes made as a result of this process.

- Develop a mechanism for the ongoing monitoring of the use of authority and power during the response phase to ensure that power and authority are not abused and that paternalistic or coercive measures are justified under the circumstances. Experience shows that solidarity and self-sacrifice often give way to disillusionment, recrimination, and litigation in the aftermath of an emergency event or disaster (Jennings and Arras 2008).

Response

Response activities address the immediate and near-term effects of the event. Response is the act of putting preparedness plans into action by mobilizing resources to save lives, stabilize the incident, and prevent further property damage or loss of assets.

The application of ethics principles in the response phase can be accomplished by the following activities (Jennings and Arras 2008):

- Monitor the use of authority and power to ensure that they are not abused and that paternalistic or coercive measures are justified under the circumstances.

- Maintain transparency in communications with the public.
  —Acknowledge uncertainty.
  —Provide follow-up information as it becomes available.
  —Advise patience and flexibility.
  —Admit mistakes and move on.
  —Provide guidance that can realistically be acted on.

- When selecting individuals for key response roles or deployment, ensure that the process is orderly, transparent, and fair and that it prevents undue family burden and personal hardship. If an individual believes an assignment is inappropriate or has been wrongly motivated, an expedient and confidential review and appeals process should be used.

Recovery

Recovery activities are designed to return the hospital to its pre-event state by restoring systems critical to the provision of care, treatment, and services. Recovery actions include compiling event documentation, conducting a critique, preparing an after-action report, performing critical incident stress debriefing, replenishing supplies, repairing or replacing equipment, addressing physical plant issues, reviewing and revising the EOP, and training or retraining personnel as necessary.

The decision to restore care or services disrupted during the emergency event should take into account the needs of the population being served as well as the resources available to resume operations. A phased approach to resuming services may be necessary—one that allows personnel mobilized during the response phase to attend to personal or family needs before returning to pre-event assignments and shift rotations. All hospital employees who participated in the emergency response, regardless of their role, have an obligation to participate in the evaluation of that response to help identify what worked well and what needs to be improved.

The application of ethics principles in the recovery phase can be accomplished by the following activities:

- Identify ethics issues and concerns during the post-event critique, and document findings and observations in the after-action report.
- Invite the hospital's ethics consultant or a member of the ethics committee (or its equivalent) to participate in post-event critique and evaluation activities.
- Review findings and observations of an ethical nature with the appropriate organizational entities (e.g., leadership, relevant committees, medical staff, department heads).
- Provide a forum for the discussion of ethics issues with all staff and relevant stakeholders.
- Review and revise the EOP, plan annexes, policies, procedures, external support agreements, and training materials to incorporate improvements to the ethical aspects of the emergency response.
- Ensure that revised training materials reinforce ethical constructs or reflect changes in processes of an ethical nature.

- Test revised processes during drills and exercises to determine if ethics issues and concerns have been adequately addressed and mitigated.
- Provide post-event medical follow-up to personnel who were exposed to harmful agents or were injured during the emergency response.
- Provide access to behavioral health support to all personnel affected by the emergency event, whether or not they were directly involved in response activities.
- Repatriate staff and patients who may have been displaced as a result of evacuation or service disruption, using processes that minimize further disruptions to personnel.

SUMMARY

Ethical values, though widely shared in American culture, are neither simple nor consistent. Although it is easy to invoke the notion of the greatest good, attempting to do the greatest good while providing universal assistance is a complex task requiring judgment and compromise. Including deliberate ethics planning as part of the emergency management construct provides a mechanism for identifying and resolving ethical issues that healthcare professionals face during emergency events—such as the duty to respond, allocation of scarce resources, and altered standards of care—and supports their professional concerns as well as the needs of the communities they serve.

REFERENCES

Agency for Healthcare Research and Quality (AHRQ). 2005. "Altered Standards of Care in Mass Casualty Events." Published April. http://archive.ahrq.gov/research/altstand/altstand.pdf.

American Nurses Association (ANA). 2008. "Adapting Standards of Care Under Extreme Conditions: Guidance for Professionals During Disasters, Pandemics, and Other Extreme Emergencies." Report prepared by the Columbia University School of Nursing Center for Health Policy. Published March. http://ana.nursingworld.org/MainMenuCategories/HealthcareandPolicyIssues/DPR/TheLawEthicsof DisasterResponse/AdaptingStandardsofCare.aspx.

Brewer, K. 2010. "Who Will Be There? Ethics, the Law, and a Nurse's Duty to Respond in a Disaster." *American Nurses Association Issue Brief* June. http://nursingworld.org/MainMenuCategories/Policy-Advocacy/Positions-and-Resolutions/Issue-Briefs/Disaster-Preparedness.pdf.

Federal Emergency Management Agency (FEMA). 2013. "Disaster Declarations by Year." Accessed April 25. www.fema.gov/tr/disasters/grid/year.

Illinois Department of Public Health. 2004. "Intergovernmental Mutual Aid Agreement for the Establishment of the Illinois Public Health Mutual Aid System (IPHMAS)." Entered June 4. www.idph.state.il.us/local/mutualaidagree_9.30.04.pdf.

International Emergency Management Group. 2013. "International Emergency Management Assistance Memorandum of Understanding." Accessed June 21. www.iemg-gigu-web.org/mou-e.asp.

Iserson, K. V., C. E. Heine, G. L. Larkin, J. C. Moskop, J. Baruch, and A. L. Aswegan. 2008. "Fight or Flight: The Ethics of Emergency Physician Disaster Response." *Annals of Emergency Medicine* 51 (4): 345–53.

Jennings, B. 2008. "Disaster Planning and Public Health." In *From Birth to Death and Bench to Clinic: The Hastings Center Bioethics Briefing Book for Journalists, Policymakers, and Campaigns,* edited by Mary Crowley, 41–44. Garrison, NY: The Hastings Center.

Jennings, B., and J. Arras. 2008. "Ethical Guidance for Public Health Emergency Preparedness and Response: Highlighting Ethics and Values in a Vital Public Health Service." White paper prepared for the Ethics Subcommittee, Advisory Committee to the Director, Centers for Disease Control and Prevention. Published October 30. www.cdc.gov/od/science/integrity/phethics/docs/White_Paper_Final_ for_Website_2012_4_6_12_final_for_web_508_compliant.pdf.

Mid-America Alliance. 2009. "Going Beyond EMAC—The Role of the Mutual Aid Project." Accessed April 25, 2013. www.unmc.edu/midamerica/index.cfm?L1_ ID=18&CONREF=18.

New York State Department of Health. 2007. "Allocation of Ventilators in an Influenza Pandemic." Planning document (draft for public comment) prepared by the New York State Workgroup on Ventilator Allocation in an Influenza Pandemic. Published March 15. www.health.ny.gov/diseases/communicable/influenza/ pandemic/ventilators/.

Phillips, S. J., and A. Knebel (eds.). 2007. *Mass Medical Care with Scarce Resources: A Community Planning Guide.* Rockville, MD: Agency for Healthcare Research and Quality.

Phillips, S. J., A. Knebel, and K. J. Johnson (eds.). 2009. *Mass Medical Care with Scarce Resources: The Essentials.* Rockville, MD: Agency for Healthcare Research and Quality.

Timbie, J. W., J. S. Ringel, D. S. Fox, D. A. Waxman, F. Pillemer, C. Carey, M. Moore, V. Karir, T. J. Johnson, N. Iyer, J. Hu, R. Shanman, J. W. Larkin, M. Timmer, A. Motala, T. R. Perry, S. Newberry, and A. L. Kellermann. 2012. "Allocation of Scarce Resources During Mass Casualty Events." AHRQ Evidence Report/ Technology Assessment Number 207. Published June. www.effectivehealthcare .ahrq.gov/search-for-guides-reviews-and-reports/?pageaction=displayproduct& productid=1152.

University of Toronto Joint Centre for Bioethics. 2005. "Stand on Guard for Thee: Ethical Considerations in Preparedness Planning for Pandemic Influenza." Report of the University of Toronto Joint Centre for Bioethics Pandemic Influenza Working Group. Published November. www.jointcentreforbioethics.ca/people/ documents/upshur_stand_guard.pdf.

US Congress. 1996. "Emergency Management Assistance Compact." Pub. L. No. 104-321, 110 Stat. 3877. Published October 19. www.gpo.gov/fdsys/pkg/PLAW-104publ321/pdf/PLAW-104publ321.pdf.

Vargas, T. 2010. "D.C. Hospital Fires 11 Nurses, 5 Staffers for Snowstorm Absences." *Washington Post* February 28. www.washingtonpost.com/wp-dyn/content/article/ 2010/02/27/AR2010022703793.html?sid=ST2010100603805.

Follow-Up on the Cases

ALTHOUGH THE CASES presented in this book have been taken from the headlines and for the most part fictionalized, even fiction has an ending. My favorite reading as a child was *What Happened Then Stories,* and the following is what actually happened or a fictional account of what most likely happened in these cases.

Recall that each of these cases is characterized by ambiguities and intertwining ethical issues, so the resolutions (or lack of resolutions) may have an impact on several people and programs in an organization or in the community in which that organization is located.

A healthcare manager is confronted with ethical dilemmas every day. Most of the time, the manager makes the right decisions unconsciously and "does the right thing." For the most part, those involved in healthcare are decent, moral individuals who are attracted to the healthcare field because they wish to contribute something positive to society. Nevertheless, they occasionally make errors in judgment, detrimental decisions, and unintentional mistakes. More often than not, mistakes are the result of the barrage of decisions that must be made by managers who are pressed for time and strained by the demands of the job. Decisions are frequently made without the benefit of thoughtful reflection or consultation with others.

The cases in this book are intended to remind healthcare managers of the untoward consequences of hasty decisions that do not consider all of the ethical dimensions involved.

PARADISE HILLS MEDICAL CENTER

The matter of the radiation overdose given to 22 oncology patients was referred to the medical center's ethics committee. Following deliberations, the committee recommended that the patients affected be informed about the errors and monitored closely for adverse effects. The medical staff and administration reviewed the committee's recommendation, but the administration decided not to follow it, maintaining that it was under no obligation to do so because the ethics committee was only advisory in nature. After review, the governing board concurred. Its decision was based on a fear of litigation and the bad publicity that was certain to follow if knowledge of the errors became public. Consequently, the patients involved were not informed about the errors. Four of the patients suffered adverse effects, the most serious of which were radiation burns.

Three months later, one of the patients learned about the errors and filed a lawsuit against the hospital for fraudulent concealment. Because the reason for the lawsuit was fraud and not malpractice, the hospital's malpractice insurance did not provide coverage. The case was settled out of court for $300,000. The lawsuit and settlement received broad news coverage both on television and in the local newspapers. As the other patients involved became aware of the incident, only a few chose to file lawsuits and settled out of court for similar amounts. The hospital considered itself lucky.

The aftermath of this experience was characterized by tension among the staff, who disagreed among themselves about how this case should have been handled. The nurses in the oncology program adamantly believed that the patients should have been told immediately about the accidental overdose. In fact, some staff members speculated that one of the nurses had informed the first patient about the errors. A prestigious oncology medical group practice, uncomfortable with all of the publicity and the inquiries from patients about the medical center's capabilities, began to disassociate itself from Paradise Hills Medical Center and to refer patients to a competing facility. Relationships between some primary care physicians and oncologists remained strained. The oncology program suffered a moderate decline in census. Some members of the governing board felt they had been misdirected by the hospital's administration. A general sense of mistrust was palpable throughout the medical center, and employees and hospital staff were chagrined that they had to defend the medical center to friends and family who were shocked by the disclosure.

QUAL PLUS HMO

Jim decided to play the game and follow the lead of his boss and the governing board. "Final" bids were requested, and the contract was awarded to Acme Construction. Jim's relationships with Brent and with the board members who had served on the facilities committee were strained. Brent began to micromanage Jim's operations, and some of Jim's responsibilities were assigned to other staff. Jim was especially offended when Brent gave oversight of the construction project to one of his coworkers. More and more, Jim felt out of the loop. His invitations to golf were declined. He began to feel slighted at social functions as well. Even Jim's wife mentioned that Brent and his wife seemed particularly cool lately.

Most of all, Jim was uncomfortable with himself. He was being eased out of the organization even though he had done what they wanted. Now he wished he had stood by his principles—and resigned, if necessary. At least he would still have his self-respect.

ROLLING MEADOWS COMMUNITY HOSPITAL

John Waverly never fully recovered from the incident at Rolling Meadows Community Hospital. He was bitter because he believed the board had treated him unfairly. He insisted he had done nothing wrong, but he believed the board was more interested in appearances than fact. They did not ask for his resignation, but John knew that he had lost credibility with them. His wife felt humiliated by his behavior and asked for a separation until things blew over. His children were openly disdainful of him. The general consensus among his colleagues, even those who liked him, was that he had been unbelievably careless.

The postgraduate fellow sought legal counsel and was told that she probably had grounds for litigation because the position was not offered to her on the basis of her gender. However, she decided not to pursue litigation. She had no difficulty finding another responsible position. Unfortunately, her experience at Rolling Meadows loomed like a shadow over her. The word was that she had threatened sexual harassment charges. Male colleagues behaved professionally toward her but kept their distance. The senior executives limited the amount of time they spent with her. She knew she had done nothing wrong, but she also believed that her experience at Rolling Meadows had hurt her career.

Some of the hospital staff congratulated themselves for knowing something was going on and imagined the most sordid of affairs. John's defenders were quick to label the postgraduate fellow as a seductress, noting that no one can trust anyone that young, attractive, and ambitious.

The incident was never made public, but word got around. The gossip was about marital infidelity. Two board members who had been among John's early supporters suggested that John might want to start looking for another position. They were apologetic but noted that the small, family-oriented community of Rolling Meadows was not very tolerant. They mentioned that another board member had even suggested that John's judgment was impaired and that he could not be trusted to make appropriate decisions in the future. John was baffled by the board's lack of compassion and support.

UNIVERSITY HOSPITAL

As expected, that afternoon the newspaper reported that a resident in training had performed unsupervised emergency surgery at University Hospital. The reporter had interviewed the patient and his family, who said that they were completely satisfied with the care they had received at University Hospital and that they had no intention of criticizing the hospital or seeking legal remedy.

The hospital staff were relieved, as were the medical staff, the surgery residency program director, the resident physician, and Dr. Spalding.

Jan was reprimanded for not calling in the surgeon on second call and for not reporting Dr. Spalding's impairment. She was found lax in her responsibility for the safe care of the patient.

Dr. Truman was reprimanded for not ordering that the surgeon on second call be notified and for not asking that the surgery residency program director be notified about the absence of an attending physician.

Following disciplinary review, Dr. Spalding had his surgical privileges suspended until he provided evidence to the credentialing committee that he had sought treatment for his drinking problem.

The publicity about the incident did not appear to harm the hospital's image. On the contrary, many thought that the patient's favorable testimonial actually helped public relations.

HILLSIDE COUNTY MEDICAL CENTER

In analyzing Hillside's overall financial situation, the CEO determined that the medical center's financial challenges had to be addressed in a manner that would ensure its long-term survivability and success. He believed that accomplishing this task would require a collaborative effort involving the input and engagement of key shareholders, such as medical staff and union leadership. In addition, he knew that the mission of the organization could not be compromised.

Accordingly, a medical staff advisory board was established. The initial responsibility of this medical advisory group (MAG) was to identify the most appropriate way to deal with the financial challenges that Hillside currently faced. The MAG identified opportunities for program and cost reductions as well as new opportunities for financial expansion. Issues such as length of stay were recognized as key opportunities for reducing operational costs. It was agreed that the MAG would continue to meet on a quarterly basis to define and develop collaborative opportunities.

At the same time, meetings were held with key union leaders to seek their input and assistance in identifying opportunities for cost reductions. Through this collaboration, significant and valuable suggestions were incorporated into the cost-reduction process. Not only was the outcome more successful, but everyone involved also gained a better understanding of the challenges that the organization faced.

This initial success may not guarantee that Hillside's financial obstacles are permanently overcome. However, it proved that Hillside could address these concerns in a collaborative manner. Collaboration, in the long run, may be the only successful way to achieve significant cost reductions.

METROPOLITAN COMMUNITY HOSPITAL

Frustrated with the lack of attention to their concerns, the nursing staff at Metropolitan began serious discussions about unionizing so that they could speak with an organized voice. The debate and dissension among the nursing staff about the desirability of this action soon spilled over into the community and made its way to the board.

The board put Eugene's feet to the fire and demanded that he quickly handle the situation before it got worse. Eugene asked Jane to resign and appointed a strong search committee that had nursing and medical staff representation. The search committee's mandate was to recruit a competent and innovative CNO as quickly as possible. The committee was successful.

The new CNO made rapid progress toward stabilizing the nursing workforce. Even retention improved. Eugene was beginning to relax when yet another staff conflict required his attention. The new CNO and the COO, Carter Sims, adamantly disagreed about whether and how the physicians' disruptive behavior should be addressed. The CNO argued that such behavior was unacceptable and that action needed to be taken immediately. Carter believed that the CNO was overreacting and argued that the medical staff were not within her purview. Eugene agreed with the CNO and knew the time had come to consider replacing Carter with a COO who could see the big picture and collaborate as part of a functional senior team. Eugene had become so far removed from operations that he knew this task was not going to be easy. He was beginning to think he had made a mistake in coming to Metropolitan.

HEARTLAND HEALTHCARE SYSTEM

Richard had been Heartland's CEO for more than 15 years and was widely credited with the success of the system. The board and the community had great confidence in his character and abilities. Richard was able to capitalize on their confidence and goodwill. He candidly admitted his hiring mistake and moved quickly to replace Jack as CIO and to terminate Les. He appointed a multidisciplinary search committee, chaired by the COO to whom the new CIO would report, and engaged the services of a nationally recognized search consultant to find a new CIO—preferably one with healthcare experience.

The board supported Richard in his efforts, and he assured the board members that once the new CIO was in place, they would receive regular reports on the objectives, metrics, and progress of information technology at Heartland. The staff at Heartland were enthusiastic about these efforts and pledged to support the incoming CIO. A year later, real IT progress had been made.

RICHLAND RIVER VALLEY HEALTHCARE SYSTEM

Within the first year following the dissolution of RRVHS, Continental Healthcare moved quickly to purchase both Trinity and Sutton Memorial, which Continental now operates as separate healthcare facilities under its national for-profit healthcare corporation.

Not wanting to labor under corporate direction and frustrated with mismanagement, a large group of prominent, highly regarded physicians in Clay County formed a physician-owned medical group practice—Richland Health Partners (RHP)—to provide primary and specialty care, urgent care, and hospital care. Continental negotiated with RHP for hospital care, and all seemed well for two years. However, the physicians were never really comfortable with the arrangement, feeling they had relinquished control and any ability to influence the delivery of healthcare in Richland. When the contracts came up for renewal, negotiations failed, the contracts were terminated, and Continental informed the physicians that they could no longer treat patients at Continental's facilities. This outcome caused much alarm in the community and prompted lawsuits between Continental and RHP.

Employees at Trinity and Sutton Memorial likewise continue to experience turmoil. When Continental took over, it implemented staff reductions to trim costs at both hospitals. Uncertainty and dissension between the medical staff and administration have exacerbated the staff's mistrust of the new management. The unions at Trinity are about to enter into contract talks with Continental and fear the worst.

Few of the original board members were retained. Both they and those who resigned have lost the respect of the community, which feels its hospitals were "sold out."

HURLEY MEDICAL CENTER

The lawsuit against Hurley Medical Center alleging racial discrimination was filed in January 2013 and was settled out of court in February 2013. The newspaper story about the settlement carried the headline "Flint Hurley Medical Center Lawsuit Settled; Nurse Glad It's a Learning Tool." Although details of the settlement were not disclosed, it was said to have been "amicably resolved" (Adams 2013). Indeed, the president and CEO of the hospital made the announcement with the plaintiffs alongside. The president said that the incident will be used in training at the hospital to prevent similar incidents from happening in the future.

The National Action Network announced that it still planned to protest outside the hospital. The political director for the Michigan chapter of the group said, "We're challenging the institution of racism that manifested itself when staff and management followed the directives of a guy that may be a Nazi" (Adams 2013). The group asked for a meeting with hospital officials.

News coverage of the event has continued throughout national media. Ten days after the lawsuit was settled, the nurse involved in the incident was interviewed by Katie Couric on ABC-TV, who was later quoted as saying she believed the nurse took appropriate action in the case (Ridley 2013).

CONCLUSION

As these sequels demonstrate, there are few winners after a breach of ethical conduct. Typically, the problems that result touch more than a few lives. For this reason and others, healthcare executives would be wise to put organizational mechanisms in place that help staff make sound ethical decisions to begin with. In the matter of ethics, as in other matters, preventing problems requires less time and energy, is less costly, and is certainly more rewarding.

REFERENCES

Adams, D. 2013. "Flint Hurley Medical Center Lawsuit Settled; Nurse Glad It's a Learning Tool." *The Flint Journal* February 22.

Ridley, G. 2013. "Nurse Sues Flint's Hurley Medical Center over Claim She Was Barred from Treating Infant Because of Her Race." *The Flint Journal* February 18.

Suggested Further Reading

Bennis, W. 2009. *On Becoming a Leader,* revised edition. New York: Perseus Books.

Bujak, J. S. 2008. *Inside the Physician Mind: Finding Common Ground with Doctors.* Chicago: Health Administration Press.

Hofmann, P. B., and F. Perry. 2005. *Management Mistakes in Healthcare: Identification, Correction, and Prevention.* New York: Cambridge University Press.

Hosmer, L. T. 1987. *The Ethics of Management,* seventh edition. New York: McGraw-Hill.

Nelson, W. A., and P. B. Hofmann. 2010. *Managing Ethically: An Executive's Guide,* second edition. Chicago: Health Administration Press.

Perry, F. 2012. *Healthcare Leadership That Makes a Difference: Creating Your Legacy.* Self-study course. Chicago: Health Administration Press.

Rice, J. A., and F. Perry. 2013. *Healthcare Leadership Excellence: Creating a Career of Impact.* Chicago: Health Administration Press.

White, K. R., and J. R. Griffith. 2010. *The Well-Managed Healthcare Organization,* seventh edition. Chicago: Health Administration Press.

Zenger, J., and J. Folkman. 2002. *The Extraordinary Leader: Turning Good Managers into Great Leaders.* New York: McGraw-Hill.

American College of Healthcare Executives Ethics Self-Assessment

Purpose of the Ethics Self-Assessment

Members of the American College of Healthcare Executives agree, as a condition of membership, to abide by ACHE's *Code of Ethics.* The *Code* provides an overall standard of conduct and includes specific standards of ethical behavior to guide healthcare executives in their professional relationships.

Based on the *Code of Ethics,* the Ethics Self-Assessment is intended for your personal use to assist you in thinking about your ethics-related leadership and actions. *It should not be returned to ACHE nor should it be used as a tool for evaluating the ethical behavior of others.*

The Ethics Self-Assessment can help you identify those areas in which you are on strong ethical ground; areas that you may wish to examine the basis for your responses; and opportunities for further reflection. The Ethics Self-Assessment does not have a scoring mechanism, as we do not believe that ethical behavior can or should be quantified.

How to Use This Self-Assessment

We hope you find this self-assessment thought provoking and useful as a part of your reflection on applying the ACHE *Code of Ethics* to your everyday activities. You are to be commended for taking time out of your busy schedule to complete it.

Once you have finished the self-assessment, it is suggested that you review your responses, noting which questions you answered "usually," "occasionally" and "almost never." You may find that in some cases an answer of "usually" is satisfactory, but in other cases such as when answering a question about protecting staff's well-being, an answer of "usually" may raise an ethical red flag.

Source: Reprinted by permission of the American College of Healthcare Executives.

We are confident that you will uncover few red flags where your responses are not compatible with the ACHE *Code of Ethics*. For those you may discover, you should use this as an opportunity to enhance your ethical practice and leadership by developing a specific action plan. For example, you may have noted in the self-assessment that you have not used your organization's ethics mechanism to assist you in addressing challenging ethical conflicts. As a result of this insight you might meet with the chair of the ethics committee to better understand the committee's functions, including case consultation activities, and how you might access this resource when future ethical conflicts arise.

We also want you to consider ACHE as a resource when you and your management team are confronted with difficult ethical dilemmas. In the About ACHE area of **ache.org,** you can access an Ethics Toolkit, a group of practical resources that will help you understand how to integrate ethics into your organization. In addition, you can refer to our regular "Healthcare Management Ethics" column in *Healthcare Executive* magazine, and you may want to consider attending our annual ethics seminar.

Source: Reprinted by permission of the American College of Healthcare Executives.

Please check one answer for each of the following questions.

	Almost Never	Occasionally	Usually	Always	Not Applicable

I. LEADERSHIP

	Almost Never	Occasionally	Usually	Always	Not Applicable
I take courageous, consistent and appropriate management actions to overcome barriers to achieving my organization's mission.	❑	❑	❑	❑	❑
I place community/patient benefit over my personal gain.	❑	❑	❑	❑	❑
I strive to be a role model for ethical behavior.	❑	❑	❑	❑	❑
I work to ensure that decisions about access to care are based primarily on medical necessity, not only on the ability to pay.	❑	❑	❑	❑	❑
My statements and actions are consistent with professional ethical standards, including the ACHE *Code of Ethics*.	❑	❑	❑	❑	❑
My statements and actions are honest even when circumstances would allow me to confuse the issues.	❑	❑	❑	❑	❑
I advocate ethical decision making by the board, management team and medical staff.	❑	❑	❑	❑	❑
I use an ethical approach to conflict resolution.	❑	❑	❑	❑	❑
I initiate and encourage discussion of the ethical aspects of management/financial issues.	❑	❑	❑	❑	❑
I initiate and promote discussion of controversial issues affecting community/patient health (e.g., domestic and community violence and decisions near the end of life).	❑	❑	❑	❑	❑
I promptly and candidly explain to internal and external stakeholders negative economic trends and encourage appropriate action.	❑	❑	❑	❑	❑
I use my authority solely to fulfill my responsibilities and not for self-interest or to further the interests of family, friends or associates.	❑	❑	❑	❑	❑
When an ethical conflict confronts my organization or me, I am successful in finding an effective resolution process and ensure it is followed.	❑	❑	❑	❑	❑

Source: Reprinted by permission of the American College of Healthcare Executives.

	Almost Never	Occasionally	Usually	Always	Not Applicable
I demonstrate respect for my colleagues, superiors and staff.	❏	❏	❏	❏	❏
I demonstrate my organization's vision, mission and value statements in my actions.	❏	❏	❏	❏	❏
I make timely decisions rather than delaying them to avoid difficult or politically risky choices.	❏	❏	❏	❏	❏
I seek the advice of the ethics committee when making ethically challenging decisions.	❏	❏	❏	❏	❏
My personal expense reports are accurate and are only billed to a single organization.	❏	❏	❏	❏	❏
I openly support establishing and monitoring internal mechanisms (e.g., an ethics committee or program) to support ethical decision making.	❏	❏	❏	❏	❏
I thoughtfully consider decisions when making a promise on behalf of the organization to a person or a group of people.	❏	❏	❏	❏	❏

II. RELATIONSHIPS

Community

	Almost Never	Occasionally	Usually	Always	Not Applicable
I promote community health status improvement as a guiding goal of my organization and as a cornerstone of my efforts on behalf of my organization.	❏	❏	❏	❏	❏
I personally devote time to developing solutions to community health problems.	❏	❏	❏	❏	❏
I participate in and encourage my management team to devote personal time to community service.	❏	❏	❏	❏	❏

Patients and Their Families

	Almost Never	Occasionally	Usually	Always	Not Applicable
I use a patient- and family-centered approach to patient care.	❏	❏	❏	❏	❏
I am a patient advocate on both clinical and financial matters.	❏	❏	❏	❏	❏
I ensure equitable treatment of patients regardless of their socioeconomic status, ethnicity or payor category.	❏	❏	❏	❏	❏
I respect the practices and customs of a diverse patient population while maintaining the organization's mission.	❏	❏	❏	❏	❏

Source: Reprinted by permission of the American College of Healthcare Executives.

	Almost Never	Occasionally	Usually	Always	Not Applicable
I demonstrate through organizational policies and personal actions that overtreatment and undertreatment of patients are unacceptable.	❏	❏	❏	❏	❏
I protect patients' rights to autonomy through access to full, accurate information about their illnesses, treatment options and related costs and benefits.	❏	❏	❏	❏	❏
I promote a patient's right to privacy, including medical record confidentiality, and do not tolerate breaches of this confidentiality.	❏	❏	❏	❏	❏

Board

	Almost Never	Occasionally	Usually	Always	Not Applicable
I have a routine system in place for board members to make full disclosure and reveal potential conflicts of interest.	❏	❏	❏	❏	❏
I ensure that reports to the board, my own or others', appropriately convey risks of decisions or proposed projects.	❏	❏	❏	❏	❏
I work to keep the board focused on ethical issues of importance to the organization, community and other stakeholders.	❏	❏	❏	❏	❏
I keep the board appropriately informed of patient safety and quality indicators.	❏	❏	❏	❏	❏
I promote board discussion of resource allocation issues, particularly those where organizational and community interests may appear to be incompatible.	❏	❏	❏	❏	❏
I keep the board appropriately informed about issues of alleged financial malfeasance, clinical malpractice and potential litigious situations involving employees.	❏	❏	❏	❏	❏

Colleagues and Staff

	Almost Never	Occasionally	Usually	Always	Not Applicable
I foster discussions about ethical concerns when they arise.	❏	❏	❏	❏	❏
I maintain confidences entrusted to me.	❏	❏	❏	❏	❏
I demonstrate through personal actions and organizational policies zero tolerance for any form of staff harassment.	❏	❏	❏	❏	❏
I encourage discussions about and advocate for the implementation of the organization's code of ethics and value statements.	❏	❏	❏	❏	❏
I fulfill the promises I make.	❏	❏	❏	❏	❏

Source: Reprinted by permission of the American College of Healthcare Executives.

	Almost Never	Occasionally	Usually	Always	Not Applicable
I am respectful of views different from mine.	❏	❏	❏	❏	❏
I am respectful of individuals who differ from me in ethnicity, gender, education or job position.	❏	❏	❏	❏	❏
I convey negative news promptly and openly, not allowing employees or others to be misled.	❏	❏	❏	❏	❏
I expect and hold staff accountable for adherence to our organization's ethical standards (e.g., performance reviews).	❏	❏	❏	❏	❏
I demonstrate that incompetent supervision is not tolerated and make timely decisions regarding marginally performing managers.	❏	❏	❏	❏	❏
I ensure adherence to ethics-related policies and practices affecting patients and staff.	❏	❏	❏	❏	❏
I am sensitive to employees who have ethical concerns and facilitate resolution of these concerns.	❏	❏	❏	❏	❏
I encourage the use of organizational mechanisms (e.g., an ethics committee or program) and other ethics resources to address ethical issues.	❏	❏	❏	❏	❏
I act quickly and decisively when employees are not treated fairly in their relationships with other employees.	❏	❏	❏	❏	❏
I assign staff only to official duties and do not ask them to assist me with work on behalf of my family, friends or associates.	❏	❏	❏	❏	❏
I hold all staff and clinical/business partners accountable for compliance with professional standards, including ethical behavior.	❏	❏	❏	❏	❏

Clinicians

	Almost Never	Occasionally	Usually	Always	Not Applicable
When problems arise with clinical care, I ensure that the problems receive prompt attention and resolution by the responsible parties.	❏	❏	❏	❏	❏
I insist that my organization's clinical practice guidelines are consistent with our vision, mission, value statements and ethical standards of practice.	❏	❏	❏	❏	❏

Source: Reprinted by permission of the American College of Healthcare Executives.

	Almost Never	Occasionally	Usually	Always	Not Applicable
When practice variations in care suggest quality of care is at stake, I encourage timely actions that serve patients' interests.	❑	❑	❑	❑	❑
I insist that participating clinicians and staff live up to the terms of managed care contracts.	❑	❑	❑	❑	❑
I encourage clinicians to access ethics resources when ethical conflicts occur.	❑	❑	❑	❑	❑
I encourage resource allocation that is equitable, is based on clinical needs and appropriately balances patient needs and organizational/clinical resources.	❑	❑	❑	❑	❑
I expeditiously and forthrightly deal with impaired clinicians and take necessary action when I believe a clinician is not competent to perform his/her clinical duties.	❑	❑	❑	❑	❑
I expect and hold clinicians accountable for adhering to their professional and the organization's ethical practices.	❑	❑	❑	❑	❑

Buyers, Payors and Suppliers

	Almost Never	Occasionally	Usually	Always	Not Applicable
I negotiate and expect my management team to negotiate in good faith.	❑	❑	❑	❑	❑
I am mindful of the importance of avoiding even the appearance of wrongdoing, conflict of interest or interference with free competition.	❑	❑	❑	❑	❑
I personally disclose and expect board members, staff members and clinicians to disclose any possible conflicts of interest before pursuing or entering into relationships with potential business partners.	❑	❑	❑	❑	❑
I promote familiarity and compliance with organizational policies governing relationships with buyers, payors and suppliers.	❑	❑	❑	❑	❑
I set an example for others in my organization by not accepting personal gifts from suppliers.	❑	❑	❑	❑	❑

Source: Reprinted by permission of the American College of Healthcare Executives.

American College of Healthcare Executives
*Code of Ethics**

PREAMBLE

The purpose of the *Code of Ethics* of the American College of Healthcare Executives is to serve as a standard of conduct for members. It contains standards of ethical behavior for healthcare executives in their professional relationships. These relationships include colleagues, patients or others served; members of the healthcare executive's organization and other organizations; the community; and society as a whole.

The *Code of Ethics* also incorporates standards of ethical behavior governing individual behavior, particularly when that conduct directly relates to the role and identity of the healthcare executive.

The fundamental objectives of the healthcare management profession are to maintain or enhance the overall quality of life, dignity and well-being of every individual needing healthcare service and to create a more equitable, accessible, effective and efficient healthcare system.

Healthcare executives have an obligation to act in ways that will merit the trust, confidence, and respect of healthcare professionals and the general public. Therefore, healthcare executives should lead lives that embody an exemplary system of values and ethics.

In fulfilling their commitments and obligations to patients or others served, healthcare executives function as moral advocates and models. Since every management decision affects the health and well-being of both individuals and communities, healthcare executives must carefully evaluate the possible outcomes of their decisions. In organizations that deliver healthcare services, they must work to safeguard and foster the rights, interests and prerogatives of patients or others served.

*As amended by the Board of Governors on November 14, 2011.

Source: Reprinted by permission of the American College of Healthcare Executives.

The role of moral advocate requires that healthcare executives take actions necessary to promote such rights, interests and prerogatives.

Being a model means that decisions and actions will reflect personal integrity and ethical leadership that others will seek to emulate.

I. THE HEALTHCARE EXECUTIVE'S RESPONSIBILITIES TO THE PROFESSION OF HEALTHCARE MANAGEMENT

The healthcare executive shall:

A. Uphold the *Code of Ethics* and mission of the American College of Healthcare Executives;

B. Conduct professional activities with honesty, integrity, respect, fairness and good faith in a manner that will reflect well upon the profession;

C. Comply with all laws and regulations pertaining to healthcare management in the jurisdictions in which the healthcare executive is located or conducts professional activities;

D. Maintain competence and proficiency in healthcare management by implementing a personal program of assessment and continuing professional education;

E. Avoid the improper exploitation of professional relationships for personal gain;

F. Disclose financial and other conflicts of interest;

G. Use this *Code* to further the interests of the profession and not for selfish reasons;

H. Respect professional confidences;

I. Enhance the dignity and image of the healthcare management profession through positive public information programs; and

J. Refrain from participating in any activity that demeans the credibility and dignity of the healthcare management profession.

II. THE HEALTHCARE EXECUTIVE'S RESPONSIBILITIES TO PATIENTS OR OTHERS SERVED

The healthcare executive shall, within the scope of his or her authority:

A. Work to ensure the existence of a process to evaluate the quality of care or service rendered;

Source: Reprinted by permission of the American College of Healthcare Executives.

B. Avoid practicing or facilitating discrimination and institute safeguards to prevent discriminatory organizational practices;

C. Work to ensure the existence of a process that will advise patients or others served of the rights, opportunities, responsibilities and risks regarding available healthcare services;

D. Work to ensure that there is a process in place to facilitate the resolution of conflicts that may arise when values of patients and their families differ from those of employees and physicians;

E. Demonstrate zero tolerance for any abuse of power that compromises patients or others served;

F. Work to provide a process that ensures the autonomy and self-determination of patients or others served;

G. Work to ensure the existence of procedures that will safeguard the confidentiality and privacy of patients or others served; and

H. Work to ensure the existence of an ongoing process and procedures to review, develop and consistently implement evidence-based clinical practices throughout the organization.

III. THE HEALTHCARE EXECUTIVE'S RESPONSIBILITIES TO THE ORGANIZATION

The healthcare executive shall, within the scope of his or her authority:

A. Provide healthcare services consistent with available resources, and when there are limited resources, work to ensure the existence of a resource allocation process that considers ethical ramifications;

B. Conduct both competitive and cooperative activities in ways that improve community healthcare services;

C. Lead the organization in the use and improvement of standards of management and sound business practices;

D. Respect the customs and practices of patients or others served, consistent with the organization's philosophy;

E. Be truthful in all forms of professional and organizational communication, and avoid disseminating information that is false, misleading or deceptive;

Source: Reprinted by permission of the American College of Healthcare Executives.

F. Report negative financial and other information promptly and accurately, and initiate appropriate action;

G. Prevent fraud and abuse and aggressive accounting practices that may result in disputable financial reports;

H. Create an organizational environment in which both clinical and management mistakes are minimized and, when they do occur, are disclosed and addressed effectively;

I. Implement an organizational code of ethics and monitor compliance; and

J. Provide ethics resources and mechanisms for staff to address ethical organizational and clinical issues.

IV. THE HEALTHCARE EXECUTIVE'S RESPONSIBILITIES TO EMPLOYEES

Healthcare executives have ethical and professional obligations to the employees they manage that encompass but are not limited to:

A. Creating a work environment that promotes ethical conduct;

B. Providing a work environment that encourages a free expression of ethical concerns and provides mechanisms for discussing and addressing such concerns;

C. Promoting a healthy work environment, which includes freedom from harassment, sexual and other, and coercion of any kind, especially to perform illegal or unethical acts;

D. Promoting a culture of inclusivity that seeks to prevent discrimination on the basis of race, ethnicity, religion, gender, sexual orientation, age or disability;

E. Providing a work environment that promotes the proper use of employees' knowledge and skills; and

F. Providing a safe and healthy work environment.

V. THE HEALTHCARE EXECUTIVE'S RESPONSIBILITIES TO COMMUNITY AND SOCIETY

The healthcare executive shall:

A. Work to identify and meet the healthcare needs of the community;

Source: Reprinted by permission of the American College of Healthcare Executives.

B. Work to support access to healthcare services for all people;

C. Encourage and participate in public dialogue on healthcare policy issues, and advocate solutions that will improve health status and promote quality healthcare;

D. Apply short- and long-term assessments to management decisions affecting both community and society; and

E. Provide prospective patients and others with adequate and accurate information, enabling them to make enlightened decisions regarding services.

VI. THE HEALTHCARE EXECUTIVE'S RESPONSIBILITY TO REPORT VIOLATIONS OF THE *CODE*

A member of ACHE who has reasonable grounds to believe that another member has violated this *Code* has a duty to communicate such facts to the Ethics Committee.

ADDITIONAL RESOURCES

Available on **ache.org** or by calling ACHE at (312) 424-2800.

1. ACHE *Ethical Policy Statements*

   "Considerations for Healthcare Executive–Supplier Interactions"

   "Creating an Ethical Culture Within the Healthcare Organization"

   "Decisions Near the End of Life"

   "Ethical Decision Making for Healthcare Executives"

   "Ethical Issues Related to a Reduction in Force"

   "Ethical Issues Related to Staff Shortages"

   "Health Information Confidentiality"

   "Impaired Healthcare Executives"

   "Promise Making, Keeping and Rescinding"

2. ACHE Grievance Procedure

3. ACHE Ethics Committee Action

4. ACHE Ethics Committee Scope and Function

Source: Reprinted by permission of the American College of Healthcare Executives.

American College of Healthcare Executives Ethical Policy Statements

CREATING AN ETHICAL CULTURE WITHIN THE HEALTHCARE ORGANIZATION

March 1992
August 1995 (revised)
November 2000 (revised)
November 2005 (revised)
November 2010 (revised)
November 2011 (revised)

Statement of the Issue

The number and significance of challenges facing healthcare organizations are unprecedented. Growing financial pressures, rising public and payor expectations, consolidations and mergers, patient safety and quality improvement issues, and healthcare reform have placed healthcare organizations under great stress—thus potentially intensifying ethics concerns and conflicts.

Healthcare organizations must be led and managed with integrity and consistent adherence to professional and ethical standards. The executive, in partnership with the board, and acting with other responsible parties such as ethics committees, must serve as a role model and foster and support a culture that not only provides high-quality, cost-effective healthcare but promotes the ethical behavior and practices of individuals throughout the organization.

Source: Reprinted by permission of the American College of Healthcare Executives.

Recognizing the significance of ethics to the organization's mission and fulfillment of its responsibilities, healthcare executives must demonstrate the importance of ethics in their own actions and seek various ways to integrate ethical practices and reflection into the organization's culture. To create an ethical culture, healthcare executives should: 1) support the development and implementation of ethical standards of behavior including ethical clinical, management, research and quality-improvement practices; 2) ensure that effective and comprehensive ethics resources, including an ethics committee, exist and are available to develop, propagate and clarify such standards of behavior when there is ethical uncertainty; and 3) support and implement a systematic and organizationwide approach to ethics training and corporate compliance.

The ability of an organization to achieve its full potential will remain dependent upon the motivation, knowledge, skills, and ethical practices and values of each individual within the organization. Thus, the executive has an obligation to accomplish the organization's mission in a manner that respects the values of individuals and maximizes their contributions.

Policy Position

The American College of Healthcare Executives believes that all healthcare executives have a professional obligation to create an ethical working environment and culture. To this end, healthcare executives should lead these efforts by:

- Demonstrating and modeling the importance of and commitment to ethics through decisions, practices and behaviors;
- Promulgating an organizational code of ethics that includes ethical standards of behavior and guidelines;
- Reviewing the principles and ideals expressed in vision, mission and value statements, personnel policies, annual reports, orientation materials and other documents to ensure congruence;
- Supporting perspectives and behaviors that reflect that ethics is essential to achieving the organization's mission;
- Using communications throughout the year to help foster an understanding of the organization's commitment to ethics;
- Communicating expectations that behaviors and actions are based on the organization's code of ethics, values and ethical standards of practice. Such expectations should also be included in orientations and position descriptions where relevant;

Source: Reprinted by permission of the American College of Healthcare Executives.

- Ensuring that individuals throughout the organization are respected and expected to behave in an ethical manner;
- Fostering an environment where the free expression of ethical concerns is encouraged and supported without retribution;
- Ensuring that effective ethics resources, such as an ethics committee, are available for discussing and addressing clinical, organizational and research ethical concerns;
- Establishing a mechanism that safeguards individuals who wish to raise ethical concerns;
- Seeking to ensure that individuals are free from all harassment, coercion and discrimination;
- Providing an effective and timely process to facilitate dispute resolution;
- Using each individual's knowledge, skills and abilities appropriately; and
- Ensuring a safe work environment exists.

These responsibilities can best be implemented in an environment in which each individual within the organization is encouraged and supported in adhering to the highest standards of ethics. This should be done with attention to the organization's code of ethics and appropriate professional codes, particularly those that stress the moral character and behavior of the executive and the organization itself.

Approved by the Board of Governors of the American College of Healthcare Executives on November 14, 2011.

Related Resources

American College of Healthcare Executives Ethics Toolkit
www.ache.org/ABT_ACHE/EthicsToolkit/ethicsTOC.cfm

Source: Reprinted by permission of the American College of Healthcare Executives.

ETHICAL DECISION MAKING FOR HEALTHCARE EXECUTIVES

August 1993
February 1997 (revised)
November 2002 (revised)
November 2007 (revised)
November 2011 (revised)

Statement of the Issue

Ethical decision making is required when the healthcare executive must address a conflict or uncertainty regarding competing values, such as personal, organizational, professional and societal values. Those involved in this decision-making process must consider ethical principles including justice, autonomy, beneficence and nonmaleficence as well as professional and organizational ethical standards and codes. Many factors have contributed to the growing concern in healthcare organizations over ethical issues, including issues of access and affordability, pressure to reduce costs, mergers and acquisitions, financial and other resource constraints, and advances in medical technology that complicate decision making near the end of life. Healthcare executives have a responsibility to address the growing number of complex ethical dilemmas they are facing, but they cannot and should not make such decisions alone or without a sound decision-making framework.

Healthcare organizations should have mechanisms that may include ethics committees, ethics consultation services, and written policies, procedures and guidelines to assist them with the ethics decision-making process. With these organizational mechanisms and guidelines in place, conflicting interests involving patients, families, caregivers, the organization, payors and the community can be thoughtfully and appropriately reviewed.

Policy Position

It is incumbent upon healthcare executives to lead in a manner that sets an ethical tone for their organizations. The American College of Healthcare Executives (ACHE) believes that education in ethics is an important step in a healthcare executive's lifelong commitment to high ethical conduct, both personally and professionally. Further, ACHE supports the development of organizational mechanisms that enable healthcare executives to appropriately and expeditiously address ethical conflicts. Whereas physicians, nurses and other caregivers may primarily address

Source: Reprinted by permission of the American College of Healthcare Executives.

ethical issues on a case-by-case basis, healthcare executives also have a responsibility to address those issues at broader organizational, community and societal levels. ACHE encourages its affiliates, as leaders in their organizations, to take an active role in the development and demonstration of ethical decision making.

To this end, healthcare executives should:

- Create a culture that fosters ethical clinical and administrative practices and ethical decision making.
- Communicate the organization's commitment to ethical decision making through its mission or value statements and its organizational code of ethics.
- Demonstrate through their professional behavior the importance of ethics to the organization.
- Offer educational programs to boards, staff, physicians and others on their organization's ethical standards of practice and on the more global issues of ethical decision making in today's healthcare environment. Further, healthcare executives should promote learning opportunities, such as those provided through professional societies or academic organizations, that will facilitate open discussion of ethical issues.
- Develop and use organizational mechanisms that reflect their organizations' mission and values and are flexible enough to deal with the spectrum of ethical concerns—clinical, organizational, business and management.
- Ensure that organizational mechanisms to address ethics issues are readily available and include individuals who are competent to address ethical concerns and reflect diverse perspectives. An organization's ethics committee, for example, might include representatives from groups such as physicians, nurses, managers, board members, social workers, attorneys, patients and/ or the community and clergy. All these groups are likely to bring unique and valuable perspectives to bear on discussions of ethical issues.
- Evaluate and continually refine organizational processes for addressing ethical issues.
- Promote decision making that results in the appropriate use of power while balancing individual, organizational and societal issues.

Approved by the Board of Governors of the American College of Healthcare Executives on November 14, 2011.

Source: Reprinted by permission of the American College of Healthcare Executives.

ETHICAL ISSUES RELATED TO A REDUCTION IN FORCE

August 1995
November 2000 (revised)
November 2005 (revised)
November 2012 (revised)

Statement of the Issue

As the result of shorter lengths of stay, the increase of ambulatory care, higher productivity, new technology and other factors, the capacity of some healthcare organizations could significantly exceed demand. As a result, these organizations may be required to reduce their workforce and related costs. Additionally, mergers and consolidations can result in further reductions and reassignments of staff. Financial pressures will continue to fuel this trend. However, patient care needs should not be compromised when determining staffing requirements.

Careful planning, diligent cost controls, effective resource management and proper consultation can lessen the hardship and stress of a reduction in force. Formal policies and procedures should be developed well in advance of the need to implement them.

The decision to reduce staff necessitates consideration of the short-term and long-term impact on all employees—those leaving and those remaining. Decision makers should consider the potential ethical conflict between formally stated organizational values and staff reduction actions.

Policy Position

The American College of Healthcare Executives recommends that specific steps be considered by healthcare executives when initiating a reduction in force process to support consistency between stated organizational values and those demonstrated before, during and after the process. Among these steps are the following:

- Recognize that cost reduction efforts must be appropriate—if they are too aggressive, the consequences for patients, staff and the organization can be as harmful as doing too little or proceeding too late;
- Explore and evaluate best practices from similar organizations which could be helpful in designing and implementing a workforce reduction plan; best practices can be identified by conducting a thorough literature review, attending seminars and speaking with colleagues;

Source: Reprinted by permission of the American College of Healthcare Executives.

- Develop a workforce reduction plan that effectively describes its rationale, objectives, implementation process, timeline and impact assessment techniques;
- Obtain input and advice from senior management and human resource leaders on the number and type of positions to be reduced, which open positions should not be filled, and when and how communication regarding the reduction plan should be made. Include other key components, such as discussing the rationale and process with the organization's governing body, medical staff leadership and, if necessary, the media;
- Consult with labor counsel;
- Provide timely, accurate, clear and consistent information—including the reasoning behind the decision—to stakeholders when staff reductions become necessary;
- Review the principles and ideals expressed in vision, mission and value statements, personnel policies, annual reports, employee orientation materials and other documents to test congruence and conformance with reduction in force decisions;
- Support, if possible, through retraining and redeployment, employees whose positions have been eliminated. Also, consider outplacement assistance, appropriate severance policies and continued service through the organization's employee assistance program, if possible; and
- Address the needs of remaining staff by demonstrating sensitivity to their potential feelings of loss, anger and survivor guilt. Also address their anxiety about the possibility of further reductions and uncertainty regarding changes in workload, work redesign and similar concerns.

Healthcare organizations encounter the same set of challenging issues associated with reductions in force as do other employers. Reduction in force decisions should reflect an institution's ethics and value statements.

Approved by the Board of Governors of the American College of Healthcare Executives on November 12, 2012.

Source: Reprinted by permission of the American College of Healthcare Executives.

ETHICAL ISSUES RELATED TO STAFF SHORTAGES

March 2002
November 2007 (revised)
November 2012 (revised)

Statement of the Issue

The effects of staff shortages are felt acutely by hospitals and other healthcare organizations. While healthcare executives have struggled with how to reduce their organization's staff responsibly, today they face an equally daunting challenge. They must fulfill their responsibility to provide high-quality, affordable patient care in the face of workforce shortages that may leave them with vacancies in many positions throughout their organization.

Alleviating workforce shortages or adapting to them is a complex problem for which there are few easy solutions. Nevertheless, healthcare executives have an ethical responsibility to address any shortages that exist within their organizations in such a way that patient care is not compromised, existing staff are not unduly burdened and financial costs do not become excessive.

Policy Position

The American College of Healthcare Executives (ACHE) recommends that healthcare executives develop responsible action plans for delivering patient care in the face of staff shortages. To this end, ACHE recommends that such plans address the following:

- Attracting and retaining qualified staff by addressing issues important to today's workforce, including strengthening the patient/clinician/executive partnership, treating each other with respect, promoting continuous quality improvement, and providing fair compensation, flexible scheduling and professional development;
- Maintaining workloads and expectations that strive to alleviate and prevent burnout;
- Examining work stream processes to ensure staff is being deployed in an effective manner to meet patient needs;
- Creating systems for job assignments and backup coverage that ensure responsibilities are appropriately matched with qualifications;

Source: Reprinted by permission of the American College of Healthcare Executives.

- Being sensitive to the financial and nonfinancial consequences of utilizing temporary personnel to fill vacancies;
- Responding to potential disasters that would significantly impact staff availability over sustained periods, requiring multilevel backup capacity;
- Conducting employee opinion surveys and exit interviews, using results to identify steps to improve job satisfaction;
- Identifying ways to engage employees to help define and address issues adversely affecting recruitment and retention objectives;
- Maintaining a diverse and culturally competent workforce;
- Analyzing departments or units with high turnover rates to determine whether management shortcomings, working conditions and/or other factors may be contributing to staff morale problems;
- Exploring, evaluating and implementing best practices from similar organizations that could be helpful in avoiding staff shortages; and
- Closing units or diverting patients if staff shortages become severe, to ensure that patient care is not compromised and high-quality care is maintained.

Healthcare executives may find it beneficial to join forces with others in their service areas to address the problem of staff shortages. Collaboration to recruit qualified staff will prove to be a more effective long-term strategy than competition for the same resources. ACHE encourages healthcare executives to collaborate on the development of creative, sustainable strategies that will benefit their respective organizations as well as help ensure that high-quality, affordable healthcare remains available in their communities.

In addition, ACHE encourages healthcare executives to work to ensure the future supply of healthcare workers. Healthcare executives should collaborate with others to expose students to careers in healthcare, including both clinical and managerial careers.

Approved by the Board of Governors of the American College of Healthcare Executives on November 12, 2012.

Source: Reprinted by permission of the American College of Healthcare Executives.

HEALTH INFORMATION CONFIDENTIALITY

February 1994
November 1997 (revised)
November 2004 (revised)
November 2009 (revised)
November 2012 (revised)

Statement of the Issue

Healthcare is among the most personal services rendered in our society; yet to deliver this care, scores of personnel must have access to intimate patient information. In order to receive appropriate care, patients must feel free to reveal personal information. In return, the healthcare provider must treat patient information confidentially and protect its security.

Maintaining confidentiality is becoming more difficult. While information technology can improve the quality of care by enabling the instant retrieval and access of information through various means, including mobile devices, and the more rapid exchange of medical information by a greater number of people who can contribute to the care and treatment of a patient, it also can increase the risk of unauthorized use, access and disclosure of confidential patient information. Within healthcare organizations, personal information contained in medical records now is reviewed not only by physicians and nurses but also by professionals in many clinical and administrative support areas.

The obligation to protect the confidentiality of patient health information is imposed by a myriad of state laws and the federal Health Insurance Portability and Accountability Act of 1996 (HIPAA) as amended under the Health Information Technology for Economic and Clinical Health Act (the "HITECH Act"). Protected health information (PHI) can only be used or disclosed by covered entities and their business associates for purposes of treatment, payment or healthcare operations without the patient's consent.

While media representatives also seek access to health information, particularly when a patient is a public figure or when treatment involves legal or public health issues, the rights of individual patients must be protected. Society's need for information rarely outweighs the right of patients to confidentiality.

In order to disclose patient information, healthcare executives must determine that patients or their legal representatives have consented to the release of information or that the use, access or disclosure sought falls within the permitted

Source: Reprinted by permission of the American College of Healthcare Executives.

purposes that do not require the patient's prior consent. Healthcare executives must implement procedures to enable them to account for such disclosures. Once health information is released, healthcare executives must keep records and implement other procedures to ensure that they are able to account to the patient for such disclosures, upon the patient's request.

Policy Position

The American College of Healthcare Executives believes that in addition to following all applicable state laws and HIPAA, healthcare executives have a moral and professional obligation to respect confidentiality and protect the security of patients' medical records. As patient advocates, executives must ensure their organization obtains proper patient authorization to release information or follow carefully defined policies and applicable laws in those cases for which the release of information without consent is indicated.

While the healthcare organization possesses the health record, outside access to the information in that record can be controlled by patients unless indicated otherwise by applicable laws and regulations. Organizations therefore must determine the appropriateness of all requests for patient information under applicable federal and state law and act accordingly.

In fulfilling their responsibilities, healthcare executives should seek to:

- Limit access to patient information to authorized individuals only.
- Ensure that institutional policies and practices with respect to confidentiality, security and release of information are consistent with regulations and laws.
- Educate healthcare personnel on confidentiality and data security requirements, take steps to ensure all healthcare personnel are aware of and understand their responsibilities to keep patient information confidential and secure, and impose sanctions for violations.
- Implement technical (including, if appropriate, the use of encryption), administrative and physical safeguards to protect medical record files and computerized data against unauthorized use, access and disclosure and ensure data confidentiality, integrity and availability.
- Conduct periodic data security audits and risk assessments.
- Develop systems that enable organizations to track (and, if required, report) the use, access and disclosure of health records.
- Provide for appropriate disaster recovery.

Source: Reprinted by permission of the American College of Healthcare Executives.

- Establish guidelines for masking patient identifiers in committee minutes and other working documents in which the identity is not necessary.
- Establish policies and procedures to provide to the patient an accounting of uses and disclosures of the patient's health information.
- Create guidelines for securing necessary permissions for the release of medical information for research, education, utilization review and other purposes.
- Adopt a specialized process to further protect sensitive information such as psychiatric records, HIV status, genetic testing information, sexually transmitted disease information or substance abuse treatment records.
- Identify special situations that require consultation with senior management prior to use or release of information.
- Obtain written agreements that detail the obligations of confidentiality and security for individuals, third parties and agencies that receive medical records information, unless the circumstances warrant an exception.
- Conduct due diligence on third parties who will receive medical records information, including a review of policies and procedures appropriate to the type of information they will possess. Ensure where applicable that such third parties adhere to the same terms and restrictions regarding PHI applicable to the organization.
- Follow all applicable policies and procedures regarding privacy of patient information even if information is in the public domain.
- Adopt procedures to address patient rights to request amendment of medical records and other rights under the HIPAA Privacy Rule.
- Educate patients about organizational policies on confidentiality and use the notice of privacy practices as required by the HIPAA Privacy Rule.
- Review applicable state and federal law related to the specific requirements for breaches involving PHI or computer systems containing PHI. Establish adequate policies and procedures to properly address these events.
- In the event of a security breach, conduct a timely and thorough investigation and notify patients promptly (and within the timeframes required under applicable law) if appropriate to mitigate harm in accordance with applicable state or federal law.
- Establish adequate policies and procedures to mitigate the harm caused by the unauthorized use, access or disclosure of health information to the extent required by state or federal law.

Source: Reprinted by permission of the American College of Healthcare Executives.

- Participate in the public dialogue on confidentiality issues such as employer use of healthcare information, public health reporting, and appropriate uses and disclosures of information in health information exchanges.

The American College of Healthcare Executives urges all healthcare executives to maintain an appropriate balance between the patient's right to confidentiality and the need to release information in the public's interest in accordance with applicable state and federal law.

Approved by the Board of Governors of the American College of Healthcare Executives on November 12, 2012.

Source: Reprinted by permission of the American College of Healthcare Executives.

IMPAIRED HEALTHCARE EXECUTIVES

February 1991
March 1995 (revised)
November 2000 (revised)
November 2005 (revised)
November 2006 (revised)
November 2012 (revised)

Statement of the Issue

The American College of Healthcare Executives recognizes that impairment is a significant problem that crosses both societal and professional boundaries. For healthcare executives, impairment can be defined as a condition that limits or diminishes a healthcare executive's ability to perform his or her responsibilities and duties in accordance with the prevailing professional standards and expectations. Some examples of causes of impairment include alcoholism, substance abuse, chemical dependency, mental/emotional instability, cognitive impairment and illness.

Impaired healthcare executives affect not only themselves and their families, they have a significant impact on their profession, their professional society, their organizations (including colleagues, patients, clients and others served), their communities, and society as a whole. Impairment typically leads to misconduct in the form of incompetence and unsafe or unprofessional behavior, which can result in substantial costs associated with loss of productivity and errors in judgment.

The impaired healthcare executive can damage the public image of his or her organization of employment. Public confidence in the organization diminishes if it appears that the organization is not being managed with consistently high standards of professional and ethical practice. This lack of public confidence may cause the community to deem the organization unworthy of its support.

Society expects healthcare executives to practice the standards of good health that they advocate for the public. Impaired healthcare executives diminish the credibility of the profession and its ability to manage society's healthcare when they are not appropriately managing their own personal health.

Policy Position

The preamble of the American College of Healthcare Executives *Code of Ethics* states, "Healthcare executives have an obligation to act in ways that will merit the

Source: Reprinted by permission of the American College of Healthcare Executives.

trust, confidence, and respect of healthcare professionals and the general public. Therefore, healthcare executives should lead lives that embody an exemplary system of values and ethics."

The American College of Healthcare Executives believes that healthcare executives who are impaired for any reason should refrain from assuming responsibilities that they may not be able to discharge effectively. Whenever there is doubt, they should seek appropriate assistance in performing their responsibilities.

Therefore, all healthcare executives have an ethical and a professional obligation to:

- Maintain a personal health that is free from impairment.
- Refrain from all professional activities if impaired.
- Seek assistance, whenever there is uncertainty, in understanding whether impairment exists.
- Expeditiously seek treatment if impairment occurs.
- Urge impaired colleagues to expeditiously seek treatment and to refrain from all professional activities while impaired.
- Support peers who identify healthcare executives in need of help.
- Intervene and report the impairment to the appropriate person(s) should the colleague refuse to seek professional assistance and should the state of impairment persist.
- Review applicable legal obligations to report the impairment to ensure compliance with federal and state requirements (such as those required by licensing boards).
- Recommend or provide, within one's employing organization, confidential avenues for reporting impairment, and either access or referral to treatment or assistance programs.
- Consider establishing an organizationwide program or committee that coordinates a reporting process and also reviews, addresses and prevents impaired executives.
- Recognize that individuals who have successfully received treatment for impairment and are no longer deemed impaired should be considered for employment opportunities for which they are qualified.
- Assist recovering colleagues when they resume their professional activities.
- Urge the community to provide information and resources for assistance and treatment of alcoholism, substance abuse, mental/emotional instability and cognitive impairment as needed and as appropriate.

Source: Reprinted by permission of the American College of Healthcare Executives.

- Raise the awareness of key stakeholders (such as employees, governing board members, etc.) on impairment issues and the resources available for assistance.

Approved by the Board of Governors of the American College of Healthcare Executives on November 12, 2012.

Source: Reprinted by permission of the American College of Healthcare Executives.

American College of Healthcare Executives
Policy Statements

CONSIDERING THE VALUE OF OLDER, EXPERIENCED HEALTHCARE EXECUTIVES

May 1992
May 1995 (revised)
December 1998 (revised)
March 2002 (revised)
November 2005 (revised)
November 2010 (revised)

Statement of the Issue

In recent decades, the world has witnessed unprecedented extensions in the longevity and well-being of citizens of developed nations. This prolongation of life is a remarkable achievement, but coping with the changes created by large numbers of long-lived people is forcing society and its institutions to make many adjustments.

Healthcare employers and employees must acknowledge the employment challenges presented by the new demographics. For employers, one challenge is overcoming unsubstantiated negative stereotypes of older, experienced employees concerning their attitudes, performance, physiological capacity, and ability to learn new techniques and skills. An opportunity for employers is to tap the extensive skills and experience of the older, experienced executive.

In 1967, the federal government enacted the Age Discrimination in Employment Act. Its purpose is protecting and promoting the employment opportunities

Source: Reprinted by permission of the American College of Healthcare Executives.

of older workers and helping to find solutions to age-related employment problems. Healthcare organizations will engender more positive regard and support from their key stakeholders by striving to embrace the spirit and the letter of the law.

Policy Position

The American College of Healthcare Executives (ACHE) encourages healthcare executives and their organizations to employ individuals without regard to their age. While overt discrimination against employment of older, experienced healthcare executives is illegal and subject to sanction under federal law, even covert discrimination against the employment of older, experienced healthcare executives is incompatible with ACHE's *Code of Ethics*.

Executive employment decisions will become increasingly complex as organizations respond to demands for staff diversity and for changing leadership and management skills. To avoid actual and perceived discrimination against older, experienced healthcare executives, ACHE advocates the following to help create equitable employment opportunities.

ACHE encourages all healthcare executives and the organizations they represent to play a significant role in addressing this issue by actively pursuing the following:

- Employers should direct executive recruiters to identify and present candidates for senior-level positions irrespective of their age, and executive recruiters should suggest that their clients consider candidates for positions irrespective of their age.
- CEOs, trustees and recruitment and retention decision makers should avoid negative stereotypes of older workers and actively recruit experienced executives for consideration, including those who are between positions.
- CEOs and trustees of healthcare organizations should establish human resources plans that provide for leadership succession and effective continuing education for older, experienced executives.

ACHE encourages older, experienced executives to actively pursue the following:

- Be flexible when seeking new positions by considering organizational settings, geographic areas, levels of responsibility and compensation structures different from those to which they may have been accustomed.

Source: Reprinted by permission of the American College of Healthcare Executives.

- Be a role model and mentor to younger executives. At the same time, accept reverse mentoring to stay attuned to the emerging leaders and foster cross-generational understanding.
- Assume responsibility for continuously maintaining and improving their leadership, management and technology skills, including use of new media such as social media, so they can contribute value to employing organizations in environments that continually change.
- Interact with colleagues and remain actively involved in professional associations at both the national and local (chapter) level.

Healthcare will continue to be regarded as a dynamic sector of the economy—one that not only offers the prospect of employment but also the opportunity to make important social contributions. Leaders in this field have an ethical responsibility to select and retain executives without regard to their age.

Approved by the Board of Governors of the American College of Healthcare Executives on November 8, 2010.

Source: Reprinted by permission of the American College of Healthcare Executives.

HEALTHCARE EXECUTIVES' ROLE IN EMERGENCY PREPAREDNESS

November 2006
November 2009 (revised)

Statement of the Issue

Due to the complex nature of emergency preparedness, it is critical that healthcare executives ensure their organization develops an all-hazards emergency operations plan relevant to their location and type of organization.

Hospitals and other healthcare delivery organizations must be prepared to care for those in need of medical services and, to the extent possible, protect staff and patients from being exposed to any further risk. The organization's emergency operations plan should recognize that a healthcare organization may be directly impacted by a disaster and still continue to operate and receive victims of the event. Such disasters include incidents of terrorism and natural occurrences such as hurricanes, tornados, floods, earthquakes or epidemics/pandemics.

It is vitally important that healthcare organizations monitor and update their emergency operations plans on an ongoing basis, maintaining a constant state of preparedness to ensure appropriate response and recovery within the shortest possible time frames. Without proper planning, an incident involving the organization may result in either a temporary or permanent failure, thus disabling a crucial community resource. The emergency operations plan also should be fully integrated with that of other organizations and appropriate agencies at the local, state, regional and national levels. This is particularly important in situations such as a pandemic that may simultaneously impact large geographic areas for several months and disrupt national and international supply chains.

Policy Position

The American College of Healthcare Executives (ACHE) believes healthcare executives should actively participate in disaster planning and preparedness activities, striving to ensure that their emergency operations plan fits within overall community plans and represents a responsible approach to the risks an organization might face. Chief executive officers should lead efforts to ensure that the plan is comprehensive, including establishing board policy that delineates the organization's responsibilities and procedures to be followed. Healthcare executives also have a unique opportunity to help educate the community about infectious disease

Source: Reprinted by permission of the American College of Healthcare Executives.

prevention and control efforts that may mitigate large-scale death during events such as a pandemic.

In developing a comprehensive emergency operations plan, ACHE encourages healthcare executives to pursue the following actions on an ongoing basis:

- Maintain a Relevant/Current Emergency/Disaster Plan: Establish a process to understand and stay current regarding applicable state and national standards for emergency preparedness, including the National Response Framework (http://www.dhs.gov/files/programs/editorial_0566.shtm) and the Hospital Preparedness Program (http://www.hhs.gov/aspr/opeo/hpp/). The plan should be updated based on actual disasters or drills as well as changes in standards.

- Focus the Plan to Address the Most Likely Scenarios: Adopt an all-hazards framework to analyze the operational issues that would arise in relevant emergency situations to cover applicable responses to a natural disaster as well as potential CBRNE (chemical, biological, radiological, nuclear and explosive) emergencies and sustained events such as a pandemic influenza.

- Develop an Incident Command System: Be prepared to adopt an incident command system and support the integration of a nationwide standardized approach to incident management and response (e.g., National Incident Management System).

- Assess Resource Availability: Coordinate and integrate organizational resources to address a full spectrum of actions (mitigation, preparedness, response and recovery), and ensure that the organization has the appropriate programs, trained and credentialed staff, staff personal protective equipment, and other supplies and equipment in place to quickly respond to events that their organization might face, as identified by the organization's all-hazards analysis. Include a determination of the impact on hospital services of a scenario that requires maximum surge capacity.

- Plan for Continuity of Operations: Ensure that the hospital can be self-sustaining for at least 96 hours and that plans are in place for obtaining critical resources such as water, electricity and just-in-time supplies that may not be available due to the emergency.

- Develop Protocols to Ensure Appropriate Resource Allocation: Ensure that services are provided equitably and impartially, consistent with ethical and legal standards relevant in a mass casualty event and based upon the vulnerability and needs of the individuals and communities affected by a disaster.

Source: Reprinted by permission of the American College of Healthcare Executives.

- Address the Safety of Employees/Patients/Families: Develop policies and processes to ensure that all reasonable efforts are made to protect employees, patients and families, as well as facilities, while maintaining quality patient care to the best of the organization's ability during a crisis. Include plans to mitigate the impact on staffing of likely scenarios, such as schools closing, public transportation closing and patients presenting with contagious/ potentially lethal illnesses. Ensure that staff members receive education that allows them to make informed decisions and to understand what the organization is doing to protect them and their families.
- Design Appropriate Communication and Coordination Protocols for Both Internal and External Audiences: Ensure active involvement in interagency planning efforts with all relevant organizations, including the development of an integrated communication plan and community-wide exercises and drills to assess effectiveness and implement improvements.
- Enhance Disease Surveillance and Reporting: Enhance clinician awareness of events, signs, symptoms or diseases that may require reporting or activation of an emergency operations plan.

As a critical component of a community's infrastructure, healthcare organizations should require proper planning for all-hazards events they may face. Healthcare executives should be active leaders in that planning and the creation of systems and processes to ensure that the emergency operating plan can be effectively and efficiently executed if ever needed.

Approved by the Board of Governors of the American College of Healthcare Executives on November 16, 2009.

Source: Reprinted by permission of the American College of Healthcare Executives.

INCREASING AND SUSTAINING RACIAL/ETHNIC DIVERSITY IN HEALTHCARE MANAGEMENT

July 1990
May 1995 (revised)
December 1998 (revised)
March 2002 (revised)
November 2005 (revised)
November 2010 (revised)

Statement of the Issue

One of the hallmarks of a democratic society is providing equal opportunity for all citizens regardless of race or ethnicity. In the healthcare sector, racially/ethnically diverse employees represent a growing percentage of all healthcare employees, but they hold only a modest percentage of top healthcare management positions. For example, according to the American Hospital Association, in 2010, 94 percent of all hospital CEOs were white[1] (non Hispanic or Latino) while 65 percent of the population is white[2] (non Hispanic or Latino), according to the most recent U.S. Census Bureau data.

This disparity persists despite two decades of success in attracting racially/ethnically diverse students to graduate study in health administration. For example, according to the Association of University Programs in Health Administration in 1990–1991, 14 percent of graduate students in healthcare management programs were racial/ethnic minorities. By the 2000–2001 academic year, the proportion rose to 30 percent and by 2009–2010, fully 42 percent of graduate students are minorities.[3]

In addition to these positive trends, a 2008 study[4] conducted jointly by the American College of Healthcare Executives (ACHE), the Asian Health Care Leaders Association, the Institute for Diversity in Health Management, the National Association of Health Services Executives, and the National Forum for Latino Healthcare Executives showed that among females, Latinos exceeded others in attaining senior-level positions. In regard to compensation levels, controlling for education and experience, black women earned similar incomes as white women. But Asian and Latino women earned about ten percent less than their white counterparts.

In the same study, the data for males shows that minority healthcare executives continue to earn less than their white counterparts. White males exceeded

Source: Reprinted by permission of the American College of Healthcare Executives.

minorities in having attained senior-level positions in healthcare organizations and earned more than other racial/ethnic groups, when controlling for experience and education.

Our country's increasingly diverse communities result in a more diverse patient population. Studies suggest that diversity in healthcare management can enhance quality of care, quality of life in the workplace, community relations and the ability to affect community health status. Achieving diversity in management will involve a commitment at all professional levels (including early entrants, middle managers, and senior executives) within the organization through the awareness of diversity issues, hiring practices that attract diverse staff, development and mentoring in educational programs and organizations, and organization wide diversity training.

Policy Position

ACHE embraces diversity within the healthcare management field and recognizes that issue as both an ethical and business imperative. ACHE urges all healthcare executives, board members, educators and policymakers to actively strive to increase diversity within healthcare management ranks, especially in regard to race and ethnic background. ACHE actively strives to increase representation of racially/ethnically diverse individuals in healthcare management and works to create a supportive, collegial environment that encourages their membership and advancement within ACHE itself. ACHE, as a founding member, also is committed to collaborating with the Institute for Diversity in Health Management and other such groups on these issues.

All stakeholders should renew and strengthen their commitment to redressing any imbalance in representation of racially/ethnically diverse individuals in leadership to enhance our profession now and in the future.

ACHE encourages all healthcare executives to play a significant role in addressing this issue by actively pursuing the following:

Recruitment

- Promote healthcare careers to diverse populations via school programs and community organizations. Encourage students to shadow healthcare executives and explore careers in healthcare.
- Develop strong outreach mechanisms to attract promising racially/ethnically diverse candidates to healthcare management careers with special

Source: Reprinted by permission of the American College of Healthcare Executives.

emphasis on increasing recruitment efforts at colleges and universities with predominately racially/ethnically diverse student enrollments.

- Offer internships, residencies and fellowships to racially/ethnically diverse students and provide mentoring to help prepare them for success in the job market.
- Advocate racial/ethnic diversity in the appointment of job search committee members and promote the provision of a diverse slate of candidates for senior management positions.
- Recruit racially/ethnically diverse individuals at every level, being transparent about hiring criteria, so as to increase current representation in management, but also to develop a pool of qualified candidates for the future.
- Recruit candidates external to the healthcare field to broaden the pool of racially/ethnically diverse candidates.
- Direct executive recruiters to identify and present racially/ethnically diverse candidates for management positions. Have them share criteria they use to recommend candidates for senior-level positions.

Promotion

- At every opportunity advocate the goal of achieving full representation of racially/ethnically diverse individuals at entry-, mid- and senior-levels in healthcare management.
- Institute policies that (1) prevent discrimination on the basis of race/ethnicity, (2) increase diversity in the recruitment and hiring of candidates, and (3) create an environment that encourages retention and promotion of qualified racially/ethnically diverse employees. Ensure that policies are well known and understood and measure and reward changes resulting from these policies.
- Consider utilizing pro-diversity initiatives to reduce social isolation through programs such as the following: appoint a manager responsible for diversity; appoint a diversity committee; adopt a diversity action plan; evaluate managers based on their diversity effectiveness; and promote social gatherings and mentoring programs.
- Publicize career advancement opportunities, such as continuing education, professional development organizations, networking events and vacancies inside the organization, in a manner that appeals to everyone, especially racially/ethnically diverse individuals.
- Encourage retention and advancement of racially/ethnically diverse individuals. Identify potential candidates to support and create clear

Source: Reprinted by permission of the American College of Healthcare Executives.

pathways for advancement from entry- to mid-level positions and from mid- to senior-level positions.

- Develop and disseminate specific criteria for advancement in management that would allow all individuals to have an equal opportunity for senior-level positions. Such criteria could be useful to racially/ethnically diverse individuals who wish to prepare themselves for senior-level positions.
- Conduct regular reviews of organizational compensation programs to ensure salaries are equitable and nondiscriminatory.

Support

- Work with organizations representing racially/ethnically diverse individuals within their communities to create sources for scholarships and fellowships.
- Advocate for governmental and private philanthropic programs that increase funding to underwrite advanced education, information dissemination and employment opportunities for racially/ethnically diverse individuals.
- Support organizations, such as the Institute for Diversity in Health Management, the Asian Health Care Leaders Association, the National Association of Health Services Executives and the National Forum for Latino Healthcare Executives that champion diverse executives through internships and other programming. Enable employed diverse executives to participate in the programs and be part of the volunteer leadership of such organizations.
- Support and assist the development of mentoring programs within healthcare organizations specifically focused on developing long-term relationships between senior healthcare managers and racially/ethnically diverse candidates.
- Provide scholarship support for employed diverse executives to participate in leadership development programs.
- Urge racially/ethnically diverse healthcare executives who are not affiliates to join ACHE and become active at both the local (via chapters) and national levels. Extend invitations to hosted events such as executive breakfasts, chapter networking events and educational programs.

In addition, ACHE encourages racially/ethnically diverse healthcare executives to actively pursue the following:

- Earn an advanced degree in healthcare management or business.
- Seek internships, fellowships and administrative development opportunities that lead to permanent positions and form a foundation for building their careers.

Source: Reprinted by permission of the American College of Healthcare Executives.

- Seek positions in organizations that offer effective pro-diversity initiatives in order to build their careers.
- Choose positions that offer new experiences and expand their skillsets and management abilities.
- Interact with colleagues and actively pursue professional development by becoming involved in professional associations.
- Seek out mentors and serve as mentors to other professionals.

ACHE advocates a variety of approaches to improve the representation and equitable treatment of racial and ethnic diversity in healthcare management.

Approved by the Board of Governors of the American College of Healthcare Executives on November 8, 2010.

References

[1]American Hospital Association, Division of Membership database. Accessed January 2010.

[2]U.S. Census Bureau, "Selected Social Characteristics in the United States." Accessed September 30, 2010. http://factfinder.census.gov

[3]Association of University Programs in Health Administration 2008–09 Academic Program Survey.

[4]American College of Healthcare Executives, "2008 Racial/Ethnic Comparison of Career Attainments in Healthcare Management." www.ache.org/PUBS/ research/Report_Tables.pdf

Related Resources

American College of Healthcare Executives Diversity Resources: www.ache.org/ policy/diversity_resources.cfm

Asian Health Care Leaders Association: www.asianhealthcareleaders.org

Institute for Diversity in Health Management: www.diversityconnection.org

National Association of Health Services Executives: www.nahse.org

National Forum for Latino Healthcare Executives: www.nflhe.org

Source: Reprinted by permission of the American College of Healthcare Executives.

PREVENTING AND ADDRESSING WORKPLACE ABUSE: INAPPROPRIATE AND DISRUPTIVE BEHAVIOR

November 1996
November 1999 (revised)
November 2002 (revised)
November 2005 (reaffirmed)
November 2010 (revised)

Statement of the Issue

Healthcare executives have a professional responsibility to create and maintain an organizational culture that promotes quality patient care and a healthy work environment that protects staff from inappropriate and disruptive behavior. Such behavior, including aggression, harassment and intimidation, can adversely affect the ability of the healthcare team to work together and can negatively impact the quality of patient care. Countering the adverse effects of inappropriate and disruptive behavior requires that healthcare executives establish an organizational code of conduct defining such behaviors, provide staff with relevant education, and implement enforceable policies and processes to identify and prevent such behaviors.

An organizational culture that clearly conveys zero tolerance for inappropriate and disruptive behaviors while providing the necessary resources and mechanisms to safeguard against such behaviors can improve teamwork, foster a sense of mutual respect, and improve communication. Not only can quality of care and patient safety be enhanced, but there is a concomitant reduction in the legal, physical and emotional repercussions of inappropriate and disruptive behavior such as loss of productivity, absenteeism, turnover, low morale, lack of trust, communication breakdowns, and long-term career and psychological damage.

Policy Position

The American College of Healthcare Executives believes that all healthcare executives have a professional and ethical responsibility to promote a healthy workplace that is free of aggression, harassment and intimidation. Healthcare executives should demonstrate zero tolerance for inappropriate and disruptive behavior, including harassment on the basis of gender, sexual orientation, age, race, ethnicity, religion, national origin, disability, or any other personal characteristic. On behalf of their employing organizations, healthcare executives must further realize that they are responsible for implementing policy and monitoring compliance among their managers. To this end, healthcare executives should model desired behaviors and promote multifaceted programs in their organizations to prevent inappropriate and disruptive behaviors. Sample program components include, but are not limited to, the following:

Clearly articulated code of conduct and policy against inappropriate and disruptive behavior. The organization should have a code of conduct that defines acceptable, disruptive and inappropriate behavior. The related policy also should define specific terms such as "harassment" (preferably as defined by the Equal Employment Opportunity Commission–EEOC) and "aggression," and reference intimidation (both verbal and non-verbal), violence (both physical and verbal) and passive aggressive behaviors. In addition, the policy should explicitly state that these behaviors are not tolerated in the organization. The policy might include examples of prohibited conduct, delineate methods for making and investigating complaints, state that retaliation is prohibited and no reprisals will be taken against any employee filing a complaint under this policy, and provide that appropriate corrective action will be taken. The code of conduct and policy should be revised on a periodic basis and incorporated into the employee handbook as well as discussed in new employee orientation.

Employee training on inappropriate and disruptive behavior and its prevention. Human resources staff or other individuals who have a technical and legal understanding of the issues, in addition to demonstrated ability to stimulate discussion about this sensitive topic should conduct training. Training should be conducted on an ongoing and regular basis with the goals of: raising awareness of harassment, intimidation and aggression; clarifying misconceptions about what constitutes these behaviors; explaining the manager's role and responsibility in providing a safe and supportive work environment; and finally, sharing the specifics of the organization's policy prohibiting inappropriate and disruptive behavior.

Procedure for reporting allegations of inappropriate and disruptive behavior. The procedure should provide as much confidentiality as possible for both the complaining employee and the person accused of these behaviors. The procedure should take into account the need of the individual accused to be presented with the specific charges so as to be able to form a defense. Employees should be protected from retaliation for filing a complaint or appearing as a witness in an investigation. Further, if the procedure requires employees to make initial complaints to their supervisors, an alternate person should be designated to handle complaints when lodged against

Source: Reprinted by permission of the American College of Healthcare Executives.

the supervisor. Supervisors should be required to report all complaints and be made aware of liability for failing to do so.

Procedure for expeditiously investigating complaints of inappropriate and disruptive behavior. According to EEOC guidelines, once an employee complains, employers should promptly investigate and take "immediate and appropriate corrective action" based upon the results of their investigation. The organization should, therefore, have a process in place for investigating complaints quickly, discreetly and completely. An objective party should conduct an investigation, and the results of the investigation should be reported to both the complaining employee and the person accused. Other staff should be informed on a "need to know" basis.

Standards for corrective action. Standards for corrective action are an essential part of any plan to prevent inappropriate and disruptive behavior. Disciplinary action should be proportionate to the severity of any behavior found. The organization's policy, as it relates to corrective action, should avoid providing specific punishments for specific actions and instead be broad enough to give the freedom to exercise appropriate action. For example, the policy might state that such behaviors may result in discipline, up to and including discharge.

In addition to the program components mentioned above, legal counsel should review policies and procedures related to inappropriate and disruptive behavior because of the potential exposure to liability.

Workplace safety and quality of patient care is dependent on teamwork, communication and a collaborative work environment. To assure quality and to promote a culture of safety, healthcare executives must address the continuum of inappropriate behaviors that threaten overall performance and patient outcomes.

Approved by the Board of Governors of the American College of Healthcare Executives on November 8, 2010.

References

American Medical Association's Opinion E-9.045

The Joint Commission Standard L.D. 03.01.01
www.jointcommission.org/NewsRoom/PressKits/Behaviors+that+Undermine +a+Culture+of+Safety/

Source: Reprinted by permission of the American College of Healthcare Executives.

The Joint Commission, Sentinel Event Alert, Issue 40
www.jointcommission.org/SentinelEvents/

Related Resources

American College of Physician Executives, "Special Report: 2009 Doctor–Nurse Behavior Survey," The Physician Executive, November/December 2009, Vol. 35, Issue 6 www.ache.org/policy/doctornursebehavior.pdf

RESPONSIBILITY FOR MENTORING

November 1994
November 1999 (revised)
November 2004 (revised)
November 2009 (revised)

Statement of the Issue

The future of healthcare management rests in large measure with those entering the field as well as with mid-careerists who aspire to new and greater management opportunities. While on-the-job experience and continuing education are critical elements for preparing tomorrow's leaders, the value of mentoring these individuals cannot be overstated. Growing through mentoring relationships is an important factor in a protégé's lifelong learning process. In turn, by sharing their wisdom, insights and experiences, mentors can give back to the profession while deriving the personal satisfaction that comes from helping others realize their potential. For the organization, mentorships can lead to more satisfied employees and the generation of new ideas and programs.

Policy Position

The American College of Healthcare Executives (ACHE) believes that healthcare executives have a professional obligation to mentor both those entering the field and mid-careerists preparing to lead the healthcare systems of tomorrow.

Experienced healthcare executives can provide guidance to others in many ways, including:

Assisting Students and Those Entering the Field

- Offer assistance by recruiting, interviewing and working with qualified students interested in pursuing healthcare management careers, including addressing their questions relative to pursuing appropriate ongoing education or a graduate degree.
- Volunteer to serve as a guest lecturer, and use this opportunity to provide students with career planning guidance and insights gleaned from past experience.
- Offer externships, internships, residencies and postgraduate fellowships.
- Provide meaningful first-job opportunities to promising graduates and counsel them along the way.

Source: Reprinted by permission of the American College of Healthcare Executives.

Engaging in and Supporting Mentoring Relationships

- Promote mentoring opportunities and an organizational culture that promotes mentoring.
- Help protégés develop clear expectations about their role so they will actively contribute to the mentoring relationship.
- Encourage development of mentoring opportunities in culturally diverse, cross-generational and group settings as well as among individuals of different genders, races and ethnicities.
- Encourage other experienced executives from across the spectrum of healthcare organizations to engage in mentoring relationships.
- Keep abreast of changes in mentoring philosophy and techniques so as to ensure continued effectiveness as a mentor in an environment characterized by profound and rapid change.
- Seek out opportunities to contribute to local independent chapters of ACHE.

By providing guidance and engaging in mentoring relationships, healthcare leaders can benefit their organizations, contribute to the future of the profession and gain the personal gratification of helping less experienced individuals grow professionally.

Approved by the Board of Governors of the American College of Healthcare Executives on November 16, 2009.

THE ROLE OF THE HEALTHCARE EXECUTIVE IN A CHANGE IN ORGANIZATIONAL OWNERSHIP OR CONTROL

November 1997
November 2000 (revised)
November 2005 (revised)
November 2010 (revised)
November 2011 (revised)

Statement of the Issue

Changes in organizational ownership or control can take several forms, including consolidations, mergers, acquisitions, affiliations, divestitures and closures. Each type of change presents special challenges for healthcare executives. In addition to potentially impacting the staff of the organization and the local economy, such changes can impact a community's access to cost-effective, quality healthcare services.

Policy Position

The American College of Healthcare Executives (ACHE) believes that CEOs, their boards and members of their senior management teams should take a comprehensive approach to assessing the benefits and risks of a change in ownership or control, including the impact on all stakeholders and the consequences for community health status. To this end, ACHE offers the following as a guide.

When initially considering a change in ownership or control:

- Identify your organization's values and goals.
- Clearly articulate the reasons for considering a potential change in ownership, the anticipated benefits, risks of not undertaking a change and the desired outcomes.
- Establish specific criteria that should be used to evaluate various proposals regarding change of ownership or control.
- Understand any legal limitations of your organization's certificate of incorporation, articles of organization, charter or other binding documents that may restrict consideration of alternatives.
- Conduct a feasibility study to assess various options for change that may be available to your organization and community, specifying the risks and

Source: Reprinted by permission of the American College of Healthcare Executives.

benefits of each option as well as their impact on the community, staff and other stakeholders.

- As early as feasible, engage the broader community in understanding the rationale for considering a change in ownership or control.
- Consider severance agreements for selected executives and employees who will assess potential community and organizational impact of the proposed change so as to remove or lessen self-interest concerns related to loss of position and income.

When considering specific proposals related to change of ownership or control:

- Establish a multi-functional team to evaluate proposals, including outside experts as needed.
- Undertake a systematic evaluation of the options in relationship to the organization's established criteria for undertaking a change, considering issues such as governance, financial, operational, legal, human resource and clinical implications, as well as community impact and fit between the organization's culture and that of a potential partner.
- Identify financial incentives that may have an undue influence on the views of board members, executives and others involved in proposing and evaluating any change in ownership or control.
- Disclose all conflicts of interest (both real and perceived), offers of future employment or future remuneration and other benefits related to the transaction.
- Gain a thorough understanding of all the terms of the proposed transaction and of all collateral agreements.

If the decision is made to proceed with a change of ownership or control:

- Establish a multi-functional team to oversee the final due diligence process and implement the transition.
- Develop and implement a phased communications plan that involves and informs all constituencies regarding the rationale for the change in ownership or control, the decision-making process that was undertaken, and the pending implementation process.
- Inform and seek approvals from the appropriate federal, state and local officials of the terms of the transaction in accordance with their requirements.

Source: Reprinted by permission of the American College of Healthcare Executives.

- In change of ownership or control situations leading to the creation of a foundation or charitable trust, obtain an independent, third-party valuation of assets being converted or restructured and ensure that control and administration will be distinct from the restructured healthcare organization.
- Develop and implement a plan that provides for fair treatment of all employees impacted by the change. Consider offering comparable severance programs to minimize the risk of friction after the merger due to inconsistent treatment of employees.
- Prohibit private inurement or personal financial gain by individuals involved in evaluating or implementing the change.

In addition, ACHE affiliates also have a personal responsibility to:

- Abide by the standards set forth in the ACHE *Code of Ethics.*
- Place community and organizational interests above personal pride, ego or gain.
- Carry out the fiduciary responsibilities of their positions.
- Conduct all negotiations with honesty and integrity.

As consolidation and related activities continue in the healthcare field, organizations and their executives will be under increased scrutiny. Executives must demonstrate through their words and actions that their business decisions are guided by professional ethics and a commitment to improving community health status.

Approved by the Board of Governors of the American College of Healthcare Executives on November 14, 2011.

Related Resources

Zuckerman, Alan M., FACHE. *Leading Your Healthcare Organization Through a Merger or Acquisition.* Chicago: Health Administration Press (2010).

"Mergers and Acquisitions: Coming Together Without Falling Apart." *Frontiers of Health Services Management,* Vol. 27, No. 4 (2011).

Source: Reprinted by permission of the American College of Healthcare Executives.

Index

American Nurses Credentialing Center, 114

anger management consultants, disruptive physician behaviors and, 117

Animal Farm (Orwell), 89

anti-retaliation protection, ethical culture and, 57–58

appeal procedures

ethical guidelines for, 218

managed care settings, 214

applied ethics, business ethics as, 206–207

Aristotle, 172–173

Arras, John, 263–265

Association of Governing Boards, 143

conflicts of interest guidelines, 47

authority, emergency management and monitoring of, 264–265

autonomy

emergency preparedness and, 263–265

job satisfaction and, 115

medical ethics and, 205

values-based decision making and principle of, 173

balance, managed care ethics and, 218–219

Baldrige, 52–53

barriers to ethical decision making, 3–5

overcoming barriers, 5–6

Beckham, D., 145

bedside care, rationing of, 209

beneficence, medical ethics and, 205–206

benefit promotion, emergency preparedness and, 263

Beth Israel Deaconess Medical Center, 70–73

bidding process, formal and fair aspects of, 48

blind bidding process, conflict of interest avoidance and, 48

Boston Globe, 37–38

bottom-line approach, values-based decision making, 178–179

Boyd v. Epstein, 216

brainstorming process, values-based decision making, 176–177

Brown, F., 146

business ethics, relevant principles of, 206–207

business practices

ethical principles in decision making and, 9–11

ethics committee's effectiveness and, 53–54

ethics integration into, 4

ethics management in, 13–15

values-based decision making and, 180

case consultation, healthcare ethics committee development of, 223–224

case studies, healthcare ethics committee program evaluation, 226–227

Center for Patient Safety, 27

Character Counts! initiative (Josephson Institute Center for Youth Ethics), 172–173

charge rates, revenue enhancement and, 101

charging programs, revenue enhancement and internal analysis of, 101

"cherry picking" of patients, managed care marketing and, 212–213

chief executive officer (CEO)

compensation ethics and, 186–187

conflict of interest avoidance and, 46–48, 130, 160–161

education of trustees by, 51–52

ethics responsibilities of, 21, 34

hospital mergers and, 166

information technology problems, 124–127, 130–133

leadership and power of, 66–68

misuse of organizational resources by, 49–51

nursing shortages and role of, 110, 112–113

in Paradise Hills case study, 19–20

partnerships with medical staff, 34–35

sexual misconduct involving, 71–73, 162

workforce reduction issues, collaboration with staff on, 96–100

chief information officer (CIO), information technology problems and, 124–127, 130–133, 165

chief operations officer (COO), conflicts of interest and, 43–48, 160–161

Christensen, Clayton, 75

Christianity, history of values and, 173

disincentives, in managed care settings, 211–213

disruptive physician behaviors
  legal perspectives on, 165
  nursing shortages and role of, 110, 115–117

distributive justice
  emergency preparedness and, 263–265
  ethical principles in decision making and, 10–11
  fee-for-service healthcare and, 208
  medical ethics and, 205–206

Dobbs, Rebecca A., 220–231, 253–267

documentation, performance evaluations, 230–231

Doing What Counts for Patient Safety: Federal Actions to Reduce Medical Errors and Their Impact report, 26

Donabedian, A., 225–226, 228–229

"do no harm" principle
  crisis management ethics and, 254
  medical ethics and, 205–206
  workforce reduction case study, 164

Dowd, Clinton H., 241–252

Drucker, Peter, 186

drug/alcohol abuse
  in healthcare professionals, 80–83, 233–238
  impairment in healthcare professionals and, 81–83
  prevalence in healthcare professionals, 234–235

Dubin, Larry, 152

duty to provide care, crisis management ethics and, 254–256

economic efficiency
  ethical principles in decision making and, 10–11
  values-based decision making and, 170–171

education initiatives, healthcare ethics committees (HECs), 222–224

electronic communication, limitations of, 196

elitist culture, physician impairment and, 87–89

emergency management
  defined, 253–254

disaster triage protocols and resource allocation, 256–258
  mitigation phase, 260–262
  phases of, 260–267
  preparedness activities, 262–265

emergency operations plan (EOP), development of, 264–265

emotional intelligence, management ethics and, 187

employee assistance programs (EAPs), impairment of healthcare professionals and, 85–86

employees
  burnout rates for, 185
  communication with, 195–196
  conflict management and, 190–194
  management ethics for, 183–200
  professional development for, 194–195
  sex discrimination and harassment and, 68–73, 161–162

employees, management ethics with. *See also* medical staff
  hospital merger case study, 143, 146–147
  nursing shortages, ethical responsibilities to, 110, 113–115
  patient satisfaction vs. hospital policies and, 150, 153–154
  principles of, 183–200
  workforce reduction issues, collaboration with, 99–100

Employment Retirement Income Security Act (ERISA), 216

Encyclopedia of American Law, 44

Enlightenment, history of values and, 173

Equal Employment Opportunity Commission (EEOC), 65, 68–73
  antidiscrimination issues and, 156

equitable treatment
  crisis management ethics and, 254
  emergency preparedness and, 263–265
  management ethics and, 187–188

errors in technology, recognition of, 133

ethical behavior
  encouragement of, 184–188
  institutional decline in, 54–58

ethical problems vs., 36
gender discrimination and, 63, 69
industrial funding of research and, 250–252
information technology problems, 124–128
leadership strategies for, 104–105
managed care incentives and disincentives, 211–213
management ethics and, 185–188
medical education and, 242–252
revenue enhancement and, 101–102
sexual harassment/misconduct settlements, 72–73
workforce reduction decisions and, 96–100
firing practices
management ethics and, 199–200
residents, 246–247
foreign countries, disaster triage protocols and resource allocation in, 258
formative program evaluation, healthcare ethics committees, 225–227
for-profit managed care systems, evolution of, 203–204
for-profit research organizations, 251–252
Fosdick, Glenn A., 91–105
Fox v. Health Net of California, 216
framing process. *See also* ethical decision-making framework
values-based decision making, 176–179
Freund, L., 6

Gable, Lance, 153–154
gender discrimination
case study in, 59–75
leadership and power and, 66–68
sexual harassment and, 68–73
Gibson, Joan McIver, 10–11, 169–181
gift giving, misuse of organizational resources for, 49–51
globalization, research ethics and, 251–252
Goold, Susan, 152
governing boards
conflict of interest avoidance and, 46–48
education of, 51–52

employee management ethics and, 183
hospital merger case study, 142–144, 166
legal perspectives on, 160–161
nursing shortages and role of, 111–112
workforce reduction issues, collaboration on, 97
government requirements, ethical principles in decision making and, 9–11
graduate medical education. *See* medical education
gratification, management ethics and importance of, 190
Greenspan, B., 189–190
Griffin, Walter P., 159–166

Hand v. Tavera, 216
harm reduction, emergency preparedness and, 263
hazard vulnerability analysis (HVA), emergency management, 261–262
Health Care and Education Reconciliation Act, 221
healthcare ethics committees (HECs)
case consultation and, 223–224
education initiatives, 222–223
evaluation of, 220–231
functions of, 222–225
internal evaluation strategies, 225, 227
organizational implications and effectiveness of, 44, 53–54
policy development, 223
practical applications of, 229–231
program evaluation, 225–227
self-assessment, 225, 227–229
Healthcare Information and Management Systems Society (HIMSS), Analytics Database, 127–128
Healthcare Leadership Excellence: Creating a Career of Impact (Rice and Perry), 3
healthcare professionals
crisis management and duty to respond, 255–256
employee management ethics involving, 183–184

hospital policy fairness toward impairment in, 86–87

impairment in, 80–83, 233–238

in managed care settings, 217–218

management's role concerning impairment in, 84–86

patient safety and, 81

professional codes of ethical conduct, impairment and, 83–84

unionization among, 197–199

Health Insurance Portability and Accountability Act, requirements of, 51–52

Hébert, P. C., E. M. Meslin, and E. V. Dunn, 32

Henry Ford Health System, 35, 52–53, 196

hiring practices, management ethics and, 188–190

Hofmann, Paul, 5

Homeland Security Presidential Directive 5, 253

honesty

business ethics and, 207

managed care information disclosure, 213

hospital administration

business ethics and, 207

healthcare ethics committees, 224–225

medical education and, 249–250

hospital merger case study, 137–148

legal perspectives on, 166

hospital policies

patient satisfaction and, 149–156

physician impairment and fairness in, 81, 86–87

hubris, unethical behavior and, 4

human dignity

business ethics and, 207

emergency preparedness and, 263–265

human events, all-hazards disaster planning approach and, 260

human resources policies, management ethics and development of, 199

human rights, emergency preparedness and, 263–265

image of nursing, in Magnet Recognition Program, 114–115

Impaired Healthcare Executives policy statement (ACHE), 83–84

impairment

defined, 233

in healthcare professionals, 80–83, 233–238

identification and reporting of, 236–237

prevalence in healthcare professionals, 234–235

improvement, managed care ethics and goal of, 218–219

inappropriate/incompetent behavior, rationalization of, 7

incentives

in managed care setting, 211–213

management ethics and, 188

inclusiveness, crisis management ethics and, 255

individual insurance agreements, revenue enhancement and analysis of, 101

individual worth

business ethics and, 207

crisis management ethics and, 254

emergency preparedness activities and, 262–265

ethical principles in decision making and, 10–11

medical ethics and, 205–206

values-based decision making and principle of, 173, 177

information

contextual frame for, 176–179

disclosure of, in managed care setting, 211, 213

information technology

case study involving, 121–135

legal perspectives on, 165

Institute of Medicine, 26–27

integrity

recruiting and hiring practices and importance of, 189

research ethics and, 250–252

values-based decision making and, 179–180

interdisciplinary relationships, nurses' role in, 115

nursing profession
  crisis management and duty to respond, 255–256
  nursing shortage case study, 107–119, 164–165
  unionization in, 197–199
Nygren, D., 147

Occupational Safety and Health Act, 57
occupational socialization, ethical issues and, 31–33
On Distinguishing Policy from Operations policy statement (AHA), 143–144
open-mindedness, information technology problems and, 134
opioid abuse, prevalence in healthcare professionals, 235
optimal health outcomes, medical ethics and, 205–206
organizational implications
  barriers to ethical decision making and, 5–6
  conflicting moral demands and, 44, 49–51
  conflict management and, 190–194
  conflicts of interest and, 46–48
  cultural issues, hospital mergers and, 145
  decline in ethical standards in, 54–58
  ethical decision-making framework in, 7–11
  ethics committees, effectiveness evaluation of, 53–54
  gender discrimination and, 61, 65–66
  information technology problems, 124, 127–128
  in Magnet Recognition Program, 114–115
  management ethics, organizational culture for, 184–188
  patient satisfaction vs. hospital policies and, 150, 155
  physician impairment and, 81, 87–89
  professional codes of ethical conduct and, 52–53
  workforce reduction case study, 96
organizational resources
  conflicting moral demands and use of, 49–51

in ethical decision-making framework, 8
Orwell, George, 89
outcome-based healthcare
  cost-containment policies vs., 215–216
  ethics and, 25
  self-assessment, healthcare ethics committees, 228–229
outsourcing, management ethics and, 186–187

patient-centered medical homes, impaired healthcare professionals and, 238
Patient Protection and Affordable Care Act, 219, 221
patient safety
  hospital policies and, 150, 153
  managed care ethics and goal of, 219
  management ethics and, 185–188
  nursing shortage case study, 110–111
  physician impairment and, 80–81
patient satisfaction
  hospital policies and, 149–156
  information technology problems and, 127–128
  revenue enhancement and internal analysis of, 101
patients' rights
  hospital policies and, 150
  managed care ethics and, 218–219
  medical ethics and, 205–206
  patient safety and, 153
  patient's right to know, 21, 25
patient volume, revenue enhancement and review of, 101
Paul-Emile, K., 151
pay for performance (P4P), in managed care setting, 212
Pegram v. Herdrich, 216
Peregrine, M. W., 147
performance evaluations
  conduct of, 230–231
  design criteria for, 230–231
  healthcare ethics committees (HECs), 220–231
  management ethics and, 190–191

public health physicians, medical ethics and, 205–206

quality control issues
    clinical care and, 102
    improvement, innovation and priorities for, 115
    information technology problems and, 127–128
    in Magnet Recognition Program, 114–115
    in managed care settings, 213–214
Quality Interagency Coordination Task Force, 25–27

racially preferred caregivers
    ethical decision-making framework and, 151–156
    workforce diversity and, 196–197
rank ordering, values-based decision making using, 178
rationing of healthcare, managed care settings and, 209
reason, values-based decision making and role of, 170–171, 173
reasonable actions, crisis management ethics and, 255
reciprocity, crisis management ethics and, 254
recovery activities, emergency management and, 266–267
recruitment
    management ethics and, 188–190
    medical education faculty, 247–248
    residents, 242–244
references, management ethics and provision of, 200
religious injunctions, ethical principles in decision making and, 9–11
Renaissance, history of values and, 173
reporting guidelines
    impaired healthcare professionals, 236–237
    performance evaluations, 230–231
    values-based decision making, 178–179
reprisals, ethical culture and fear of, 55–58
research activity

ethical issues in, 250–252
    medical education and decline in, 242
residency ethics, 241–252
    recruitment issues, 242–244
    resident evaluation and, 244–245
    retention and discipline issues, 245–247
Residency Review Committees (RRCs), 243
resources
    business ethics and management of, 207
    disaster triage and allocation of, 256–258
    in ethical decision-making framework, 8
    healthcare rationing and, 209
    managed care allocation of, 214
    management ethics and, 186
    staff shortages and availability of, 115
responsiveness
    crisis management ethics and, 255
    emergency management and, 265–266
retention policies
    medical education faculty, 248–249
    medical residents, 245–247
revenue enhancement, initiatives for, 101–102
role modeling
    employee management ethics and, 184–188
    team building and, 194
root-cause analysis, medical errors case study, 37–38
Rubin, Richard H., 203–219
Russell, J., 189–190

sanctity of life, values-based decision making and principle of, 173
Sarbanes-Oxley Act, 57–58
SARS (severe acute respiratory syndrome) outbreak, ethical decision-making and, 254
Scanlan, L., 145
Schlichting, Nancy, 35, 53, 196
science, values-based decision making and, 170–171, 173
selective marketing, managed care ethics and, 212–213
self-assessment
    executives, 5, 52

triage, disaster planning and, 256–258

trust

    crisis management ethics and, 255

    managed care ethics and, 219

    partnerships with medical staff and, 34–35

    sexual harassment/misconduct issues and,
    72–73

trustees. *See* governing boards

truth telling

    disclosure of information and, 211

    justice and fairness and, 22–24

    managed care ethics and, 217–218, 219

    medical ethics and, 205–206

    values-based decision making and, 174

*Unaccountable: What Hospitals Won't Tell You
    and How Transparency Can Revolutionize
    Health Care* (Makary), 29

Unamuno, Miguel de, 169

unions

    management ethics and working with,
    197–199

    workforce reduction issues, collaboration on,
    97–99

United States, history of values in, 172–173

universal rules, ethical principles in decision
    making and, 10–11

University of Toronto Joint Centre for
    Bioethics, 254

university settings, medical education in,
    241–242

unrealistic expectations, promotion of, 6–7

US Bureau of Labor Statistics, 197–199

US News & World Report, Best Hospitals list,
    115

utilitarian benefits, ethical principles in decision
    making and, 9–11

values base, values-based decision making
    using, 178

values-based decision making, 169–181

    contextual approach to, 174–179

theory and history, 170

tools for, 180–181

values sources and types, 170–174

values statement, adherence to, 21, 25–29

    conflicting moral demands and, 44

    gender discrimination and, 61, 64

    governing board education about, 51–52

    information technology problems, 124,
    128–129

    nursing shortage case study, 110–112

    physician impairment and, 81

    workforce reduction case study, 96

veracity

    disclosure of information and, 211

    medical ethics and, 205–206

Volcker, Paul, 186

wages and salaries

    management ethics and inequities in,
    186–188, 190

    residency retention and, 245–247

Walters, Barbara, 37–38

weighing process, values-based decision
    making and, 178

weighted multiple voting, values-based
    decision making using, 178

Western culture, history of values in, 172–174

whistle-blowing, ethical issues and, 57–58

Wickline v. California, 215–216

Williams, Juan, 15

Woodstock Theological Center, 206–207, 219

work environment

    conflict management in, 190–194

    management ethics and, 185–188

workforce diversity, 151–156, 196–197

workforce reduction case study, 91–105

    alternatives to reduction, 99–100

    legal perspectives on, 164

    management ethics and, 186

    problem resolution, participants in, 96–100

    revenue enhancement alternatives, 101–102

Workplace Ethics in Transition report, 54–55

About the Author

Frankie Perry, RN, MA, LFACHE, has held senior positions in both nursing and hospital administration. She served as assistant medical center director of Hurley Medical Center in Flint, Michigan, for several years. In addition to her hospital experience, she served as executive vice president of the American College of Healthcare Executives (ACHE) and as a national and international healthcare consultant with engagements in Cairo, Egypt; Doha, Qatar; and Mumbai, India, among other locations. She has published many articles on ethics and healthcare management and in 1984 received ACHE's Edgar C.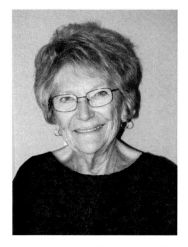
Hayhow Award for Article of the Year. Her book *Management Mistakes in Healthcare: Identification, Correction, and Prevention,* coedited with Paul B. Hofmann, DrPH, FACHE, was published by Cambridge University Press in 2005. Her self-study course *Healthcare Leadership That Makes a Difference: Creating Your Legacy* was published by Health Administration Press in 2012, and *Healthcare Leadership Excellence: Creating a Career of Impact,* coauthored with James A. Rice, PhD, FACHE, was published by Health Administration Press in 2013. She currently serves as faculty for the University of New Mexico. In addition, she teaches an online seminar, "Management Mistakes, Moral Dilemmas and Lessons Learned," for ACHE. In 2008, she received a Regent's Award in recognition of significant contributions to the achievement of the goals of ACHE and the advancement of healthcare management. In 2011, she was the first female recipient of ACHE's Lifetime Service Award. She is a past member of the board of directors of the Commission on Accreditation of Healthcare Management Education.

About the Contributors

Melissa Cole, MSW, FACHE, is president of Cole Consulting LLC, where she leverages her passion for patient safety, technology, and patient engagement in supporting healthcare facilities in the adoption and optimization of technology and health information technology (IT). Ms. Cole was named as one of the 12 Powerful Players in Healthcare Innovation by MedCity News in October 2012 and is among Healthcare IT News's Top 100 to Follow on Twitter for health IT information. She serves as the immediate past president of the New Mexico Chapter of the American College of Healthcare Executives and is an active member of the Healthcare Information and Management Systems Society. She holds a master of social work degree from the University of Michigan and earned her bachelor degree in nursing at Hope College in the Hope-Calvin department of nursing.

Rebecca A. Dobbs, RN, PhD, CEM, CHEP, FACHE, is an independent consultant with experience in critical care nursing, aeromedical evacuation, nursing administration, and health services administration in both the government and private sectors. She has extensive experience in emergency management program development, oversight, and evaluation and frequently serves as a subject matter expert in the areas of healthcare contingency planning, hospital emergency management program development and evaluation, and exercise program development. She is a Certified Emergency Manager, a Certified Healthcare Emergency Professional, and a past American College of Healthcare Executives Regent for New Mexico.

Clinton H. Dowd, MD, FRCS©, FACOG, is emeritus professor of obstetrics-gynecology at the Michigan State University College of Human Medicine. While at the Michigan State University College of Human Medicine, he was also residency program director for obstetrics-gynecology at Hurley Medical Center and undergraduate coordinator of obstetrics-gynecology at the Flint, Michigan, campus from 1976 to 1996. During this time, he started and remained closely involved in the obstetrical perinatal program at Hurley Medical Center. He is currently clinically involved in the Women's Health Division of William Beaumont Army Hospital at Fort Bliss in El Paso, Texas.

Glenn A. Fosdick, MHSA, FACHE, has had a distinguished career in hospital and health system administration spanning more than 30 years. Since 2001 he has been president and chief executive officer of The Nebraska Medical Center in Omaha, Nebraska. Previously, he served as executive vice president and chief operating officer and then as president and chief executive officer of Hurley Medical Center in Flint, Michigan. He also held administrative positions at The Buffalo General Hospital in Buffalo, New York, and the Genesee Memorial Hospital in Batavia, New York. He earned a bachelors in business administration at the State University of Buffalo, New York, and a masters in health services administration at the University of Michigan–Ann Arbor. He is a Fellow of the American College of Healthcare Executives (ACHE) and is currently the ACHE Regent for Nebraska. He has received numerous awards, including the Management Excellence Award bestowed by the Regents of ACHE for Michigan in 1998. He holds the rank of major in the US Army Retired Reserve, Medical Service Corps and educational appointments as a member of the Dean's Advisory Council in the School of Management at the State University of Buffalo, New York; as a member of the Clarkson College board of directors in Omaha, Nebraska; and as senior associate dean at the University of Nebraska Medical Center College of Medicine in Omaha, Nebraska.

Walter P. Griffin, JD, maintains a general practice, including personal injury law, mediation, business law, and general litigation. He attended Tulane University of Louisiana and is a graduate of the Wayne State University School of Law. He was first lieutenant in the Judge Advocate General's Corps of the US Air Force. He maintains memberships in the Genesee County Bar Association (of which he is past president), the State Bar of Michigan (of which he is past chairperson of the Negligence Law Section), the American Bar Association, and the Michigan Defense Trial Counsel (of which he is past president) and is a Fellow of the American College of Trial Lawyers. He was the recipient of the 2001 Michigan Trial Lawyers Association Respected Advocate Award for Defense Counsel and was named the 2007 Distinguished Case Evaluator of the Year by the Genesee County Bar Association.

Joan McIver Gibson, PhD, is a philosopher and consultant in applied ethics, bioethics, and values-based decision making. She has more than 30 years of teaching, training, consulting, and administrative experience in a variety of settings, including universities, business, state and federal government, healthcare, community, and research organizations. She has written several books and articles, most recently the book *Pause: How to Turn Tough Choices into Strong Decisions*.

Richard H. Rubin, MD, FACP, is professor emeritus of medicine at the University of New Mexico School of Medicine. He was a coeditor of *Medicine: A Primary Care Approach* (W. B. Saunders, 1996), a textbook of primary care medicine directed at a medical student readership. He received the Arnold P. Gold Foundation Humanism in Medicine Award (selected by the students of the University of New Mexico School of Medicine) in 2006 and the Laureate Award from the New Mexico Chapter of the American College of Physicians in 2007. He is currently a member of the volunteer teaching faculty at the Oregon Health and Science Center in Portland.

Pete Shelkin, CISSP, FHIMSS, is president of Shelkin Consulting, LLC, where he provides interim management, strategic planning, and other health information technology–related consulting services to healthcare organizations nationwide. He has extensive experience providing information technology leadership for health plans, hospital systems, academic medical and research centers, and clinic groups in chief information officer, chief technology officer, and consulting roles. He has also lectured as an adjunct instructor for The Ohio State University's School of Allied Medical Professions and serves on the board of directors of the Healthcare Information and Management Systems Society.

J. Mitchell Simson, MD, is an associate professor of internal medicine at the University of New Mexico School of Medicine. Previously he was in private practice and worked for the New Mexico Department of Health as a staff physician at Turquoise Lodge, an alcohol and drug inpatient rehabilitation program. He is board certified in internal medicine and addiction medicine.

Technical assistance was provided by Kristine M. Meurer, PhD.